50% OFF
PMHNP Test Prep Course!

Dear Customer,

Thank you for your purchase of this PMHNP Study Guide. Included with your purchase is **discounted access to our online PMHNP Prep Course.** Many Psychiatric and Mental Health Nurse Practitioner courses are needlessly expensive and don't deliver enough value. Our course provides the best PMHNP prep material, and with discounted access, you only pay half price.

We have structured our online course to perfectly complement your printed study guide. The PMHNP Test Prep Course contains **in-depth lessons** that cover all the most important topics, **700 practice questions** to ensure you feel prepared, more than **550 flashcards** for studying on the go, and over **30 instructional videos**.

Online PMHNP Prep Course

Topics Covered:

- Scientific Foundation
  - Advanced Pathophysiology
  - Neurodevelopment
- Advanced Practice Skills
  - Health Promotion and Disease Prevention
  - Risk Assessment
- Diagnosis and Treatment
  - Diagnostic Impression
  - Therapeutic Frameworks
- Psychotherapy and Related Theories
  - Grief and Loss
  - Developmental Theories
- Ethical and Legal Principles
  - Patient's Bill of Rights
  - Transition and Continuum of Care
- And More!

Course Features:

- PMHNP Study Guide
  - Get access to content from the best reviewed study guide available.
- Track Your Progress
  - Our customized course allows you to check off content you have studied or feel confident with.
- 4 Full-Length Practice Tests
  - With 700 practice questions and lesson reviews, you can test yourself again and again to build confidence.
- PMHNP Flashcards
  - Our course includes a flashcard mode consisting of over 550 content cards to help you study.

To lock in your discounted access, visit mometrix.com/university/pmhnp/ or simply scan this QR code with your smartphone. At the checkout page, enter the discount code: **PMHNP50OFF**

If you have any questions or concerns, please contact us at support@mometrix.com.

Mometrix
TEST PREPARATION

SCAN HERE

ACCESS YOUR ONLINE RESOURCES

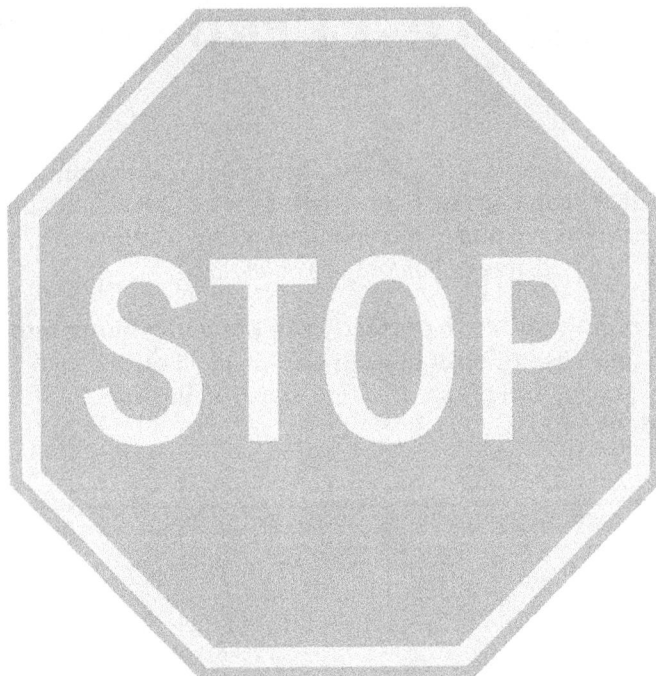

STOP

DON'T MISS OUT ON THE ONLINE RESOURCES INCLUDED WITH YOUR PURCHASE!

Your purchase of this product unlocks access to our Online Resources page. Elevate your study experience with our **interactive practice test interface**, along with all of the additional resources that we couldn't include in this book.

Flip to the Online Resources section at the end of this book to find the link and a QR code to get started!

Mometrix
TEST PREPARATION

Mometrix
TEST PREPARATION

Psychiatric-Mental Health Nurse Practitioner Exam Secrets Study Guide

PMHNP Certification Review 2025-2026 with Practice Test Questions

3rd Edition

Written and edited by Matthew Bowling

Printed in the United States of America

This paper meets the requirements of ANSI/NISO Z39.48-1992 (Permanence of Paper).

Mometrix offers volume discount pricing to institutions. For more information or a price quote, please contact our sales department at sales@mometrix.com or 888-248-1219.

Mometrix Media LLC is not affiliated with or endorsed by any official testing organization. All organizational and test names are trademarks of their respective owners.

Paperback
ISBN 13: 978-1-5167-2781-0
ISBN 10: 1-5167-2781-9

DEAR FUTURE EXAM SUCCESS STORY

First of all, **THANK YOU** for purchasing Mometrix study materials!

Second, congratulations! You are one of the few determined test-takers who are committed to doing whatever it takes to excel on your exam. **You have come to the right place.** We developed these study materials with one goal in mind: to deliver you the information you need in a format that's concise and easy to use.

In addition to optimizing your guide for the content of the test, we've outlined our recommended steps for breaking down the preparation process into small, attainable goals so you can make sure you stay on track.

We've also analyzed the entire test-taking process, identifying the most common pitfalls and showing how you can overcome them and be ready for any curveball the test throws you.

Standardized testing is one of the biggest obstacles on your road to success, which only increases the importance of doing well in the high-pressure, high-stakes environment of test day. Your results on this test could have a significant impact on your future, and this guide provides the information and practical advice to help you achieve your full potential on test day.

Your success is our success

We would love to hear from you! If you would like to share the story of your exam success or if you have any questions or comments in regard to our products, please contact us at **800-673-8175** or **support@mometrix.com**.

Thanks again for your business and we wish you continued success!

Sincerely,
The Mometrix Test Preparation Team

Need more help? Check out our flashcards at:
http://mometrixflashcards.com/NP

TABLE OF CONTENTS

Introduction

Thank you for purchasing this resource! You have made the choice to prepare yourself for a test that could have a huge impact on your future, and this guide is designed to help you be fully ready for test day. Obviously, it's important to have a solid understanding of the test material, but you also need to be prepared for the unique environment and stressors of the test, so that you can perform to the best of your abilities.

For this purpose, the first section that appears in this guide is the **Secret Keys**. We've devoted countless hours to meticulously researching what works and what doesn't, and we've boiled down our findings to the five most impactful steps you can take to improve your performance on the test. We start at the beginning with study planning and move through the preparation process, all the way to the testing strategies that will help you get the most out of what you know when you're finally sitting in front of the test.

We recommend that you start preparing for your test as far in advance as possible. However, if you've bought this guide as a last-minute study resource and only have a few days before your test, we recommend that you skip over the first two Secret Keys since they address a long-term study plan.

If you struggle with **test anxiety**, we strongly encourage you to check out our recommendations for how you can overcome it. Test anxiety is a formidable foe, but it can be beaten, and we want to make sure you have the tools you need to defeat it.

Review Video Directory

As you work your way through this guide, you will see numerous review video links interspersed with the written content. If you would like to access all of these review videos in one place, click on the video directory link found on the online resources page: **mometrix.com/resources719/nppmh-27810**

1

Secret Key #1 – Plan Big, Study Small

There's a lot riding on your performance. If you want to ace this test, you're going to need to keep your skills sharp and the material fresh in your mind. You need a plan that lets you review everything you need to know while still fitting in your schedule. We'll break this strategy down into three categories.

Information Organization

Start with the information you already have: the official test outline. From this, you can make a complete list of all the concepts you need to cover before the test. Organize these concepts into groups that can be studied together, and create a list of any related vocabulary you need to learn so you can brush up on any difficult terms. You'll want to keep this vocabulary list handy once you actually start studying since you may need to add to it along the way.

Time Management

Once you have your set of study concepts, decide how to spread them out over the time you have left before the test. Break your study plan into small, clear goals so you have a manageable task for each day and know exactly what you're doing. Then just focus on one small step at a time. When you manage your time this way, you don't need to spend hours at a time studying. Studying a small block of content for a short period each day helps you retain information better and avoid stressing over how much you have left to do. You can relax knowing that you have a plan to cover everything in time. In order for this strategy to be effective though, you have to start studying early and stick to your schedule. Avoid the exhaustion and futility that comes from last-minute cramming!

Study Environment

The environment you study in has a big impact on your learning. Studying in a coffee shop, while probably more enjoyable, is not likely to be as fruitful as studying in a quiet room. It's important to keep distractions to a minimum. You're only planning to study for a short block of time, so make the most of it. Don't pause to check your phone or get up to find a snack. It's also important to **avoid multitasking**. Research has consistently shown that multitasking will make your studying dramatically less effective. Your study area should also be comfortable and well-lit so you don't have the distraction of straining your eyes or sitting on an uncomfortable chair.

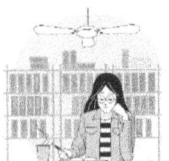

The time of day you study is also important. You want to be rested and alert. Don't wait until just before bedtime. Study when you'll be most likely to comprehend and remember. Even better, if you know what time of day your test will be, set that time aside for study. That way your brain will be used to working on that subject at that specific time and you'll have a better chance of recalling information.

Finally, it can be helpful to team up with others who are studying for the same test. Your actual studying should be done in as isolated an environment as possible, but the work of organizing the information and setting up the study plan can be divided up. In between study sessions, you can discuss with your teammates the concepts that you're all studying and quiz each other on the details. Just be sure that your teammates are as serious about the test as you are. If you find that your study time is being replaced with social time, you might need to find a new team.

Secret Key #2 – Make Your Studying Count

You're devoting a lot of time and effort to preparing for this test, so you want to be absolutely certain it will pay off. This means doing more than just reading the content and hoping you can remember it on test day. It's important to make every minute of study count. There are two main areas you can focus on to make your studying count.

Retention

It doesn't matter how much time you study if you can't remember the material. You need to make sure you are retaining the concepts. To check your retention of the information you're learning, try recalling it at later times with minimal prompting. Try carrying around flashcards and glance at one or two from time to time or ask a friend who's also studying for the test to quiz you.

To enhance your retention, look for ways to put the information into practice so that you can apply it rather than simply recalling it. If you're using the information in practical ways, it will be much easier to remember. Similarly, it helps to solidify a concept in your mind if you're not only reading it to yourself but also explaining it to someone else. Ask a friend to let you teach them about a concept you're a little shaky on (or speak aloud to an imaginary audience if necessary). As you try to summarize, define, give examples, and answer your friend's questions, you'll understand the concepts better and they will stay with you longer. Finally, step back for a big picture view and ask yourself how each piece of information fits with the whole subject. When you link the different concepts together and see them working together as a whole, it's easier to remember the individual components.

Finally, practice showing your work on any multi-step problems, even if you're just studying. Writing out each step you take to solve a problem will help solidify the process in your mind, and you'll be more likely to remember it during the test.

Modality

Modality simply refers to the means or method by which you study. Choosing a study modality that fits your own individual learning style is crucial. No two people learn best in exactly the same way, so it's important to know your strengths and use them to your advantage.

For example, if you learn best by visualization, focus on visualizing a concept in your mind and draw an image or a diagram. Try color-coding your notes, illustrating them, or creating symbols that will trigger your mind to recall a learned concept. If you learn best by hearing or discussing information, find a study partner who learns the same way or read aloud to yourself. Think about how to put the information in your own words. Imagine that you are giving a lecture on the topic and record yourself so you can listen to it later.

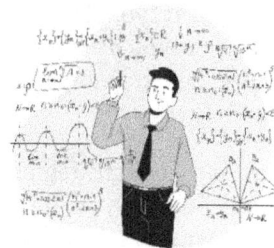

For any learning style, flashcards can be helpful. Organize the information so you can take advantage of spare moments to review. Underline key words or phrases. Use different colors for different categories. Mnemonic devices (such as creating a short list in which every item starts with the same letter) can also help with retention. Find what works best for you and use it to store the information in your mind most effectively and easily.

Secret Key #3 – Practice the Right Way

Your success on test day depends not only on how many hours you put into preparing, but also on whether you prepared the right way. It's good to check along the way to see if your studying is paying off. One of the most effective ways to do this is by taking practice tests to evaluate your progress. Practice tests are useful because they show exactly where you need to improve. Every time you take a practice test, pay special attention to these three groups of questions:

- The questions you got wrong
- The questions you had to guess on, even if you guessed right
- The questions you found difficult or slow to work through

This will show you exactly what your weak areas are, and where you need to devote more study time. Ask yourself why each of these questions gave you trouble. Was it because you didn't understand the material? Was it because you didn't remember the vocabulary? Do you need more repetitions on this type of question to build speed and confidence? Dig into those questions and figure out how you can strengthen your weak areas as you go back to review the material.

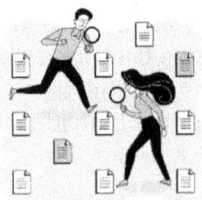

Additionally, many practice tests have a section explaining the answer choices. It can be tempting to read the explanation and think that you now have a good understanding of the concept. However, an explanation likely only covers part of the question's broader context. Even if the explanation makes perfect sense, **go back and investigate** every concept related to the question until you're positive you have a thorough understanding.

As you go along, keep in mind that the practice test is just that: practice. Memorizing these questions and answers will not be very helpful on the actual test because it is unlikely to have any of the same exact questions. If you only know the right answers to the sample questions, you won't be prepared for the real thing. **Study the concepts** until you understand them fully, and then you'll be able to answer any question that shows up on the test.

It's important to wait on the practice tests until you're ready. If you take a test on your first day of study, you may be overwhelmed by the amount of material covered and how much you need to learn. Work up to it gradually.

On test day, you'll need to be prepared for answering questions, managing your time, and using the test-taking strategies you've learned. It's a lot to balance, like a mental marathon that will have a big impact on your future. Like training for a marathon, you'll need to start slowly and work your way up. When test day arrives, you'll be ready.

Start with the strategies you've read in the first two Secret Keys—plan your course and study in the way that works best for you. If you have time, consider using multiple study resources to get different approaches to the same concepts. It can be helpful to see difficult concepts from more than one angle. Then find a good source for practice tests. Many times, the test website will suggest potential study resources or provide sample tests.

4

Practice Test Strategy

If you're able to find at least three practice tests, we recommend this strategy:

UNTIMED AND OPEN-BOOK PRACTICE

Take the first test with no time constraints and with your notes and study guide handy. Take your time and focus on applying the strategies you've learned.

TIMED AND OPEN-BOOK PRACTICE

Take the second practice test open-book as well, but set a timer and practice pacing yourself to finish in time.

TIMED AND CLOSED-BOOK PRACTICE

Take any other practice tests as if it were test day. Set a timer and put away your study materials. Sit at a table or desk in a quiet room, imagine yourself at the testing center, and answer questions as quickly and accurately as possible.

Keep repeating timed and closed-book tests on a regular basis until you run out of practice tests or it's time for the actual test. Your mind will be ready for the schedule and stress of test day, and you'll be able to focus on recalling the material you've learned.

Secret Key #4 – Pace Yourself

Once you're fully prepared for the material on the test, your biggest challenge on test day will be managing your time. Just knowing that the clock is ticking can make you panic even if you have plenty of time left. Work on pacing yourself so you can build confidence against the time constraints of the exam. Pacing is a difficult skill to master, especially in a high-pressure environment, so **practice is vital**.

Set time expectations for your pace based on how much time is available. For example, if a section has 60 questions and the time limit is 30 minutes, you know you have to average 30 seconds or less per question in order to answer them all. Although 30 seconds is the hard limit, set 25 seconds per question as your goal, so you reserve extra time to spend on harder questions. When you budget extra time for the harder questions, you no longer have any reason to stress when those questions take longer to answer.

Don't let this time expectation distract you from working through the test at a calm, steady pace, but keep it in mind so you don't spend too much time on any one question. Recognize that taking extra time on one question you don't understand may keep you from answering two that you do understand later in the test. If your time limit for a question is up and you're still not sure of the answer, mark it and move on, and come back to it later if the time and the test format allow. If the testing format doesn't allow you to return to earlier questions, just make an educated guess; then put it out of your mind and move on.

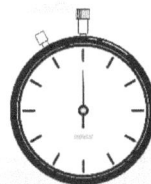

On the easier questions, be careful not to rush. It may seem wise to hurry through them so you have more time for the challenging ones, but it's not worth missing one if you know the concept and just didn't take the time to read the question fully. Work efficiently but make sure you understand the question and have looked at all of the answer choices, since more than one may seem right at first.

Even if you're paying attention to the time, you may find yourself a little behind at some point. You should speed up to get back on track, but do so wisely. Don't panic; just take a few seconds less on each question until you're caught up. Don't guess without thinking, but do look through the answer choices and eliminate any you know are wrong. If you can get down to two choices, it is often worthwhile to guess from those. Once you've chosen an answer, move on and don't dwell on any that you skipped or had to hurry through. If a question was taking too long, chances are it was one of the harder ones, so you weren't as likely to get it right anyway.

On the other hand, if you find yourself getting ahead of schedule, it may be beneficial to slow down a little. The more quickly you work, the more likely you are to make a careless mistake that will affect your score. You've budgeted time for each question, so don't be afraid to spend that time. Practice an efficient but careful pace to get the most out of the time you have.

6

Secret Key #5 – Have a Plan for Guessing

When you're taking the test, you may find yourself stuck on a question. Some of the answer choices seem better than others, but you don't see the one answer choice that is obviously correct. What do you do?

The scenario described above is very common, yet most test takers have not effectively prepared for it. Developing and practicing a plan for guessing may be one of the single most effective uses of your time as you get ready for the exam.

In developing your plan for guessing, there are three questions to address:

- When should you start the guessing process?
- How should you narrow down the choices?
- Which answer should you choose?

When to Start the Guessing Process

Unless your plan for guessing is to select C every time (which, despite its merits, is not what we recommend), you need to leave yourself enough time to apply your answer elimination strategies. Since you have a limited amount of time for each question, that means that if you're going to give yourself the best shot at guessing correctly, you have to decide quickly whether or not you will guess.

Of course, the best-case scenario is that you don't have to guess at all, so first, see if you can answer the question based on your knowledge of the subject and basic reasoning skills. Focus on the key words in the question and try to jog your memory of related topics. Give yourself a chance to bring the knowledge to mind, but once you realize that you don't have (or you can't access) the knowledge you need to answer the question, it's time to start the guessing process.

It's almost always better to start the guessing process too early than too late. It only takes a few seconds to remember something and answer the question from knowledge. Carefully eliminating wrong answer choices takes longer. Plus, going through the process of eliminating answer choices can actually help jog your memory.

Summary: Start the guessing process as soon as you decide that you can't answer the question based on your knowledge.

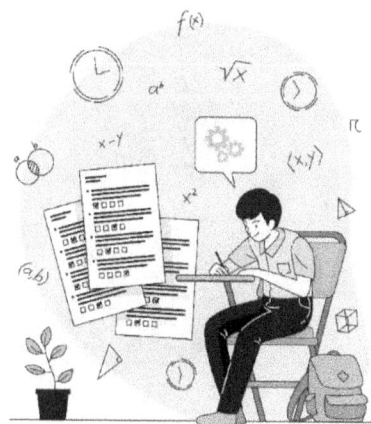

7

How to Narrow Down the Choices

The next chapter in this book (**Test-Taking Strategies**) includes a wide range of strategies for how to approach questions and how to look for answer choices to eliminate. You will definitely want to read those carefully, practice them, and figure out which ones work best for you. Here though, we're going to address a mindset rather than a particular strategy.

Your odds of guessing an answer correctly depend on how many options you are choosing from.

Number of options left	5	4	3	2	1
Odds of guessing correctly	20%	25%	33%	50%	100%

You can see from this chart just how valuable it is to be able to eliminate incorrect answers and make an educated guess, but there are two things that many test takers do that cause them to miss out on the benefits of guessing:

- Accidentally eliminating the correct answer
- Selecting an answer based on an impression

We'll look at the first one here, and the second one in the next section.

To avoid accidentally eliminating the correct answer, we recommend a thought exercise called **the $5 challenge**. In this challenge, you only eliminate an answer choice from contention if you are willing to bet $5 on it being wrong. Why $5? Five dollars is a small but not insignificant amount of money. It's an amount you could afford to lose but wouldn't want to throw away. And while losing $5 once might not hurt too much, doing it twenty times will set you back $100. In the same way, each small decision you make—eliminating a choice here, guessing on a question there—won't by itself impact your score very much, but when you put them all together, they can make a big difference. By holding each answer choice elimination decision to a higher standard, you can reduce the risk of accidentally eliminating the correct answer.

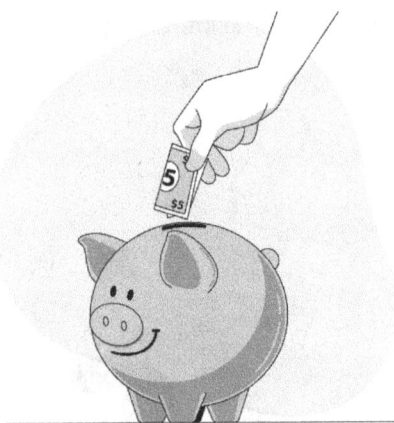

The $5 challenge can also be applied in a positive sense: If you are willing to bet $5 that an answer choice *is* correct, go ahead and mark it as correct.

Summary: Only eliminate an answer choice if you are willing to bet $5 that it is wrong.

Which Answer to Choose

You're taking the test. You've run into a hard question and decided you'll have to guess. You've eliminated all the answer choices you're willing to bet $5 on. Now you have to pick an answer. Why do we even need to talk about this? Why can't you just pick whichever one you feel like when the time comes?

The answer to these questions is that if you don't come into the test with a plan, you'll rely on your impression to select an answer choice, and if you do that, you risk falling into a trap. The test writers know that everyone who takes their test will be guessing on some of the questions, so they intentionally write wrong answer choices to seem plausible. You still have to pick an answer though, and if the wrong answer choices are designed to look right, how can you ever be sure that you're not falling for their trap? The best solution we've found to this dilemma is to take the decision out of your hands entirely. Here is the process we recommend:

Once you've eliminated any choices that you are confident (willing to bet $5) are wrong, select the first remaining choice as your answer.

Whether you choose to select the first remaining choice, the second, or the last, the important thing is that you use some preselected standard. Using this approach guarantees that you will not be enticed into selecting an answer choice that looks right, because you are not basing your decision on how the answer choices look.

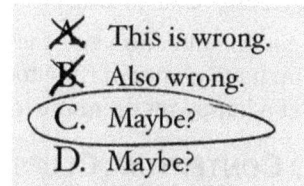

This is not meant to make you question your knowledge. Instead, it is to help you recognize the difference between your knowledge and your impressions. There's a huge difference between thinking an answer is right because of what you know, and thinking an answer is right because it looks or sounds like it should be right.

Summary: To ensure that your selection is appropriately random, make a predetermined selection from among all answer choices you have not eliminated.

Test-Taking Strategies

This section contains a list of test-taking strategies that you may find helpful as you work through the test. By taking what you know and applying logical thought, you can maximize your chances of answering any question correctly!

It is very important to realize that every question is different and every person is different: no single strategy will work on every question, and no single strategy will work for every person. That's why we've included all of them here, so you can try them out and determine which ones work best for different types of questions and which ones work best for you.

Question Strategies

☑ READ CAREFULLY

Read the question and the answer choices carefully. Don't miss the question because you misread the terms. You have plenty of time to read each question thoroughly and make sure you understand what is being asked. Yet a happy medium must be attained, so don't waste too much time. You must read carefully and efficiently.

☑ CONTEXTUAL CLUES

Look for contextual clues. If the question includes a word you are not familiar with, look at the immediate context for some indication of what the word might mean. Contextual clues can often give you all the information you need to decipher the meaning of an unfamiliar word. Even if you can't determine the meaning, you may be able to narrow down the possibilities enough to make a solid guess at the answer to the question.

☑ PREFIXES

If you're having trouble with a word in the question or answer choices, try dissecting it. Take advantage of every clue that the word might include. Prefixes can be a huge help. Usually, they allow you to determine a basic meaning. *Pre-* means before, *post-* means after, *pro-* is positive, *de-* is negative. From prefixes, you can get an idea of the general meaning of the word and try to put it into context.

☑ HEDGE WORDS

Watch out for critical hedge words, such as *likely, may, can, often, almost, mostly, usually, generally, rarely,* and *sometimes*. Question writers insert these hedge phrases to cover every possibility. Often an answer choice will be wrong simply because it leaves no room for exception. Be on guard for answer choices that have definitive words such as *exactly* and *always*.

☑ SWITCHBACK WORDS

Stay alert for *switchbacks*. These are the words and phrases frequently used to alert you to shifts in thought. The most common switchback words are *but, although,* and *however*. Others include *nevertheless, on the other hand, even though, while, in spite of, despite,* and *regardless of*. Switchback words are important to catch because they can change the direction of the question or an answer choice.

☑ FACE VALUE

When in doubt, use common sense. Accept the situation in the problem at face value. Don't read too much into it. These problems will not require you to make wild assumptions. If you have to go beyond creativity and warp time or space in order to have an answer choice fit the question, then you should move on and consider the other answer choices. These are normal problems rooted in reality. The applicable relationship or explanation may not be readily apparent, but it is there for you to figure out. Use your common sense to interpret anything that isn't clear.

Answer Choice Strategies

⊘ ANSWER SELECTION

The most thorough way to pick an answer choice is to identify and eliminate wrong answers until only one is left, then confirm it is the correct answer. Sometimes an answer choice may immediately seem right, but be careful. The test writers will usually put more than one reasonable answer choice on each question, so take a second to read all of them and make sure that the other choices are not equally obvious. As long as you have time left, it is better to read every answer choice than to pick the first one that looks right without checking the others.

⊘ ANSWER CHOICE FAMILIES

An answer choice family consists of two (in rare cases, three) answer choices that are very similar in construction and cannot all be true at the same time. If you see two answer choices that are direct opposites or parallels, one of them is usually the correct answer. For instance, if one answer choice says that quantity x increases and another either says that quantity x decreases (opposite) or says that quantity y increases (parallel), then those answer choices would fall into the same family. An answer choice that doesn't match the construction of the answer choice family is more likely to be incorrect. Most questions will not have answer choice families, but when they do appear, you should be prepared to recognize them.

⊘ ELIMINATE ANSWERS

Eliminate answer choices as soon as you realize they are wrong, but make sure you consider all possibilities. If you are eliminating answer choices and realize that the last one you are left with is also wrong, don't panic. Start over and consider each choice again. There may be something you missed the first time that you will realize on the second pass.

⊘ AVOID FACT TRAPS

Don't be distracted by an answer choice that is factually true but doesn't answer the question. You are looking for the choice that answers the question. Stay focused on what the question is asking for so you don't accidentally pick an answer that is true but incorrect. Always go back to the question and make sure the answer choice you've selected actually answers the question and is not merely a true statement.

⊘ EXTREME STATEMENTS

In general, you should avoid answers that put forth extreme actions as standard practice or proclaim controversial ideas as established fact. An answer choice that states the "process should be used in certain situations, if…" is much more likely to be correct than one that states the "process should be discontinued completely." The first is a calm rational statement and doesn't even make a definitive, uncompromising stance, using a hedge word *if* to provide wiggle room, whereas the second choice is far more extreme.

⊘ BENCHMARK

As you read through the answer choices and you come across one that seems to answer the question well, mentally select that answer choice. This is not your final answer, but it's the one that will help you evaluate the other answer choices. The one that you selected is your benchmark or standard for judging each of the other answer choices. Every other answer choice must be compared to your benchmark. That choice is correct until proven otherwise by another answer choice beating it. If you find a better answer, then that one becomes your new benchmark. Once you've decided that no other choice answers the question as well as your benchmark, you have your final answer.

11

⊘ PREDICT THE ANSWER

Before you even start looking at the answer choices, it is often best to try to predict the answer. When you come up with the answer on your own, it is easier to avoid distractions and traps because you will know exactly what to look for. The right answer choice is unlikely to be word-for-word what you came up with, but it should be a close match. Even if you are confident that you have the right answer, you should still take the time to read each option before moving on.

General Strategies

⊘ TOUGH QUESTIONS

If you are stumped on a problem or it appears too hard or too difficult, don't waste time. Move on! Remember though, if you can quickly check for obviously incorrect answer choices, your chances of guessing correctly are greatly improved. Before you completely give up, at least try to knock out a couple of possible answers. Eliminate what you can and then guess at the remaining answer choices before moving on.

⊘ CHECK YOUR WORK

Since you will probably not know every term listed and the answer to every question, it is important that you get credit for the ones that you do know. Don't miss any questions through careless mistakes. If at all possible, try to take a second to look back over your answer selection and make sure you've selected the correct answer choice and haven't made a costly careless mistake (such as marking an answer choice that you didn't mean to mark). This quick double check should more than pay for itself in caught mistakes for the time it costs.

⊘ PACE YOURSELF

It's easy to be overwhelmed when you're looking at a page full of questions; your mind is confused and full of random thoughts, and the clock is ticking down faster than you would like. Calm down and maintain the pace that you have set for yourself. Especially as you get down to the last few minutes of the test, don't let the small numbers on the clock make you panic. As long as you are on track by monitoring your pace, you are guaranteed to have time for each question.

⊘ DON'T RUSH

It is very easy to make errors when you are in a hurry. Maintaining a fast pace in answering questions is pointless if it makes you miss questions that you would have gotten right otherwise. Test writers like to include distracting information and wrong answers that seem right. Taking a little extra time to avoid careless mistakes can make all the difference in your test score. Find a pace that allows you to be confident in the answers that you select.

⊘ KEEP MOVING

Panicking will not help you pass the test, so do your best to stay calm and keep moving. Taking deep breaths and going through the answer elimination steps you practiced can help to break through a stress barrier and keep your pace.

12

Final Notes

The combination of a solid foundation of content knowledge and the confidence that comes from practicing your plan for applying that knowledge is the key to maximizing your performance on test day. As your foundation of content knowledge is built up and strengthened, you'll find that the strategies included in this chapter become more and more effective in helping you quickly sift through the distractions and traps of the test to isolate the correct answer.

Now that you're preparing to move forward into the test content chapters of this book, be sure to keep your goal in mind. As you read, think about how you will be able to apply this information on the test. If you've already seen sample questions for the test and you have an idea of the question format and style, try to come up with questions of your own that you can answer based on what you're reading. This will give you valuable practice applying your knowledge in the same ways you can expect to on test day.

Good luck and good studying!

Four-Week Study Plan

On the next few pages, we've provided an optional study plan to help you use this study guide to its fullest potential over the course of four weeks. If you have eight weeks available and want to spread it out more, spend two weeks on each section of the plan.

Below is a quick summary of the subjects covered in each week of the plan.

- Week 1: Scientific Foundation & Advanced Practice Skills
- Week 2: Diagnosis and Treatment
- Week 3: Psychotherapy and Related Theories & Ethical and Legal Principles
- Week 4: Practice Tests

Please note that not all subjects will take the same amount of time to work through.

Two full-length practice tests are included in this study guide. We recommend saving any additional practice tests until after you've completed the study plan. Take these practice tests without any reference materials a day or two before the real thing as practice runs to get you in the mode of answering questions at a good pace.

Week 1: Scientific Foundation & Advanced Practice Skills

INSTRUCTIONAL CONTENT

First, read carefully through the Scientific Foundation & Advanced Practice Skills chapters in this book, checking off your progress as you go:

- ❏ Advanced Pathophysiology
- ❏ Advanced Pharmacology and Psychopharmacology
- ❏ Neurodevelopment
- ❏ Psychogenomics
- ❏ Clinical Interviewing
- ❏ Health Promotion and Disease Prevention
- ❏ Mental Health Screening
- ❏ Tool Selection and Interpretation
- ❏ Family Assessment
- ❏ Substance Use Screening
- ❏ Abuse and Domestic Violence
- ❏ Emergency Situations and Crisis Management
- ❏ Psychoeducation

As you read, do the following:

- Highlight any sections, terms, or concepts you think are important
- Draw an asterisk (*) next to any areas you are struggling with
- Watch the review videos to gain more understanding of a particular topic
- Take notes in your notebook or in the margins of this book

After you've read through everything, go back and review any sections that you highlighted or that you drew an asterisk next to, referencing your notes along the way.

Week 2: Diagnosis and Treatment

INSTRUCTIONAL CONTENT

First, read carefully through the Diagnosis and Treatment chapter in this book, checking off your progress as you go:

- ❏ Diagnostic Impression
- ❏ Diagnostic and Laboratory Tests
- ❏ Psychiatric Disorders and Diagnosis
- ❏ Evidence-Based Practice
- ❏ Treatment Planning
- ❏ Therapeutic Frameworks
- ❏ Group Therapy
- ❏ Family Therapy
- ❏ Psychopharmacotherapeutic Management
- ❏ Complimentary Interventions
- ❏ Evaluating Intervention Effectiveness

As you read, do the following:

- Highlight any sections, terms, or concepts you think are important
- Draw an asterisk (*) next to any areas you are struggling with
- Watch the review videos to gain more understanding of a particular topic
- Take notes in your notebook or in the margins of this book

After you've read through everything, go back and review any sections that you highlighted or that you drew an asterisk next to, referencing your notes along the way.

Week 3: Psychotherapy and Related Theories & Ethical and Legal Principles

INSTRUCTIONAL CONTENT

First, read carefully through the Psychotherapy and Related Theories & Ethical and Legal Principles chapters in this book, checking off your progress as you go:

- ❏ Psychotherapy Principles and Theoretical Frameworks
- ❏ Grief and Loss
- ❏ Developmental Theories
- ❏ Therapeutic Alliance Development and Management
- ❏ Patient's Bill of Rights
- ❏ Ethics in Clinical Decision Making
- ❏ Scope and Standards of Practice
- ❏ Standards of Advanced Practice
- ❏ Laws and Regulations
- ❏ Transition and Continuum of Care
- ❏ Interdisciplinary Collaboration
- ❏ Cultural and Spiritual Competence

As you read, do the following:

- Highlight any sections, terms, or concepts you think are important
- Draw an asterisk (*) next to any areas you are struggling with
- Watch the review videos to gain more understanding of a particular topic
- Take notes in your notebook or in the margins of this book

After you've read through everything, go back and review any sections that you highlighted or that you drew an asterisk next to, referencing your notes along the way.

Week 4: Practice Tests

Your success on test day depends not only on how many hours you put into preparing, but also on whether you prepared the right way. It's good to check along the way to see if your studying is paying off. One of the most effective ways to do this is by taking practice tests to evaluate your progress. Practice tests are useful because they show exactly where you need to improve. Every time you take a practice test, pay special attention to these three groups of questions:

- The questions you got wrong
- The questions you had to guess on, even if you guessed right
- The questions you found difficult or slow to work through

This will show you exactly what your weak areas are, and where you need to devote more study time. Ask yourself why each of these questions gave you trouble. Was it because you didn't understand the material? Was it because you didn't remember the vocabulary? Do you need more repetitions on this type of question to build speed and confidence? Dig into those questions and figure out how you can strengthen your weak areas as you go back to review the material.

PRACTICE TEST #1

Now that you've read over the instructional content, it's time to take a practice test. Complete Practice Test #1. Take this test with **no time constraints**, and feel free to reference the applicable sections of this guide as you go. Once you've finished, check your answers against the provided answer key. For any questions you answered incorrectly, review the answer rationale, and then **go back and review** the applicable sections of the book. The goal in this stage is to understand why you answered the question incorrectly, and make sure that the next time you see a similar question, you will get it right.

PRACTICE TEST #2

Next, complete Practice Test #2. This time, give yourself **3.5 hours** to complete all of the questions. You should again feel free to reference the guide and your notes, but be mindful of the clock. If you run out of time before you finish all of the questions, mark where you were when time expired, but go ahead and finish taking the practice test. Once you've finished, check your answers against the provided answer key, and as before, review the answer rationale for any that you answered incorrectly and then go back and review the associated instructional content. Your goal is still to increase understanding of the content but also to get used to the time constraints you will face on the test.

As you go along, keep in mind that the practice test is just that: practice. Memorizing these questions and answers will not be very helpful on the actual test because it is unlikely to have any of the same exact questions. If you only know the right answers to the sample questions, you won't be prepared for the real thing. **Study the concepts** until you understand them fully, and then you'll be able to answer any question that shows up on the test.

Scientific Foundation

Advanced Pathophysiology

NEURONS

The neuron, or **nerve cell**, is instrumental in thought processes and behavior. Most of the neurons that a human will ever have are present at birth. It is possible for neurons to regenerate throughout life. Most neurons have three basic components: dendrites, cell body (soma), and axon:

- The **dendrites** are like arms that receive information in the form of electrical impulses from other cells and relay it to the soma.
- The **cell body (soma)** then processes that information and passes it to the axon, which may then pass it along to other cells. Neurons typically have one axon which divides into a few branches, called collaterals.
- **Axons** are covered by a thin, fatty substance known as the *myelin sheath*, which accelerates the conduction of nerve impulses. The process through which electrical impulses are passed within a cell is called *conduction*; communication between cells is performed through the release of neurotransmitting chemicals between the cells (in a gap known as a *synapse*).

> **Review Video: Function of the Nervous System**
> Visit mometrix.com/academy and enter code: 708428

CROSS SECTION OF A NEURON

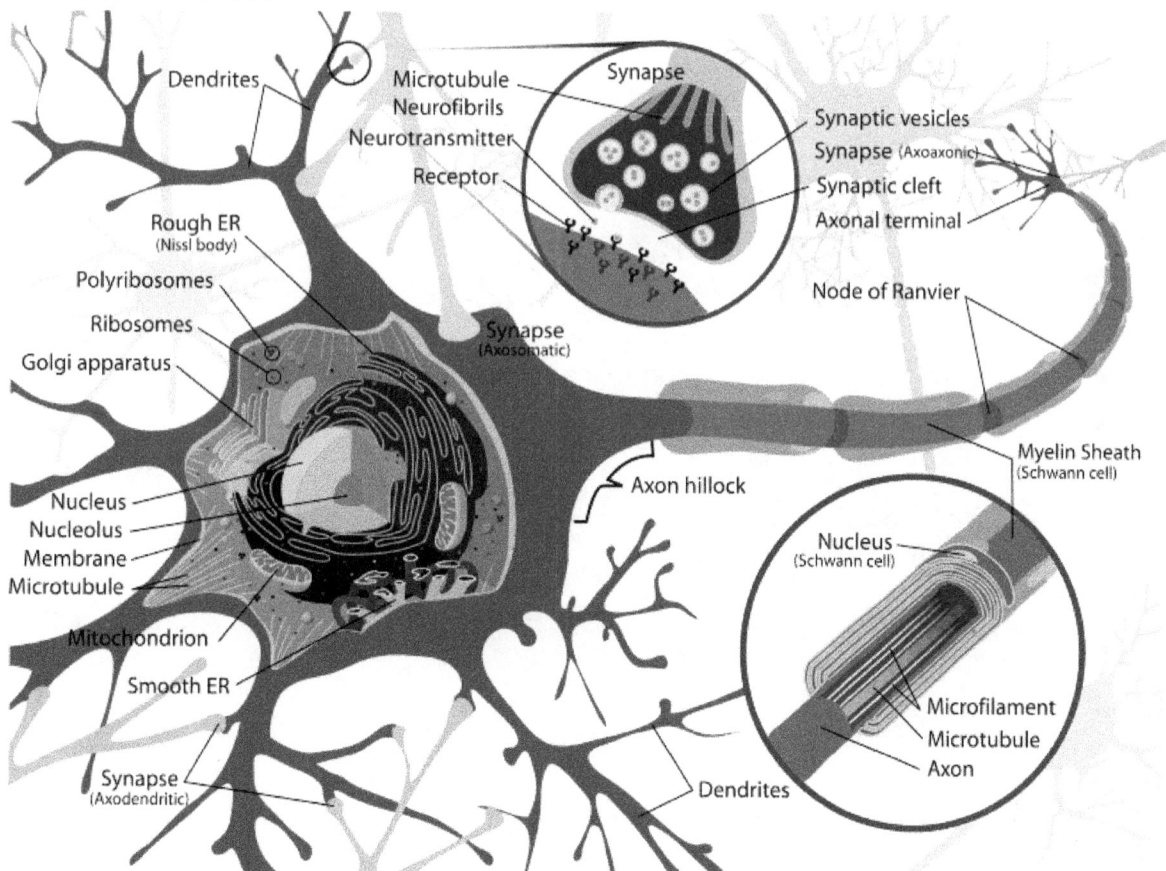

NEUROTRANSMITTERS

ACETYLCHOLINE

Acetylcholine (**ACh**) is a neurotransmitter found in both the peripheral and central nervous systems. When it is released into the neuromuscular junction by the peripheral nervous system, it contracts the muscles. In the central nervous system, ACh is responsible for REM sleep, the maintenance of the circadian rhythm, and memory. The memory deficits associated with Alzheimer's disease and other illnesses result from the degeneration of ACh cells in the entorhinal cortex (EC) and other regions of the brain that communicate with the hippocampus.

There are two sorts of receptors for these cells: **nicotinic receptors** are excitatory, while **muscarinic receptors** are inhibitory. Nicotine in tobacco products creates alertness by mimicking ACh at receptor sites.

GENERIC NEUROTRANSMITTER SYSTEM

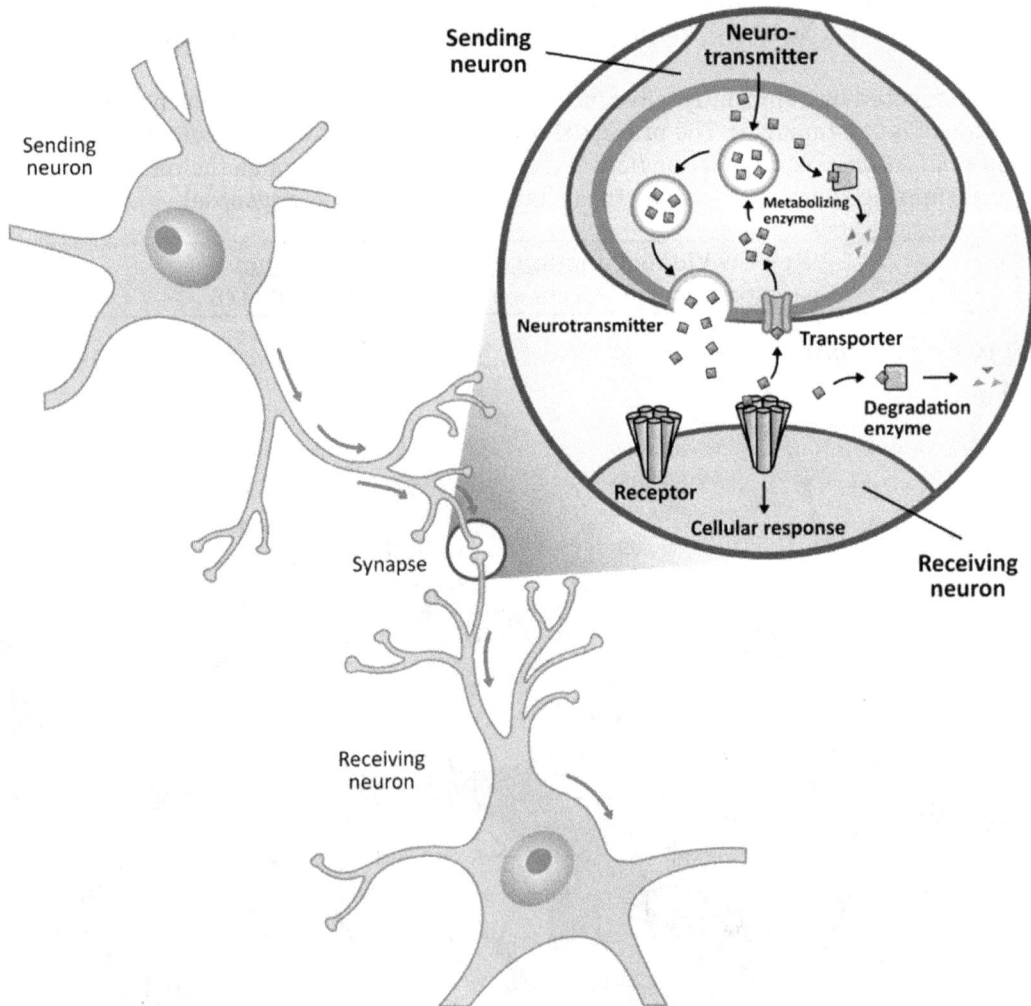

20

GABA, GLUTAMATE, AND ENDORPHINS

Gamma-aminobutyric acid, or **GABA**, is an inhibitory neurotransmitter that influences sleep, eating, seizure, and anxiety disorders. The development of Huntington's disease is in part due to the degeneration of the cells in the basal ganglia that are responsible for secreting GABA. **Glutamate**, on the other hand, is an excitatory neurotransmitter involved in learning and the formation of long-term memories. When glutamate receptors are overexcited, the result can be seizures and/or brain damage. **Endorphins** are not neurotransmitters but neuromodulators; they have analgesic properties and are thought to lower the sensitivity of postsynaptic neurons to neurotransmitters.

CATECHOLAMINES AND SEROTONIN

The group of neurotransmitters known as the **catecholamines** includes **norepinephrine, epinephrine (adrenaline)**, and **dopamine**. Catecholamines affect personality, mood, memory, and sleep. **Dopamine** is instrumental in regulating movement, and in reinforcing substance addiction. Elevated levels of dopamine in the mesolimbic areas of the brain are associated with the pleasant feelings engendered by stimulants, opiates, alcohol, and nicotine. Another important neurotransmitter (which is not a member of the catecholamines) is **serotonin**. Serotonin is inhibitory in general, and implicated in a broad range of serotonin disorders like depression, schizophrenia, and Parkinson's disease. Serotonin deficiencies have been one of the factors to blame for ailments such as anorexia, bulimia, obsessive compulsive disorders, migraines, social phobias, and schizophrenia.

CENTRAL NERVOUS SYSTEM

The central nervous system contains the brain and the spinal cord. There are **five basic stages** in the development of the central nervous system:

1. **Proliferation** (begins at ~2.5 weeks), in which new cells are produced inside the neural tube
2. **Migration** (~8 weeks), in which the young neurons move to the appropriate place in the brain and begin to form structures
3. **Differentiation**, in which the neurons begin to develop axons and dendrites
4. **Myelination**, in which glial cells form an insulating and protective sheath around the axons of some cells
5. **Synaptogenesis**, in which the synapses form (occurs at various periods, depending on both the brain's internal schedule and factors of experience after birth)

SPINAL CORD

The spinal cord is composed of **axons, dendrites, cell bodies**, and **interneurons**. The job of the spinal cord is to carry information between the brain and the peripheral nervous system, coordinate the right and left sides of the body, and control all of the simple reflexes that do not involve the brain. The nerve fibers in the superior portion of the spinal cord carry sensory messages, while the nerve fibers in the inferior portion transmit motor messages. There are 31 sections to the spinal cord, divided into five groups. From top to bottom, in order, these five sections are the **cervical, thoracic, lumbar, sacral**, and **coccygeal**.

SPINAL CORD DAMAGE

When the spinal cord is damaged at the **cervical level**, the result is **quadriplegia**; when it is damaged at the **thoracic level**, the result is **paraplegia**. When a spinal cord injury is complete, there will be a total lack of sensation and voluntary movement below the site of the injury. When the injury is incomplete, some sensory and motor function below the level of injury will be maintained. If the flow of cerebrospinal fluid (CSF) to and from the four cerebral ventricles is obstructed, then a condition called **hydrocephalus** may develop in which fluid backs up and there is an enlargement of the ventricles, destroying brain tissue. A similar enlargement of the ventricles has been observed in individuals with schizophrenia.

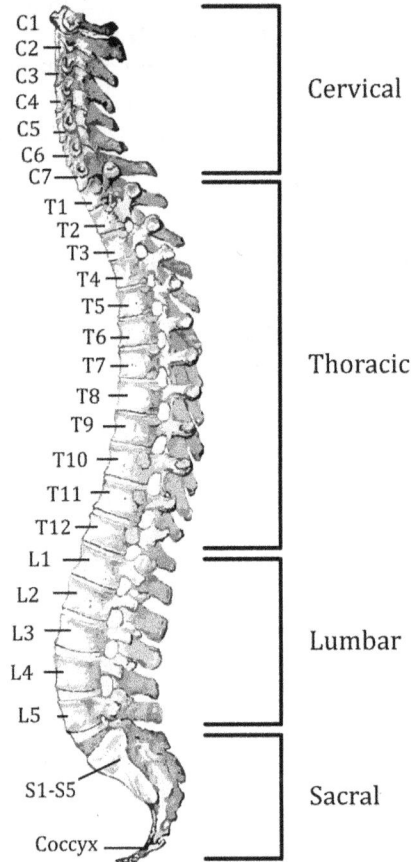

THE BRAIN

MIDBRAIN

The midbrain is made up of the **reticular formation**, which extends from the spinal cord through the hindbrain and midbrain into the hypothalamus structure in the forebrain. It contains over 90 groups of neurons, with functions ranging from respiration, to coughing, to posture and locomotion. The **reticular activating system (RAS)** is essential to consciousness, arousal, and wakefulness. It regulates sensory input, especially during sleep. When it detects important information, it alerts other parts of the brain. If an individual suffers damage to his or her reticular formation, his or her sleep-wake cycle may be disrupted; it is even possible to fall permanently asleep as a result of damage to this area. Some anesthetics work by depressing the RAS so that sharp pains do not wake the person up.

HINDBRAIN

The medulla and the pons, which are located at the base of the brain near the spinal cord, combine with the cerebellum to form the hindbrain. The **medulla** regulates the flow of information between the spinal cord and the brain, and coordinates a number of important processes like swallowing, coughing, sneezing, and heart rate. The **pons** bridges the two halves of the brain and is instrumental in coordinating movements between the right and left sides of the body. The **cerebellum** makes balance and posture possible and contributes to the performance of coordinated and refined motor movements. Autistic individuals have been found to have smaller than normal cerebellums. A damaged cerebellum may result in **ataxia**, a condition involving slurred speech, tremors, and a loss of balance.

THALAMUS, HYPOTHALAMUS, AND SUPRACHIASMATIC NUCLEUS

The forebrain is composed of both cortical and subcortical structures. The subcortical structures are the thalamus, hypothalamus, basal ganglia, and limbic system. The **thalamus** takes sensory input (except for olfactory input) and directs it to the appropriate part of the brain. Korsakoff syndrome is associated with atrophy in the thalamus.

The **hypothalamus** is linked to hunger, thirst, sex, sleep, body temperature, movement, and emotional reactions; if it is damaged, the emotions can be out of control. The hypothalamus also maintains homeostasis by regulating the pituitary and other glands. The **suprachiasmatic nucleus** is located in the hypothalamus and controls the circadian rhythm.

BASAL GANGLIA, AMYGDALA, AND HIPPOCAMPUS

The structure of the brain known as the **basal ganglia** includes the caudate nucleus, putamen, globus pallidus, and substantia nigra. The basal ganglia plan voluntary movements, and control the amplitude and direction of movement. The basal ganglia are also responsible for various facial movements that indicate emotional states, like smiling or frowning. Parkinson's disease, Tourette's syndrome, Huntington's disease, mania, depression, and psychosis all may stem from abnormalities in the basal ganglia. The **amygdala** directs motivational and emotional functions, and deals with emotionally-charged memories. The **hippocampus** processes spatial, verbal, and visual information, and consolidates declarative memories.

CEREBRAL CORTEX
FRONTAL LOBE

The **cerebral cortex**, otherwise known as the neocortex, is the largest part of the brain. It is divided into a right and left hemisphere, each of which is further divided into four lobes. The **frontal lobe** includes **motor**, **premotor**, and **prefrontal** areas. The **primary motor cortex** controls voluntary movements, while the **premotor cortex** contains the region known as Broca's area, which helps produce speech. Damage to Broca's area results in a condition called aphasia, in which a person cannot produce spoken or written language. The **prefrontal cortex** is involved in memory, emotion, self-awareness, and the so-called executive (sophisticated cognitive) functions. Damage to the prefrontal cortex can cause pseudodepression, pseudopsychosis, and trouble with abstract thinking.

PARIETAL LOBE

The parietal lobe of the cerebral cortex includes the somatosensory cortex, which controls the sensations of pressure, pain, temperature, gustation, and proprioception. If the **parietal lobe** is damaged, the individual may suffer spatial disorientation, apraxia (the inability to perform sophisticated motor movements), and somatosensory agnosia. This last condition includes tactile agnosia (the inability to recognize familiar items by touch), anosognosia (the inability to recognize one's own brain disorder), and asomatognosia (the inability to recognize parts of one's own body). If the **right** side of the parietal lobe is damaged, the individual may lose the ability to conceive of or control the left side of the body. If the **left** side is damaged, the individual may develop ideational apraxia, the inability to follow a simple set of directions

OCCIPITAL LOBE

The occipital lobe of the cerebral cortex includes the visual cortex, a region in which visual perception, visual recognition, and visual memory are managed. If an individual suffers damage to his or her **occipital lobe**, then he or she may suffer visual hallucinations, visual agnosia (the inability to recognize familiar objects by sight), or cortical blindness. In some cases, damage to the left occipital lobe can result in simultagnosia, or the inability to see either more than one thing or more than one aspect of a thing at a time. Individuals who suffer lesions at the intersection of the occipital, temporal, and parietal lobes may suffer from prosopagnosia, an inability to recognize the faces of familiar people.

TEMPORAL LOBE

The temporal lobe of the cerebral cortex contains several parts. The **auditory cortex** processes audible sensations. If a person sustains damage to the auditory cortex, he or she may suffer auditory hallucinations, auditory agnosia, and other disturbances. Another part of the temporal lobe is called **Wernicke's area**; this region is responsible for the comprehension of language. Damage to Wernicke's area can cause a form of aphasia in which there are severe problems with language comprehension and production. There are other, smaller areas of the temporal lobe involved in the encoding, storage, and retrieval of long-term memories. Interesting studies have been performed in which electrical stimulation of these regions caused people to recall long-forgotten events.

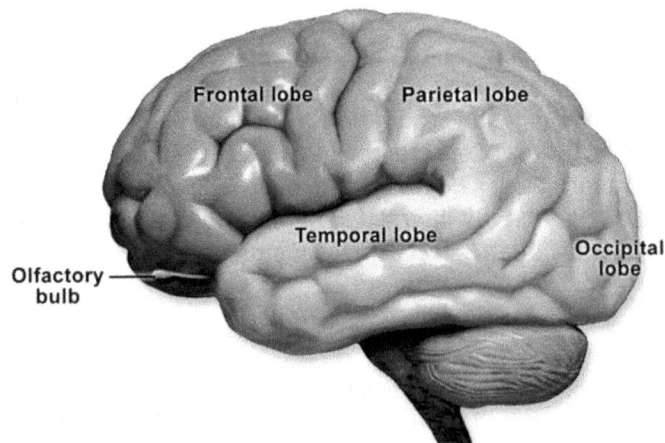

HEMISPHERIC SPECIALIZATION

The two hemispheres of the brain are somewhat specialized in their functions. For almost all people, the **right hemisphere** manages spatial relationships, face recognition, and creativity, while the **left hemisphere** takes care of language, analytical thinking, and logic. Scientists first discovered this phenomenon in studies of so-called "split-brain" patients, individuals whose corpus callosum had been severed as a treatment for epilepsy. Besides greatly reducing the frequency of seizures, the procedure produced some amazing insights. Although the brain retained its levels of intelligence, memory, and motivation, in some areas it behaved quite differently. For instance, the patients were unable to say the name of a familiar object when it was placed in their left visual field, though they could do so easily when it was in the right visual field.

CONTRALATERAL REPRESENTATION

Contralateral function refers to the fact that for almost all sensory and motor functions, the left side of the body is controlled by the right side of the brain, and vice versa. For example, all of the movements in the right leg are controlled by the motor cortex in the left hemisphere. There are only a few places in the brain where the two hemispheres are connected. One of these is a large bundle of fibers known as the **corpus callosum**. The fibers of the corpus callosum relay information that is sent from the body to both hemispheres. Fascinating studies have been made in which the corpus callosum is severed, causing the brain to act as two autonomous entities.

> **Review Video: Brain Anatomy**
> Visit mometrix.com/academy and enter code: 222476

PERIPHERAL NERVOUS SYSTEM

The peripheral nervous system (PNS) is composed of nerves in distal parts, not in the spinal cord or brain. Its function is to transmit messages between the central nervous system and the sensory organs, muscles, and glands. There are 12 pairs of cranial nerves and 31 sets of sensory and motor nerves that link to the spinal cord. The PNS is divided into the **somatic nervous system (SNS)** and the **autonomic nervous system (ANS)**.

The SNS controls voluntary motions by relaying messages from the sense receptors to the CNS; the ANS is primarily concerned with involuntary motions, and connects the viscera to the CNS. The **sympathetic branch** of the ANS is associated with arousal and the discharge of energy, while the **parasympathetic branch** is concerned with relaxation and digestion.

Review Video: The Autonomic Nervous System
Visit mometrix.com/academy and enter code: 598501

Key
● Structure
▲ Function

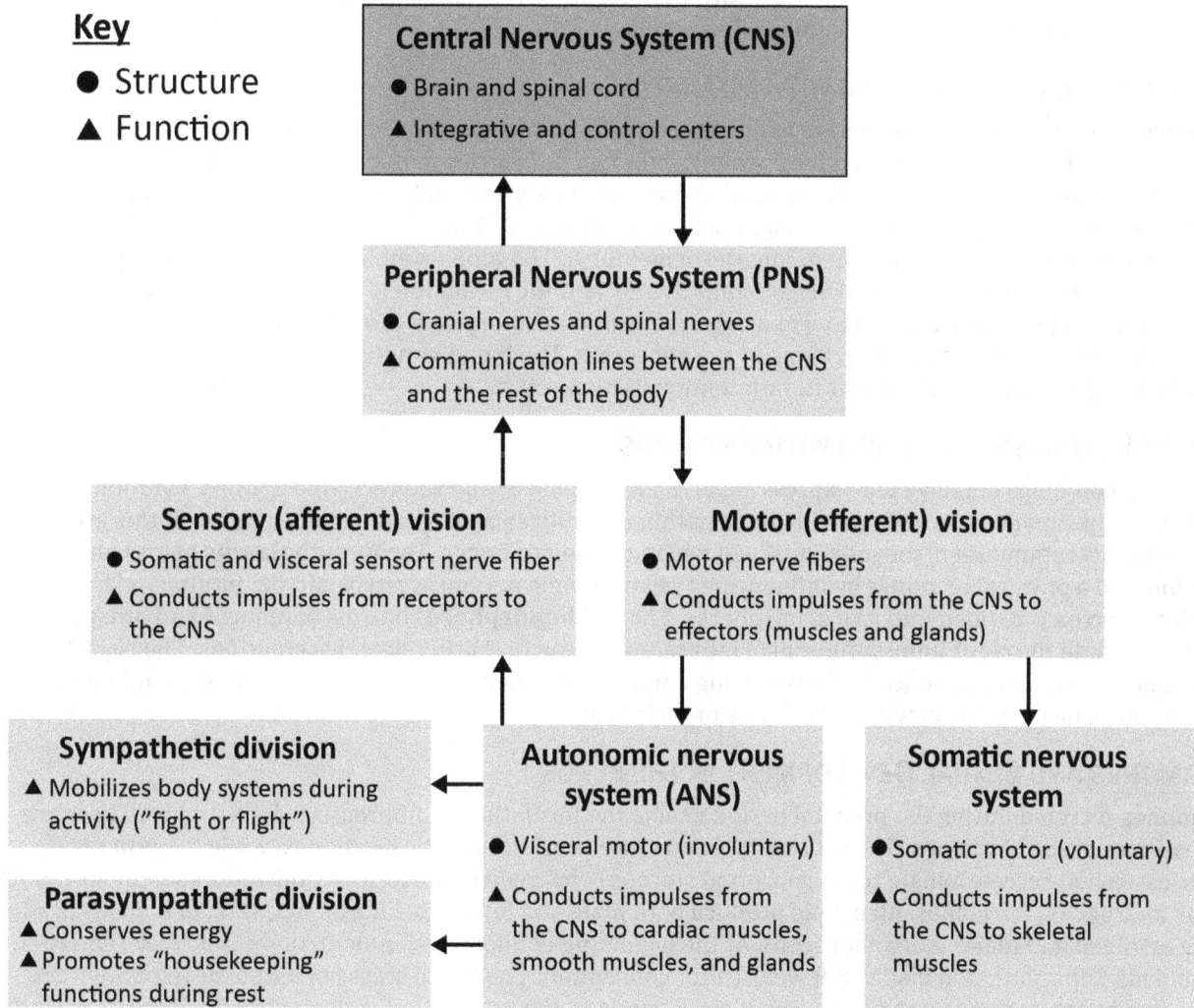

Central Nervous System (CNS)
● Brain and spinal cord
▲ Integrative and control centers

Peripheral Nervous System (PNS)
● Cranial nerves and spinal nerves
▲ Communication lines between the CNS and the rest of the body

Sensory (afferent) vision
● Somatic and visceral sensort nerve fiber
▲ Conducts impulses from receptors to the CNS

Motor (efferent) vision
● Motor nerve fibers
▲ Conducts impulses from the CNS to effectors (muscles and glands)

Sympathetic division
▲ Mobilizes body systems during activity ("fight or flight")

Parasympathetic division
▲ Conserves energy
▲ Promotes "housekeeping" functions during rest

Autonomic nervous system (ANS)
● Visceral motor (involuntary)
▲ Conducts impulses from the CNS to cardiac muscles, smooth muscles, and glands

Somatic nervous system
● Somatic motor (voluntary)
▲ Conducts impulses from the CNS to skeletal muscles

CUTANEOUS SENSES

The cutaneous (skin) senses are pressure, warmth, cold, and pain. Sensory information is carried from cutaneous receptors to nerves and into the spinal cord. The place where the nerve enters the spinal cord is the **dorsal root**. The dorsal root of a particular section of spinal column is known as the **dermatome**. Adjacent dermatomes overlap, so when a nerve is damaged the result is typically diminished sensation, rather than the extinction of sensation altogether. Several kinds of stimulus cause pain: Heat, pressure, and cold. An individual's perception of pain may be amplified by depression or anxiety. The **gate control theory**, proposed by Melzack, suggests that the nervous system can handle a limited amount of information at any given time, and excess sensory information is blocked by cells in the spinal column. One way to reduce pain, then, is to apply more sensory input, like heat or cold

NEURAL MECHANISMS INVOLVED WITH MEMORY

Scientists acquired much information about the neural mechanisms that affect human memory by studying sea slugs. One of the general insights is that short-term memory formation is shown by neurochemical changes at already existing synapses, while long-term memories necessitate the creation of more synapses and a change in the overall synaptic structure. **Long-term potentiation (LTP)** is the increased responsivity of a postsynaptic neuron to low-intensity stimulation for a while after it has been subject to high-frequency stimulation. LTP causes changes in the number and shape of dendrites, and increases glutamate receptors. Protein synthesis increases during memory formation. Genetic research has linked the apolipoprotein E gene (apoE4 on Chromosome 19) to Alzheimer's disease.

BRAIN MECHANISMS INVOLVED WITH MEMORY

Recent advances in neuroimaging have made it possible to locate specific areas of memory within the brain. The **temporal lobes** are involved in the encoding, storage, and retrieval of long-term declarative memories; the **right temporal lobe** is primarily engaged in nonverbal memory, while the **left temporal lobe** handles verbal memory. The **hippocampus** manages the consolidation of long-term declarative memory (that is, it transfers memories from short-term to long-term memory). The hippocampus also is involved in spatial memory. The **amygdala** is involved in fear conditioning and the formation of emotional memories. The **prefrontal cortex** helps with short-term memory, episodic memory, and prospective memory. The **thalamus** processes information and passes it along to the neocortex. The **basal ganglia**, **cerebellum**, and **motor cortex** all help with procedural and implicit (non-intentional) memory.

BRAIN MECHANISMS INVOLVED WITH EMOTIONS

The **amygdala** helps perceive and express anger, fear, happiness, and sadness, among other emotions. One function of the amygdala is to determine the emotional significance of incoming information. If this area is given electrical stimulation, the individual will become afraid or angry. The **hypothalamus** helps convert emotion into a physical response by influencing the autonomic nervous system and the pituitary gland. The **cerebral cortex** is divided into two hemispheres. The **left hemisphere** controls happiness and other positive emotions, while the **right hemisphere** manages sadness, fear, and other negative emotions. The right hemisphere is typically in control of recognizing emotions in other people, and indeed, most people tend to express more facial emotion with the left side of their face.

HORMONES AND SEXUAL DEVELOPMENT IN THE FETUS

Hormones secreted during the prenatal period enable the formation of differentiated sex organs. There are two sources of sex hormones: The **pituitary gland** secretes gonadotropic hormones, while the **gonads** (ovaries, testes) secrete female (estrogen, progesterone) and male (testosterone and androstenedione, known as the androgens) hormones. All people produce both male and female sex hormones, though females produce more estrogen and males more androgens. At the beginning of fetal development, there is no differentiation in the gonads. Differentiation begins 6-8 weeks after conception. The initial stages of sexual development are motivated by the chromosomes, but without sex hormones, the process will not get very far. If there is a lack of androgen, for instance, both females and males will develop female sex characteristics.

HORMONES AND SEXUAL DEVELOPMENT DURING PUBERTY AND ADULTHOOD

The beginning of **puberty** is heralded by an increase in **gonadal hormones**, which stimulate the emergence of secondary sex characteristics. Basically, the hypothalamus secretes chemicals that instruct the anterior pituitary gland to release hormones, stimulating the production of testosterone and sperm in the male, and ovulation and the production of estrogen in the female. The age at which puberty begins is influenced by genetic and environmental factors like nutrition, exercise, and temperature. For humans, there is less connection between adult sexual behavior and hormones than there is for lower animals. In fact, research has shown that there is not a predictable relationship between estrogen and sexual interest in females, though there does seem to be some connection between testosterone and sex drive in males.

Impact of Dimorphism and Spinal Injuries on Sexuality

Sexual dimorphism is sex-based differences in appearance. The human brain is sexually dimorphic; males and females have differently-sized corpus callosa, hippocampi, and SCNs. Most researchers believe that these differences in brain structure are the result of varying exposure to androgens during the prenatal and early postnatal periods.

Individuals who suffer **spinal cord injuries** are likely to retain sexual interest, and many are still able to have intercourse. Men that have complete lesions of the spinal cord, however, are unlikely to be able to ejaculate. Spinal cord injuries create even less of an obstacle to female sexual activity. Most women with spinal injuries report arousal and lubrication, though they have varying success reaching orgasm.

Physiological Reactions to Stress

There is a universal human response to stress, which was dubbed the **general adaptation syndrome (GAS)** by Selye. There are three stages to GAS response, which are managed by the adrenal and pituitary glands:

- **Stimulation**: The hypothalamus stimulates the adrenal medulla to release epinephrine (adrenaline). The glucose level rises and the heart and respiration rates increase as the individual becomes alarmed.
- **Resistance**: The body resists the stress by returning respiration and heart rates to baseline. The hypothalamus commands the pituitary gland to release ACTH, a hormone that causes the adrenal cortex to release cortisol, a chemical that maintains high levels of blood glucose.
- **Exhaustion**: The pituitary and adrenal glands fatigue, and the physiological processes break down. It is this sort of prolonged stress that is most destructive to health.

Sleep

Stages of Sleep

Electroencephalograms distinguish five stages of sleep:

- **Stage 1**: The EEG is mostly composed of **alpha** waves, and is similar to that of a relaxed, awake person.
- **Stage 2**: The EEG is composed mainly of **theta** waves, indicating relaxation, though there are some bursts of activity known as K complexes or sleep spindles.
- **Stage 3**: The EEG mainly records long, slow **delta** waves.
- **Stage 4**: In deep sleep, **delta** waves continue to predominate with fewer interruptions from K complexes and sleep spindles. Muscle activity decreases from stage 1 to stage 3, and then increases markedly during stage 4 sleep. This is the period in which sleepwalking and night terrors may occur.
- **Stage 5**: **Rapid eye-movement (REM)** sleep occurs, the period of the most elaborate and vivid dreams.

REM Sleep

Dreams are typically remembered if the individual is woken up during REM (rapid eye movement) phase of sleep, but if he or she is woken up just a few minutes after exiting this phase of sleep the dreams are likely to be forgotten. EEG readings taken during REM sleep are remarkably similar to those of stages 1 and 2, and indeed the physiological activity during REM sleep is almost identical to the wake state. Heart rate and respiration are both elevated, and sexual arousal may occur. Paradoxically, though, when individuals are in REM sleep they are almost entirely paralyzed. An individual typically runs through all five stages of sleep every 90-100 minutes and does this three or four times a night.

Sleep Patterns and Results of Sleep Deprivation

In the first 2-3 months of life, infants begin their **sleep cycle** in REM sleep, and slowly progress into non-REM, or NREM, sleep. Eventually, this sequence will reverse, and total sleep time will decrease. In these first couple of months, about half of all sleep time is spent in REM sleep, while as an adult only about 20% of sleep is REM sleep. It is a common fallacy that older people need less sleep; it is true, however, that they often have a harder time falling asleep and wake more often during the night. There are only mild adverse consequences of **sleep deprivation** lasting less than 48 hours. Any more than that, however, can result in hallucinations, personality changes, and disorientation. When people are deprived specifically of REM sleep, they tend to have a harder time learning new information.

OPEN-HEAD INJURY AND CLOSED-HEAD CEREBRAL TRAUMA

An open-head cerebral trauma occurs when the skull is penetrated. A closed-head cerebral trauma (concussion) occurs when a severe impact damages the brain without penetrating the skull. A closed-head injury often includes damage both at the site of the impact and at the opposite side of the brain, as the brain was pushed against the skull wall. There may be bleeding (hemorrhage) and a buildup of fluid (edema). Transient loss of consciousness and/or coma associated with closed-head injury results from strain on the nerve fibers in the brain stem. Patients who wake from a coma are likely to endure a period of **post-traumatic amnesia (PTA)**, in which there are memory deficits, intellectual impairments, personality change, and motor deficit. If these problems last longer than 24 hours, then they are probably permanent.

SYMPTOMS OF CLOSED-HEAD TRAUMA

Closed-head injuries often cause a small period of **retrograde amnesia**. Recovery from retrograde amnesia usually begins with the patient regaining the most remote memories. Patients who suffer severe closed-head injuries recover the most during the first three months post trauma. In most cases, it is easier to recover cognitive functions, rather than social adjustment and personality.

Postconcussion syndrome is diagnosed in the presence of the following:

- A history of head trauma, including cerebral concussion
- Disturbances in attention or memory
- At least three of these symptoms:
  - Fatigue
  - Depression
  - Affective liability
  - Personality change
  - Disordered sleep
  - Apathy
  - Lack of spontaneity

LANGUAGE AS IT RELATES TO BRAIN ASYMMETRY

Though the **left hemisphere** is typically dominant in the production and comprehension of language, there is increasing evidence that the **right hemisphere** also plays a role in these processes. Studies of patients who lost use of their left hemisphere indicate the right hemisphere will take over linguistic functions. Brain damage may result in a few different kinds of **aphasia**, impairments in the production and/or comprehension of language.

BROCA'S APHASIA

In Broca's aphasia, an individual will only be able to speak slowly and with great difficulty. Individuals with this form of aphasia will often suffer from anomia, the inability to name familiar objects. Broca's aphasia, unlike other impairments, does not include a lack of self-awareness, so individuals are likely to become very frustrated by their deficits and impairments.

WERNICKE'S APHASIA, CONDUCTION APHASIA, AND TRANSCORTICAL APHASIA

Wernicke's aphasia is caused by damage to the left temporal lobe. It is characterized by difficulty understanding and generating meaningful language. People with **Wernicke's aphasia** are capable of talking quite fluently, but will be unable to say anything consequential. **Conduction aphasia** is a condition that includes anomia and impaired repetition. **Transcortical aphasia** is caused by lesions that disconnect Broca's and Wernicke's areas from other parts of the brain. If Broca's area is isolated, then the patient labors to speak, may be unable to speak spontaneously, and may suffer from anomia. If Wernicke's area is isolated, the patient may have deficits in comprehension, anomia, and fluent but meaningless speech.

CEREBRAL STROKE

A stroke is a disruption in the supply of blood to the brain. Stroke can have a sudden onset (aneurysm) or gradual onset (atherosclerosis). There are three major causes of stroke:

- An **embolism** is the sudden blockage of an artery by material from somewhere else in the blood stream.
- A **thrombosis** is the gradual blockage of an artery by a blood clot.
- A **hemorrhage** is bleeding from trauma or a congenitally weak-walled blood vessel.

Risk factors for stroke include hypertension (high blood pressure), atherosclerosis (hardening of the arteries), smoking, and diabetes. Symptoms of stroke are contralateral hemiplegia, hemianesthesia of the face, arms, and legs, and contralateral visual field loss.

EPILEPSY

Epilepsy is the most widely known seizure disorder. Seizures are caused by an electrical storm in the brain. The patient may have an **aura** (sight, smell, sound, or feeling denoting an impending seizure), then loss of consciousness, and finally, abnormal movement.

- A **generalized seizure** is one that occurs in both hemispheres of the brain and does not have a focal onset.
- **Tonic-clonic (grand mal)** seizures have three stages:
  o Muscle contraction (tonic)
  o Rhythmic shaking of the limbs (clonic)
  o Depression/confusion combined with amnesia (ictal)
- **Absences (petit mal seizures)** are brief attacks in which consciousness is lost without motor symptoms being present. A person undergoing an absence seizure stares blankly ahead.

All other kinds of seizures are partial, beginning on one side of the brain and only affecting one side of the body. **Simple** partial seizures do not result in loss of consciousness; **complex** partial seizures do.

> **Review Video: Seizures**
> Visit mometrix.com/academy and enter code: 977061

PSYCHOPHYSIOLOGICAL DISORDERS
HYPERVENTILATION

Psychophysiological disorders are those in which the physical symptoms are initiated or amplified by emotional factors. Most of them only involve one system of organs, especially the autonomic nervous system. **Hyperventilation** is a psychophysiological disorder. The individual breathes rapidly from fear, anxiety, or anger. Carbon dioxide levels in the bloodstream drop, which leads to respiratory alkalosis and cerebral hypoxia. An impending hyperventilation episode may be heralded by chest pain, tingling and numbness in the hands and feet, dizziness, impaired concentration, and tinnitus (ringing ears). For many people, anxiety is compounded by the fact that the symptoms of hyperventilation are quite similar to those of certain coronary conditions.

MIGRAINE HEADACHE

Migraine headaches are severe, recurrent headaches that are usually restricted to one side of the head. **Migraine headaches** throb and are frequently accompanied by nausea, vomiting, diarrhea or constipation, and extreme sensitivity to light, noise, and odors. Any motion tends to make the headache much worse.

- A **classic migraine** begins with an aura, or focal onset, which alerts the individual that a migraine is about to occur.
- A **common migraine** does not have an aura, but may be preceded by gastrointestinal difficulties.

The cause of migraines is unknown. Most research suggests that they arise out of problems with the constriction and dilation of blood vessels in the brain. NSAIDs, beta blockers, SSRI antidepressants, anticonvulsants, triptans, ergots, butalbital, Botox, antihistamines, and feverfew are used to treat migraines.

HEADACHES OTHER THAN MIGRAINES

A **cluster headache** is characterized by excruciating, burning pain that occurs in clusters over a 2-to 3-month period. The pain is often centered behind one of the eyes, though it may spread to the face and/or temple. **Tension headaches** are characterized by non-pulsating pain on both sides of the head, at the back of the neck, and/or in the face. A tension headache may feel like a band of pressure around the head, almost like a tight hat. Although the traditional view was that tension headaches were caused by stress and muscle tension, it is now believed that they may also be caused by the dilation of blood vessels in the skull. The final kind of non-migraine headache is the **sinus headache**, which feels like pressure in the sinus cavity. This kind of headache may be caused by infection of the frontal sinuses.

HYPERTENSION AND FIBROMYALGIA

Optimal blood pressure is 120/80 mmHg. There are three kinds of hypertension (high blood pressure):

- **Primary (essential) hypertension**: The cause of the high blood pressure is unknown, but it is linked to smoking, sodium intake, stress, and old age. Primary hypertension has few symptoms and is often undiagnosed ("The Silent Killer").
- If primary hypertension is not treated, it can lead to **malignant hypertension** (diastole >120 mmHg). Malignant hypertension causes blindness, strokes, heart failure, aneurysm, transient ischemic attacks (TIA), and kidney failure.
- **Secondary hypertension**: High blood pressure related to a known condition, such as diabetes or kidney disease.

Fibromyalgia is a non-specific condition characterized by general muscle aches, tenderness, stiffness, fatigue, and sleep disturbances. The condition is more common among women, and though it may have a physical cause, it is often attributed to psychological factors.

ENDOCRINE DISORDERS

PITUITARY GLAND

The **endocrine system** is composed of the ovaries, testicles, adrenals, thyroid, parathyroid, hypothalamus, pancreas, pineal, and pituitary glands. Endocrine glands are ductless and secrete hormones directly into the bloodstream, where they are carried to the various organs of the body. The exception is the pancreas, an exocrine and endocrine gland that has a duct. The pituitary gland secretes **antidiuretic hormone (ADH)** and **somatotropic growth hormone**. Deficiency of ADH causes excessive water loss from diabetes insipidus. Children who do not produce enough somatotropic hormone have dwarfism. Children who produce excess somatotropic hormone have gigantism. Adults who produce excess somatotropic hormone develop acromegaly, in which the hands, feet, and facial features become grotesquely enlarged.

THYROID GLAND AND PANCREAS

The thyroid gland secretes thyroxine to maintain metabolism. If too much thyroxine is secreted, the result is hyperthyroidism, also known as goiter or **Graves' disease**. Patients with Graves' disease suffer accelerated metabolism, bulging eyes, pyrexia (high body temperature around 38 °C), heat intolerance, rapid weight loss, nervousness, and tachycardia (accelerated heart rate). If the thyroid produces too little thyroxine, hypothyroidism results. Patients with hypothyroidism suffer slowed metabolism, low body temperature (less than 37 °C), weight gain, depression, hair loss, fatigue, and impaired cognitive function (myxedema).

The pancreas secretes insulin, a hormone instrumental in taking up and using glucose and amino acids. If there is too much insulin, the blood sugar gets dangerously low (**hypoglycemia**). If the pancreas does not produce enough insulin, **diabetes mellitus** results.

MENTAL HEALTH DISORDERS DUE TO RENAL AND HEPATIC DYSFUNCTION

Renal or uremic encephalopathy is an **organic brain disorder** that results from increased toxins in the blood because of acute or chronic renal failure and a GFR of less than 15 mL/min. BUN and creatinine levels are markedly increased. Symptoms vary from fatigue to seizures and coma and may include confusion, impaired memory, emotional lability, somnolence, and asterixis (common) although the cause is unclear. Some medications, such as lithium and digoxin, may accumulate because of reduced renal function, contributing to encephalopathy. Treatment is dialysis, anemia reversal, and regulation of electrolytes.

Hepatic encephalopathy is a **metabolic brain disorder** that is most often associated with cirrhosis of the liver and acute liver failure and results from increased levels of ammonia, which impair function of neurotransmitters and cause damage to astrocytes, inducing swelling of the astrocytes and cerebral edema. Symptoms are progressive, usually beginning with confusion and lethargy. Patients become increasingly somnolent and disoriented, then stuporous, and finally comatose with decerebrate posturing. Motor activity decreases as the disease progresses, and asterixis is usually present. Treatment focuses on reducing hyperammonemia.

MENTAL HEALTH DISORDERS ASSOCIATED WITH METABOLIC DYSFUNCTION

Severe mental health disorders, such as schizophrenia and mood disorders, are associated with **metabolic dysfunction**, referred to as **metabolic syndrome**. This disorder is characterized by insulin resistance and glucose intolerance, obesity, high blood pressure, hyperlipidemia, and hyperuricemia. Patients with metabolic syndrome are at increased risk of diabetes mellitus and cardiovascular disease. Patients with severe mental illness often have high levels of cortisol as a reaction to stress, and this has been associated with increased visceral obesity, a contributing factor to diabetes and hypertension. Studies have shown that patients with schizophrenia tend to have **increased rates of obesity**, especially visceral obesity. Other studies indicate that those undergoing psychotic stress have impairment of beta-cell function in the pancreas and increased insulin sensitivity, and those with depression have increased risk of diabetes. Patients with bipolar also have increased rates of diabetes and high rates of obesity.

Advanced Pharmacology and Psychopharmacology

PSYCHOPHARMACOLOGY

Most psychiatric patients receive some sort of psychopharmacology treatment. With increased public education on many mental health disorders, pharmacological treatments are on the rise. Psychiatric medications mainly affect the **central nervous system**. More specifically, these medications affect actions at the cellular and synaptic level. Many times, drug therapy is used in conjunction with other therapies such as counseling or behavior modification.

The role of the nurse in psychopharmacology is very important. The nurse must understand each medication and what effects it may have on the patient. **Documentation** of a complete patient assessment is vital to the evaluation process of any medication. An **assessment** should be performed before initiation of treatment to determine the patient's baseline. An assessment should also be performed during treatment to evaluate for any change in symptoms or presence of side effects. The nurse also has an important role in **patient education**. Many psychiatric medications can have extreme side effects that the patients themselves must monitor. Education should also include, benefits, dosage, frequency, lifestyle effects, and whom to contact for any problems.

METABOLISM OF PSYCHIATRIC MEDICATIONS

Many of the mediations used to treat mental illness are taken orally. These medications are absorbed by the gastrointestinal (GI) tract and then move on to the **liver** for metabolism. The liver alters much of the medication causing it to be unavailable for use by the body. More specifically, many of these medications are metabolized by a specific enzyme in the liver called **CYP 450**. Certain medications are greatly affected by the **first pass effect**. The first pass effect is when an organ in the body acts to greatly reduce the effectiveness of the drug by decreasing the drugs availability for systemic circulation. Drug levels in the body are determined by the body's ability to metabolize these medications.

ROLE OF A RECEPTOR SITE IN PHARMACOTHERAPY

Most medications are developed for use by a specific receptor site within the body. Receptors are located on the cellular membrane and act to allow molecules to affect the action of the cell. Naturally occurring **neurotransmitters** or medications acting as neurotransmitters modify the body's receptor site by bonding with them. A drug that acts as an **agonist** produces the same effects as the neurotransmitter and stimulates this receptor. When a drug acts as an **antagonist**, it blocks the receptor site, therefore inhibiting the action of the cell by other agonists.

SELECTIVITY, AFFINITY, AND INTRINSIC ACTIVITY OF MEDICATIONS

A medication has the ability to bond with a particular receptor site due to its selectivity, affinity, or intrinsic activity.

- **Selectivity** refers to the medications ability to bond only with specific receptors. It selects the target receptor type from all others. It will not interact with unwanted cells of other organs or tissues and can help reduce certain side effects.
- **Affinity** describes the intensity of the attraction between the medication and its receptor site. If the drug has a high affinity, its effects will last longer and it is less likely that another drug will knock it off of its receptor site.
- The **intrinsic activity** of a drug describes its ability to produce the desired physiologic response. An example of a drug that would not produce an intrinsic response is an antagonist. It bonds selectively and may have strong affinity but does not act to produce a physiologic response. It acts to block one.

FACTORS THAT AFFECT SYSTEMIC DRUG AVAILABILITY

There are many factors that may affect drug availability within the body. The **route** through which a medication is given can determine systemic availability of that medication. The availability of a drug given **orally** can be reduced by a high first pass effect or diminished absorption of the drug in the GI tract due to increased or decreased motility or altered nutritional status. Conversely, medications that are given by **IV or IM** often have higher systemic availability because they are not subject to the same type of absorption or metabolism effects seen with oral medications. Often times the same medication is given at greatly reduced dosages when given by IV or IM when compared to the oral dosage.

DEVELOPMENT OF TOLERANCE, DEPENDENCY, AND WITHDRAWAL SYMPTOMS

A person can develop a **tolerance** to a particular medication when that medication is used over a period of time. The effects of the medication diminish and can lead to a need to increase the dosage to achieve the same response. Sometimes dependency and withdrawal symptoms can be seen along with the development of tolerance. **Dependency** can be psychological or physical in nature. The **withdrawal** of this medication can produce stress or anxiety along with real physical symptoms. The medication will often have to be weaned by slowly decreasing the dosage. In severe cases, abrupt discontinuation of the medication can lead to death.

POTENCY AND EFFICACY OF MEDICATION

The potency and efficacy of a medication helps to guide health care providers with medication choices.

- The **potency** of a medication is determined by how much drug produces the desired effect and is an important consideration when comparing medications. One medication may produce the same response as another but utilizes less medication to achieve it. This would make the drug more potent than the other.
- The **efficacy** of a drug is its ability to elicit a physiologic response from the receptor. A medication with increased efficacy will produce a greater response than one with low efficacy. A medication may be very potent but have low efficacy.

PHASES OF PHARMACOLOGICAL TREATMENT

There are four main phases of pharmacological treatment. These include **initiation, stabilization, maintenance**, and **discontinuation**. The nurse is involved in all phases of this treatment process and patient assessment during all phases is vital. It must be determined if the patient is actually taking the medication as it was prescribed and if the desired effect is achieved. Careful assessment and documentation will provide insight into which phase the patient is in and if the patient is progressing as expected. Alterations of the medication can be made based upon the patient's response during any of these phases.

INITIATION PHASE

The initiation phase involves a complete **assessment and patient history**. A complete picture of the patient must be obtained to assist in determining which medication should be utilized. Lab work such as blood chemistry, complete blood count, and liver, kidney, and thyroid function tests should be obtained. Certain medication dosages may need to be adjusted based on these results. The presence of any physical condition should also be ruled out as a cause of symptoms. The inpatient should be closely monitored with the first dose of any medication for adverse reactions.

STABILIZATION PHASE

The stabilization phase is the time in which the **proper dosage of medication** is determined. There may need to be increases or decreases in dosage to achieve the desired response with minimal side effects. There should be an ongoing assessment process. This should include physical and psychological assessments along with re-evaluation of certain lab values or drug levels. The patient should be closely monitored for any unwanted side effects of adverse reactions such as abnormal muscle movements or elevated blood pressure or temperature.

The initial medication chosen may not produce the desired response and it may require the addition of another medication or be discontinued altogether. The patient should be closely monitored for any drug interactions.

MAINTENANCE PHASE

During the maintenance phase, a medication is utilized to **prevent reoccurrence** of the unwanted symptoms. Occasionally, these symptoms may reappear even though the medication is continued. This can occur because of a change in metabolism caused by the medication, development of tolerance, physical illness, stress, or use of additional prescription or over the counter medications. Some side effects may not be evident until the patient has been on the medication for a period of time. It is very important that patients are educated about the potential side effects and possible decrease in their drug's efficacy. They should be able to recognize red flag signs of symptoms of each of these. They should understand the importance of follow-up visits and testing to evaluate their particular medication regime.

DISCONTINUATION PHASE

The discontinuation phase of drug therapy is when a particular medication is **stopped**. Most psychiatric medications are not stopped abruptly, but require the dose to be slowly decreased over time. During the time the drug is being weaned off, the patient should be closely monitored for reappearance of the unwanted symptoms. By weaning off the medication, withdrawal symptoms can also be avoided. Some diagnoses, such as schizophrenia, require mediation to continue throughout the patient's life. Support, reassurance, and education are vital to the successful discontinuation of many psychiatric medications.

ETHNIC, CULTURAL, AND GENDER CONSIDERATIONS WITH DRUG THERAPY

Cultural and ethnic beliefs can affect an individual's attitudes and practices concerning health care. Communication and assessment of the patient can be complicated by language and social considerations. It may be difficult to get the patient to open up and verbalize their symptoms. The provider should be knowledgeable, respectful, and sensitive to an individual's cultural beliefs and how they affect their treatment regime. Along with the **social considerations** of different ethnic and cultural backgrounds come the **biological differences**. The biological differences between race, culture, and gender can affect the efficacy of the medication. There can be biologic, genetic, and hormonal differences that affect how a person responds to medications at a cellular level.

EFFECTS OF MEDICATIONS ON SEXUALITY

There are many different types of medications that can lead to **sexual dysfunction**. Medications such as antihypertensives, anticholinergics, neuroleptics, antiseizure, benzodiazepines, antipsychotics, and SSRIs are all examples of medication types that can cause sexual dysfunction. With anticholinergics and antiseizure medications, the side effects can include a decreased libido or orgasmic disorders in both men and women. SSRIs can cause a disruption in any phase of the sexual response. Women commonly complain of anorgasmia or delayed orgasm. Men also complain of anorgasmia plus additional problems with ejaculation. Many of these side effects lead to patient noncompliance and they will stop taking their medications in order to avoid these side effects. Many times, the medication or dosage can be changed to help combat these side effects.

PEDIATRIC PHARMACOLOGY

There are a number of pediatric pharmacology concerns. Pediatric doses are calculated according to the child's **weight** in kilograms, but other factors may affect dosage. Weight is estimated by age (although actual weight is safer):

$$\text{50th percentile weight (kg)} = (\text{age} \times 2) + 9$$

Only **pediatric medications** should be prescribed if possible. Adult pills, for example, should not be cut for use for a child as even small variations in dosage may have adverse effects. Dosages should always be checked. Drug therapy in children may sometimes require adult dosages due to the increased ability of children to metabolize the medications quickly. Children may also exhibit unusual responses (e.g., paradoxical effects) or side effects to drugs compared to adults and should be very closely evaluated and frequently assessed.

GERONTOLOGICAL PHARMACOLOGY

A number of issues can affect gerontological pharmacology, which are listed below:

- **Antidepressants** are associated with excess sedation, so typical doses are only 16–33% of a younger adult's dose. Although selective serotonin reuptake inhibitors are safest, fluoxetine (Prozac) may cause anorexia, anxiety, and insomnia and should be avoided.
- **Older antipsychotics**, such as haloperidol, have a high incidence of side effects. Atypical antipsychotics appear to be safer; risperidone (< 2 mg daily), for example, has the fewest adverse effects. The lowest possible dose should be tried first with careful monitoring of any antipsychotic.
- **Adverse effects of drugs** are two to three times more common in older patients than younger patients, which is often related to polypharmacy.
- Drugs may impact **nutrition** by impairing appetite. Interactions may also alter the pharmacokinetics of nutrients or drugs, interfering with absorption, distribution, metabolism, and elimination.

SPECIAL CONSIDERATIONS IN DRUG THERAPY WHEN USED IN CHILDREN AND THE ELDERLY

Medications can affect the very old, the very young, pregnant and breastfeeding women, and people from different cultures in a variety of ways. Dosages are usually less for the **elderly population**. Medical disease processes may affect the metabolism and clearance of many medications and they may also take many other medications that can lead to drug-drug interactions. Drug therapy in **children** will often require adult dosages due to their increased ability to quickly metabolize the medications. Children may also exhibit more unusual responses or side effects to drugs than adults and should be very closely evaluated and frequently assessed.

ADMINISTERING MEDICATIONS

When administering medications, the nurse should verify the **five rights** (i.e., patient, medicine, dose, route, time). Medications in unit-dose packaging should be placed in medicine cups and the packaging opened in the patient's presence. **Liquid medications** should be carefully measured in appropriate medicine cups. **Oral medications** should be taken in the presence of nursing staff followed by at least 60 cc of fluid to ensure that the medications have been swallowed. **Procedures** may vary within different facilities. If hoarding is a problem, patients may be asked to open their mouths for examination after taking medications. If medications are mixed with food or fluids, this should first be discussed with the interdisciplinary team and documented as to reasons (e.g., confusion); this is done to avoid the legal implications of coercion as this practice may be misconstrued as administration of hidden medications.

TRIAL PERIOD FOR NEW MEDICATION

When initiating any sort of pharmaceutical treatment for mental disorders, it is important to have an adequate trial period for new medication before switching to alternative therapies due to unresponsiveness. Generally speaking, a medication, such as an antipsychotic, is tested for **8 weeks** before switching. However, **4–6 weeks** is sufficient for stimulants before opting for a second-line treatment. Before switching medications, one should check with a pharmacist to ensure the dose of the current therapy has been optimized. It is not uncommon for agents to be prescribed in doses that fail to optimize the drug. **Drug optimization** may occur at either a lower or higher dose for an individual patient than the dose commonly prescribed. Dose optimization is one of the many reasons why upward and downward titrations are important.

PATIENT EDUCATION ASSOCIATED WITH TAKING PRESCRIPTION MEDICATIONS

Patient education is vital to the success and safety of taking prescribed medications. Patient education should include both the generic and brand name of the drug, indications for use, expected actions of the drug, dosage, route, duration of effects, what to do when a dose is missed, any associated precautions such as operating machinery or diet restrictions, any associated side effects, and when to call the prescribing medical practitioner or seek help. Patients should also be educated on ways to help decrease side effects. They should be given written information including drug name, dosage, action, side effects, purpose, and any other pertinent information about the specific medication. All patient education should be documented and include his or her understanding of the information, evaluation of the patient's ability to administer the medication, and his or her ability to obtain the medication.

Neurodevelopment

PRE-SCHOOL AGED CHILDREN
NORMAL PHYSICAL DEVELOPMENT

Children in **early childhood** range in age from 1-5 years. This age group makes great strides in their **cognitive and physical development**. Normal healthy children in this age group develop mentally, physically, and emotionally at different rates. Toddlers include 1- to 3-year-olds, and preschoolers include 3- to 5-year-olds. By age 2 most children can run, jump in place, and stand on their tip-toes. By age 3, the child has greatly improved fine motor skills and balance. They can perform tasks such as walking up steps, riding a tricycle, picking up small objects, and placing shapes through appropriate holes. By age 4 most children can run, kick a ball, get dressed, and eat without assistance. By the end of their fourth year, they can draw and cut simple shapes with scissors. By keeping regular checkup appointments with the pediatrician, many developmental delays can be identified in early childhood, and proper evaluation and treatment can be started. In 24 hours, toddlers require 11-14 hours of sleep (including naps), and preschoolers require 10-13 hours of sleep (including naps).

NORMAL COGNITIVE DEVELOPMENT

Most pre-school aged children learn from what they see others do around them and thrive in environments full of stimuli. A child's personality, sex, age, and siblings are all factors that can affect **language and cognitive development** during this time. By age 2, most children begin to become aware that they are separate from others. They can speak simple 2- to 3-word phrases and are able to communicate simple needs. By age 3, speech becomes clearer and children can often form short phrases consisting of 3-5 words. They begin to engage in imaginary and social situational play. By their fourth birthday, the child usually has a vocabulary of approximately 1500 words and can easily form sentences using 4-5 words. Memory has increased and they can begin to recall stories or events.

SCHOOL-AGED CHILDREN
NORMAL PHYSICAL DEVELOPMENT

School-aged children are considered to be between the ages of 5-12 years. By the age of 7, most children have continued **slow steady development**. Balance continues to improve. Most children of this age can balance on one foot, catch a ball, use simple tools, do some simple gymnastics, tie their shoes, and print words or short sentences. They start to lose their baby teeth and permanent teeth begin to appear. They may appear gawky due to long arms and/or legs. Older children from age 7 on to adolescence have greatly developed many of the fine motor and large muscle skills. Eyes reach maturity in both size and function, however, extended time viewing small print or screens can cause eye strain. School-aged children need approximately 10 hours of sleep per night.

NORMAL COGNITIVE DEVELOPMENT

School-aged children continue to have slow and steady **cognitive growth**. By age 8, most children have moved out of fantasy play and are more interested in real life scenarios. They have increased attention spans and enjoy working on tasks with friends or in groups. Following the rules and completion of these tasks becomes very important. They enjoy collecting things. They often make a best friend or establish a group of friends. They typically write clearly, however, they may reverse some letters. Their reading skills increase due to the fact that they can understand more complex stories. They are able to understand time in days and weeks. From age 9 on to adolescence, peer groups and social acceptance become increasingly important. They begin to understand and talk about the distant future. Daydreaming or fantasizing are not uncommon. They have continued interest in reading and often enjoy fictional books.

ADOLESCENT CHILDREN
NORMAL PHYSICAL DEVELOPMENT

Adolescence occurs between the ages of 12 and 18. **Physical development** occurs rapidly during the teen years and is commonly called **puberty**. It is during this time that secondary sex characteristics develop and the child becomes a mature adult able to reproduce. The physical changes that occur during this time include hormonal and brain development. In males, the hormonally induced physical changes include development of facial, underarm, and pubic hair, changing of the voice, and penile development. In girls, these changes include breast and genital development, onset of menses, and increased growth of underarm and pubic hair. Both boys and girls experience rapid weight gain and increased production of oils and sweat gland activity, often leading to the development of acne. **Brain development** continues throughout the teen years. Neurons responsible for the maturation of emotions continue to develop. Many teens experience difficulty controlling their emotions or impulses, often leading to risky behaviors.

NORMAL COGNITIVE DEVELOPMENT

As teens move through the adolescent years, they begin to mature in their thought processes and develop a sense of identity. They begin to develop advanced reasoning and abstract thinking skills. Many adolescents have a greatly increased sense of self-consciousness. They often feel as if everyone is watching and judging them. A preoccupation with their appearance, behaviors, and feelings can develop. They begin to develop the ability to think about how they feel and how others perceive them. Many teens develop a sense of immortality and participate in many high-risk activities such as unsafe sex or reckless driving. They believe that nothing bad will happen to them. Confidentiality is also very important during this developmental stage, and they may be hesitant to share information.

AGE CATEGORIES OF THE ELDERLY

The elderly population can be divided into three groups. The age group ranging from 65-74 years is considered the **young-old**, 75-84 are considered the **middle-old**, and 85 and older are considered **old-old**. There are many physical and psychological changes that occur as someone moves through these age groups. As this population increases in size, so does the number of those with mental illness. The mental health problems of this particular population are largely **undertreated**. Many rely on their primary health care provider to treat their mental health problems as well as their medical disease processes. Many of their medical diseases can lead to a loss of independence and feelings of helplessness, depression, and anxiety. These feelings may result in individuals leaving their careers or losing friends.

CHANGES ASSOCIATED WITH AGING
BIOLOGICAL CHANGES

As people move from the young-old to the old-old, many **physical and biological changes** occur throughout their bodies. Organs and tissues such as the kidneys, liver, heart, GI tract, and brain begin to decline, and some, such as the ovaries and uterus, fall into disuse and atrophy. Dysfunction of the **kidneys and liver** is of particular importance because these organs are responsible for drug metabolism. This population may also experience peripheral neuropathy, decreased reaction times, and decreased balance due to changes in the nervous system. There can also be a decline in the five senses. Changes in vision and hearing can affect performance on many of the assessment tools used to evaluate this population for mental health issues such as depression, delirium, dementia, or anxiety.

PSYCHOLOGICAL CHANGES

Psychological changes can occur in cognition, learning capacity, and memory. These changes can lead to **decreased continued development** and can **change relationships** with family and friends. Many of the cognitive changes are brought about by a general atrophy in the brain. The aging process does not impair a person's state of consciousness; however, there can be a generalized decrease in concentration, attention span, and reaction times, leading to poor performance on many assessment tools. Learning may be diminished simply because the elderly person may lack motivation.

Significant **memory loss** is not a natural part of the aging process. Memory loss can occur for a variety of reasons such as disease processes, medications, substance abuse, or depression.

SOCIOCULTURAL CHANGES

The elderly may experience many social changes such as changes in functional independence, employment, and social experiences with groups and friends. As the individual moves from young-old to old-old, many of the things that they were able to **do for themselves** will diminish. This can range from fixing household problems to basic activities of daily living (ADLs) such as bathing and dressing. This population also enters retirement and daily life may become less organized, and they may experience financial stress and anxiety. With retirement, this population may also have a reduction in healthcare benefits inhibiting them from seeking needed assistance. Debilitating medical conditions may also inhibit their social activities and lead to feelings of isolation.

AGING PROCESS AS IT RELATES TO MENTAL HEALTH

The elderly are becoming a larger proportion of the national population as advancements in health care increase longevity. **Mental health problems** among the elderly are also on the rise. Some of these mental health problems can be attributed to developmental issues. The elderly must adjust to having grandchildren, retirement, loss of activity levels, and the death of a loved one. The normal aging process is distinct from pathological aging that occurs from illness and disease. The distinction can readily be seen in the gradual progression of life transitions over long periods of time, as opposed to sudden, catastrophic illness. The elderly person may have a deficit in the form of a physical impairment, emotional deficiency, social issue, or financial inability to sustain a cherished lifestyle.

COMMONALITIES AND DISPARITIES BETWEEN THE ELDERLY AND THE YOUNG

Age-related disease or illness can cause an elderly person to experience a variety of **physical impairments**. A person who is incapacitated may experience **mental health complications**. The combination of these two problems can cause a state of **clinical pathology** to occur. The provider may find that the deviations from normal make it difficult to provide a differential diagnosis. Erikson's life span developmental theory indicates that the elderly must achieve a sense of integrity at this stage of life or fall into despair. Butler theorized that the elderly find a sense of integrity by verbalizing stories about life events. The stories predominantly seek to give them meaning and purpose through a life well-lived. If a person cannot do this, the result may be a depressive state of being.

HOW THE ELDERLY DEAL WITH LIFE TRANSITIONS

Typically, the elderly population seeks to cope with whatever problem comes their way without the benefit of mental health care. In 1991, Butler and Lewis developed a definition for **loss** in relation to the elderly. The elderly can experience a range of emotions whenever loss or death occurs. Examples of loss could be loss of friends, loss of significant others or spouse, loss of social roles within the community, loss of work or career, loss of a prestigious role, loss of income, loss of physical vigor, or loss of health. Some may experience personality changes or changes in sexual appetites. Elderly people may have a situational crisis that puts a strain on their resources. The resiliency of this population is evident by the large number of seniors who live independently with only a little support. Only 4-5% are institutionalized, and 10-15% receive homecare.

DISORDERS EXPERIENCED BY THE ELDERLY

The elderly population is highly susceptible to **anxiety disorders** for a variety of reasons. Depression may be underreported because of its complexity. Some elderly suffer with severe cognitive impairments attributable to **organic brain disorders**. Organic brain disorders include Alzheimer's disease and dementia senilis. Most who suffer an organic brain disorder are also afflicted by depression and psychosis. Drug and alcohol abuse are often reported inaccurately because it is difficult to differentiate substance abuse from major neurocognitive disorder (formerly dementia), and other health problems. Many of the elderly also experience sleep disorders and insomnia.

PROPENSITY TO MENTAL HEALTH DISORDERS EXPERIENCED BY THE ELDERLY

For a long time, the elderly were assumed to have a high incidence of untreated mental health problems, but the studies of Gatz and Smyer in 1992 reviewed the data and determined that this was not true. In fact, only one third of the elderly population requires mental health services at all. Many older members of the population that do receive mental health services were previously diagnosed with severe depression, bipolar disorders, and affective disorders. The most significant problems experienced by the elderly are anxiety, severe cognitive impairment, and mood disorders. **Anxiety** is the most prevalent of these problems. These numbers may be skewed by the fact that the elderly may not be seeking help when needed. Sadly, **suicide** rates are higher in this population than in any other population. The older a person gets, the higher the rate of suicide. Anxiety and depression can cause much suffering in the elderly.

FACTORS PREVENTING THE ELDERLY FROM RECEIVING MENTAL HEALTH SERVICES

There are a number of factors that **prevent the elderly from receiving mental health services**. Part of the problem lies in the strong values which guide the elderly to solve their own problems. Other seniors feel they should keep quiet about private issues. Still others feel a negative connotation from past stigmas attached to those who needed mental health care. Baby boomers approaching old age have been bombarded with literature on psychology and healthy lifestyles. Therefore, the baby boomer generation may take on a healthier attitude about receiving the appropriate mental health care for their needs. A limited number of counselors and therapists are trained in geriatric care. Providers for the elderly have difficulties working with payment policies and insurance companies. In addition, seeing the client's aging problems may cause unpleasant personal issues about aging to surface for the provider.

Psychogenomics

FOUNDATIONAL CONCEPTS OF GENETICS

Distinguishing the genetic influence on psychiatric disorders relies on an understanding of the following foundational concepts of genetics:

- **Genes**: Genes are the basic biological unit of inheritance. A gene is a section of deoxyribonucleic acid (DNA) that contains the equation for specific cell formation and building. Genes are found in specific sites on the chromosomes.
- **Alleles**: An allele is one or more alternate forms of a gene.
- **Genome**: This is the complete person's genes and alleles, containing all hereditary factors.
- **Genotype**: A genotype is the sum of a person's genetic constitution and alleles. One's genotype is unique to the individual and determines the type species.
- **Phenotype**: A phenotype is the observable characteristics or behaviors (physical, biochemical, and physiological) of an individual. Physical characteristics include height, weight, and eye color. Likewise, the phenotype may include one's expressions, responses to stimuli, and other behaviors. Phenotype is influenced by both genetics and environment.

GENETICS AND MENTAL ILLNESS

Genetic inheritance has a profound effect on the development of some mental illnesses, especially schizophrenia and depression. Most psychiatric disorders are caused by a combination of factors, such as genetic makeup, peripartum stressors and influences, environmental influences, and family and social stressors. Eliciting **family history of mental illness** is a very important aspect of case management as it may expose a genetic predisposition for illness, particularly if a first-degree relative has a disorder. An individual may have a high level of genetic risk if mental illness is prevalent in the family, or a low level of genetic risk if it is absent. If genetic risk is present, that individual is much more susceptible to developing mental illness as he or she ages, experiences life stressors, or is negatively influenced by environmental interactions.

DIATHESIS-STRESS MODEL

The diathesis-stress model is a theoretical psychological principal in which genes and environment interact to bring about mental illness. In other words, mental illness is a product of both nature and nurture. The diathesis-stress model theorizes that in the presence of **genetic predisposition, environmental stress** may trigger mental illness. The intensity of the stress and the severity of genetic predisposition may vary. For example, someone who has a weak genetic predisposition for mental illness may only develop the illness if he or she is exposed to extreme stress. On the other hand, an individual who has a strong genetic predisposition for mental illness may develop illness in the presence of a little stress. It is important to note, however, that an individual may have underlying genetic predisposition for mental illness but may never develop illness, regardless of stress.

HERITABILITY AND MENTAL ILLNESS

Heritability is the genetic contribution to a **phenotype** in a specific population of individuals. This genetic contribution is affected by maternal and paternal genetic contributions and allelic and dominance variations. Heritability may be estimated by statistical means that take into account both genetic and environmental variances on a given population. Heritability may be estimated using **regression and correlation models** (comparison of close relatives, siblings, twins, parents, and offspring) or **analysis of variance** (equations and coefficients of variance). Because mental illness is often directly correlated with genetic predisposition, predicted heritability patterns may expose a genetic predisposition for illness, such as schizophrenia or chronic depression, before symptoms present. In some cases, patients may express concern about their offspring inheriting mental illness. Research indicates that genetic variations can markedly increase the risk of developing mental illness in relation to stress and other environmental issues.

Advanced Practice Skills

Clinical Interviewing

OBTAINING A PATIENT HISTORY AND DATA FROM MULTIPLE SOURCES

During the admissions assessment, the nurse gathers information about the **patient's history**. The interview should occur in a space that allows for privacy, but it should not be isolated in case the patient becomes violent or threatening. Asking open-ended questions in a nonjudgmental manner (e.g., What problem brings you to the hospital?) is more effective than asking yes or no questions. Questions should focus on one problem or symptom at a time (e.g., Tell me about your sleeping habits.). Depending on the patient's condition, information may be obtained by:

- Directly interviewing the patient
- Observing the patient's behavior and interactions with others
- Reviewing previous hospitalization and discharge records
- Interviewing family or caregivers, ideally without the patient present so caregivers can speak freely (The nurse must be careful to not violate the patient's right to privacy and should ask the patient's permission to speak with others.)
- Interviewing police (if involved) and requesting a copy of police reports
- Interviewing EMS personnel and reviewing their written reports

SUBJECTIVE AND OBJECTIVE INFORMATION

There are two types of information that medical providers will receive from patients: subjective and objective. Information obtained through these means is what the health care provider will utilize in documentation.

- **Subjective information** includes what the patient tells the provider. This information is based on their description or opinion and is usually received verbally or through writing.
- **Objective information** is what the health care provider actually observes. This includes patient behaviors as well as any findings during physical assessment.

INTERVIEWING PRE-SCHOOL AGED PATIENTS

In most cases, it is better to interview the parent and child **separately**, though this may occur in the company of one another before the child is of school-age. Children can usually give better information about what they are feeling, and parents give better information on their external behavior. When talking with young children, speak in simple terms and short sentences. Convey a neutral attitude. Most children between the ages of 1-4 understand more than they can communicate. Children may not be able to communicate **absolute ideas**. Assessing the child during **play** may give insight into real world experiences that the child cannot verbalize through questions alone. Play will often allow for evaluation of physical and cognitive development, adaptability, social and moral development, and coping abilities. It may give great insight into the child's perceptions of social relationships and family. Play may include drawing, dolls, puppets, dress up clothes, or modeling clay.

INTERVIEWING SCHOOL-AGED PATIENTS

The interview of the school-aged patient usually takes place with the patient sitting on the exam table or in a chair. Talking with the patient is the best way to build rapport. At this age, children are gaining more **independence** and it is important to respect that. Starting the interview with a casual conversation about school and their interests, such as their friends or video games, can help to lighten the mood. Asking about their favorite subjects in school and what they like the most and least about school can open the door to gaining some insight on their school performance. Most school-aged patients can provide their own medical history, depending upon the severity of their illness. At this age, the parent or guardian of the patient should be present to confirm or clarify any medical history to ensure it is accurate. The patient's history of academic performance, including any disciplinary issues at school, should be confirmed with the parent or guardian.

INTERVIEWING ADOLESCENT PATIENTS

Establishing a healthy rapport with the adolescent patient is essential in order to obtain an open, honest history. The patient can sit on the exam table or in a chair and the interviewer should sit to place themselves at the **same level** as the patient. Initially, **patient confidentiality** should be explained to the adolescent patient and specifically what can and cannot be kept confidential. Any statements about wanting to hurt themselves or someone else cannot be kept confidential. The majority of the visit with an adolescent patient should be done without the parent or guardian present unless it is necessary. The interview should contain open-ended questions that cover their home life, education or employment, activities alone and with friends, any drug use or dieting habits, sexuality, suicide and depression, and safety issues. When discussing any drug use with the adolescent patient, make sure to ask about their friends' habits, also.

INTERVIEWING ADULT PATIENTS

Within the first few minutes of the interview of the adult patient, it is important that introductions are completed and are clear. Try to sit during the interview to not seem to be towering over the patient and place yourself at the **same level** as them. Provide **active listening** to the patient's concerns, empathy for these concerns, and concern for the patient as an individual. When a patient knows that that their concerns are taken seriously, they are more likely to be more active in their healthcare. Ask about job satisfaction, involvement in community activities, and social support to evaluate for possible signs of depression. Providing reassuring touch or a shared silence with the patient may put them more at ease and let them know that their problems matter. It is important to not be quick to move onto the next question, and rather, let the patient fully answer a question without interrupting them. Finally, while some of the problems expressed by the patient may not seem medically significant, they should still be addressed to some degree to validate them.

INTERVIEWING ELDERLY PATIENTS

The interview of the elderly patient differs from that of the adult patient because the interviewer is trying to identify what the patient can do versus what they should be able to do or would like to be able to do. In order to gather this information, it is important to spend the time necessary with the patient and provide patience in listening to their **complete history**. Hearing loss, vision changes, and dementia can affect communication with the patient, so more **time** may need to be spent with these patients and/or their family members. Important elements to consider in the interview process are the general health status of the patient, their mental health status, the activities of daily living, their social support system, the future outlook, and any family concerns they may have. Identifying their reliance on community services that are available can help to identify the patient's ability to care for themselves. There is a high incidence of depression and dementia amongst the elderly, and identification of these symptoms can help to determine in which area of living they need assistance.

MEDICATION RECONCILIATION

When obtaining an in-home medication list, known as a medication reconciliation, the first step is to ask if the patient has a list of medications or has brought current medications. If so, the nurse should review each medication, including the **dose and frequency**. If the medicine is available, the nurse should check the **date** on the medicine bottle as patients often keep medications for long periods of time and should assess the amount of remaining medication in relation to the dispensing date. If necessary, the nurse should ask the patient, family, or caregivers to provide information about medication, asking detailed questions about the drugs. Other questions can include the duration of treatment, reasons for taking the drugs, names of prescribing physicians, and the dispensing pharmacies. The nurse should specifically question any complementary treatments (e.g., vitamins, probiotics) and over-the-counter medications, asking about specific categories of drugs (e.g., pain medicines, antacids, laxatives, stool softeners, antihistamines) used both frequently and infrequently.

Health Promotion and Disease Prevention

HEALTH BELIEF MODEL

The Health Belief Model (HBM) is a model used to predict health behavior with the understanding that people take a health action to avoid negative consequences, if the person expects that the negative outcome can be avoided and that he/she is able to do the action. The HBM, as modified, is based on 6 basic perceptions:

- **Susceptibility**: Belief that the person may get a negative condition
- **Severity**: Understanding of how serious a condition is
- **Benefit**: Belief that the action will reduce risk of getting the condition
- **Barriers**: Direct and psychological costs involved in taking action
- **Action cues**: Strategies used to encourage action, such as education
- **Self-efficacy**: Confidence in the ability to take action and achieve positive results

This model attempts to encourage people to make changes or take action (such as stopping smoking) in order to avoid negative consequences, so this model—when used for education—focuses on the negative consequences (such as quitting smoking to avoid cardiovascular and pulmonary disease).

> **Review Video: What is the Health Belief Model?**
> Visit mometrix.com/academy and enter code: 954833

THEORY OF REASONED ACTION

The Theory of Reasoned Action, developed in 1975 by Fishbein and Ajzen, is based on the idea that the actions people take voluntarily can be predicted according to their personal attitude toward the action and their perception of how others will view their doing the action. There are three basic concepts to the theory:

- **Attitudes**: These are all of the attitudes about an action, and they may be weighted (some more important than others).
- **Subjective norms**: People are influenced by those in their social realm (family, friends) and their attitudes toward particular actions. The influence may be weighted. For example, the attitude of a spouse may carry more weight than the attitude of a neighbor.
- **Behavioral intention**: The intention to take action is based on weighing attitudes and subjective norms (opinions of others), resulting in a choice to either take an action or avoid the action.

HEALTHY PEOPLE 2030

The goals of *Healthy People 2030* are to allow people to have longer and healthier lives, to reduce health disparities, to create environments that promote health, and to improve the quality of life and health across all age groups. *Healthy People 2030* has 62 topic areas with 355 total objectives divided across five sections:

- Health Conditions
- Health Behaviors
- Populations
- Settings and Systems
- Social Determinants of Health

The Mental Health and Mental Disorders topic is included within the Health Conditions section and aims to utilize preventive measures, screening, assessment tools, and mental health services to improve mental health, particularly the access to and pursuit of treatment for those with mental illness. Goals include:

- Increase the proportion of adults with mental illness who seek treatment to 68.8% (currently 64.1%)

- Increase the proportion of children with mental illness who seek treatment to 82.4% (currently 73.3%)
- Reduce the suicide rate to 12.8/100,000 (currently 14.2/100,000), focusing on disparities by sex and age
- Reduce suicide attempts by adolescents to 1.8/100 (currently 2.4/100), focusing on disparities in obesity, sex, school grade, race, and ethnicity
- Increase the proportion of adolescents experiencing major depressive episodes who seek treatment to 46.4% (currently 41.4%), focusing on disparities by location, insurance status, sex, race and ethnicity, age, income, and country of birth
- Increase the proportion of adults experiencing major depressive episodes who seek treatment to 69.5% (currently 64.8%) focusing on disparities by location, age, and education

Other goals include expanding treatment for children and adults and increasing depression screening.

TYPES OF PREVENTIVE MEASURES IN MENTAL HEALTH

Gerald Caplan's (1964) **model for prevention** in mental health includes three types of preventive measures:

- **Primary**: The focus is on helping people to cope with stress and decreasing stressors in the environment, specifically targeting at-risk groups. Examples include teaching parenting skills to parents; providing support services to the unemployed; providing food, shelter, and other services to the homeless; and teaching about the harmful effects of drugs and alcohol to schoolchildren.
- **Secondary**: The focus is on identifying problems early and beginning treatment in order to shorten the duration of the disorder. Examples include follow-up for patients at risk for recurrence, staffing rape crisis centers, providing suicide hotlines, and providing referrals as needed.
- **Tertiary**: The focus is on preventing complications and promoting rehabilitation through teaching patients socially-appropriate behaviors. Examples include teaching the patient to manage daily living skills, monitoring effectiveness of outpatient services, and referring patients to support services.

HEALTH PROMOTION ACTIVITIES SPECIFIC TO MENTAL ILLNESS

Mental health screening, exercise, and patient education are especially important when promoting health specific to mental illness:

- **Mental health screenings** need to start at the physician's office. Most of these screenings can be performed by the nursing staff. These include depression screens to identify early signs of depression, dementia screenings, and suicide risk questionnaires.
- Patients with serious mental health issues are at risk for chronic disease due to a sedentary lifestyle and may have increased risk for diabetes and cardiovascular disease. **Exercise** can help to improve mood and provide an outlet for stress relief. It can also reduce social withdrawal.
- **Education** should be done at the individual level and community-wide. There has been a push to educate the general public on the symptoms of depression and to help identify those who are at increased risk for suicide. There have also been efforts to decrease the stigma associated with seeking treatment for mental health issues so that more people will come forward to receive the help they need.

MENTAL HEALTH PROMOTION AT THE COMMUNITY LEVEL

Mental health promotion at the community level focuses on helping people maintain optimal levels of health and wellbeing, providing preventive measures, and assessing risks and protective factors associated with mental health. **Promotion efforts** may include:

- Programs for children and adolescents, such as through mentoring or education, to help children learn coping and problem-solving skills
- 12-step programs to help people maintain sobriety/abstinence through peer support

46

- Early childhood intervention programs that help teach good parenting skills
- Support programs for people with mental illness to help them learn skills needed to live independently
- Sheltered workshops to provide opportunity for skill acquisition and employment for people with mental impairment
- Anti-bullying campaigns targeting all ages
- Programs to support the LGBT community and prevent abuse and prejudice
- Senior citizens' programs to provide services and social activities
- Primary, secondary, and tertiary preventive measures
- Boys' and girls' clubs to promote social interaction in a safe environment

SELF-CARE PROMOTION FOR THOSE WITH PSYCHIATRIC ILLNESS

Self-care promotion for those with psychiatric illness is imperative. The following should be taught and reinforced to these patients in order to maximize quality of life and minimize exacerbations of their illness:

- Stress management and relaxation techniques
- Exercise
- Medication education
- Pursuing healthy hobbies
- Establishing a support network that encourages a healthy lifestyle
- Prioritizing adequate and quality sleep
- Redirecting negative thinking
- Recognizing signs/symptoms of relapse/episodes/exacerbation
- Healthy eating
- Knowing when to seek professional help

ANTICIPATORY GUIDANCE TO IMPROVE CARE

Anticipatory guidance is a method of educating the patient and/or family about the diagnosis, prognosis, and future care. Anticipatory guidance allows patients and their parents/guardians to formulate realistic expectations with regard to the treatment plan. Anticipatory guidelines are a catalyst for bringing forth questions and concerns regarding patient development, treatment progress, disease progression, therapy outcomes, rehabilitation or palliation, and follow-up or community care. As with all communications, the NP ensures anticipatory guidance is **clear and concise** by:

- Asking patients and/or families if they have any questions
- Offering them a business card so they can phone with any questions they think of later
- Giving written anticipatory guidance handouts so the patient and family have reference information available at home (Often, they will not retain verbal information due to the initial shock that the diagnosis and prognosis causes.)
- Directing them to a reputable patient support group and arranging for the team's social worker to help them
- Asking if they would like the chaplain to visit

USUAL ANTICIPATORY GUIDANCE VS. TARGETED ANTICIPATORY GUIDANCE

Usual anticipatory guidance is the practice of disseminating a generic set of guidelines to a certain patient population. For example, parents of a toddler may receive pamphlets and/or physician-directed education on milestones, socialization, toilet training, and discipline that are standard issue for the institution or catchment area.

Targeted anticipatory guidance is when a healthcare provider specifically speaks to the individual questions and concerns of a patient and/or the parents/guardian.

There are pros and cons to both types of guidance. For example, usual anticipatory guidance covers a larger spectrum of topics and concerns, but may not touch on the one troubling behavior that is of specific concern to the parent, such as tantrums or combative behavior. Targeted anticipatory guidance covers the primary concern thoroughly, but fails to provide guidance on other topics that may become concerns in the interim before their next visit.

NEUROPROTECTIVE STRATEGIES

Neuroprotective strategies are those used to prevent damage to the brain. Strategies include:

- **Substance use disorder programs**: Dual diagnosis is common, but substance abuse may worsen symptoms and interfere with recovery or maintenance, so patients should be referred to substance use disorder programs specifically intended for those with mental illness.
- **Medication choice**: Atypical antipsychotics are less likely to result in extrapyramidal adverse effects than typical but more likely to result in metabolic effects and weight gain, which may lead to cardiovascular disease and diabetes. Patients should be maintained on drugs for psychotic episodes at least one year and many may need drugs indefinitely. Patients must learn to recognize signs of relapse. Restarting medications immediately on relapse can prevent symptoms from becoming severe.
- **Cognitive behavioral therapy**: Can help patients learn to control symptoms and recognize hallucinations and delusions, allowing them to function better in society.
- **Early intervention**: The prognosis for mental disorders is better if treatment is instituted early, with the first episode, rather than delayed.
- **Support programs**: Programs to support patients in the community increase compliance with treatment.

HHS GUIDELINES FOR HELPING SMOKERS QUIT

The US Department of Health and Human Services guidelines for **helping smokers quit** includes the following information:

- **Ask** about and record smoking status at every visit.
- **Advise** all smokers to quit and explain health reasons why quitting is beneficial.
- **Assess** readiness to quit by questioning and if willing, provide resources. If the patient is not willing, provide support and attempt to motivate the person to quit with information.
- **Assist** smokers with a plan that sets a date (within 2 weeks), removes cigarettes, enlists family and friends, reviews past attempts, and anticipates challenges during the withdrawal period. The NP must give advice about the need for abstinence and discuss the association of smoking with drinking. Medications to help control the urge to smoke (patches, gum, lozenges, prescriptions) and resources should be provided.
- **Follow-up monitoring** should be done to evaluate progress and reinforce the program.

EXERCISE

Daily exercise is an important component of good health practices but should be age-appropriate, and some health conditions may pose restrictions. Toddlers and young children usually get exercise by running and playing and do not need organized activities, but others benefit from **planned exercise**:

- **4- to 5-year-olds** may participate in dancing, skating and other supervised activities but lack coordination and judgment about safety.
- **6- to 12-year-olds** are still growing and muscles are short, so they do best with non-competitive sports, such as bicycling and swimming, until about age 10. Team sports should be supervised to ensure children are not straining muscles. Weight lifting may be done at 11 to build strength. Gymnastics may begin but children should be monitored for eating disorders.

- **12- to 18-year-olds** can participate in any sports activity unless limited by illness or disability. Exercise should be done at least 3 times weekly for 30 minutes.
- **Adults**: Exercise should be done at least 30 minutes daily or 150 minutes/week.

EMERGENCY CONTRACEPTION

Females who have had unprotected sexual intercourse, consensual or rape, are at risk for pregnancy and may desire **emergency contraception**. Emergency contraception inhibits ovulation and prevents pregnancy rather than aborting a pregnancy. Because the medications contain hormones (such as ethinyl estradiol and norgestrel or levonorgestrel) in differing amounts, this treatment is contraindicated in those with a history of thromboembolia or severe migraine headaches with neurological symptoms. The criteria for administration of emergency contraception include:

- ≤72 hours since unprotected sexual intercourse
- Negative pelvic exam
- Negative pregnancy test

The regimen involves taking a first dose of 1-20 pills (depending upon the brand and concentration of hormones) and then a second dose of 1-20 pills 12 hours later. A follow-up pregnancy test should be done if the person does not menstruate within 3 weeks as the failure rate is about 1.5%. Side effects include nausea (relieved by taking medication with meals or with an antiemetic), breast tenderness, and irregular bleeding.

PREVENTION OF SEXUALLY TRANSMITTED INFECTIONS

The **Centers for Disease Control and Prevention (CDC)** has developed 5 strategies to prevent and control the spread of sexually transmitted infections (STIs):

- Educate those at risk about how to make changes in sexual practices to prevent infection
- Identify symptomatic and asymptomatic infected persons who may not seek diagnosis or treatment
- Diagnose and treat those who are infected
- Prevent infection of sex partners through evaluation, treatment, and counseling
- Provide pre-exposure vaccination for those at risk

Practitioners are advised to obtain sexual histories of patients and to assess risk. The **5-P approach** to questioning is advocated.

- **Partners**: Gender and number
- **Pregnancy prevention**: Birth control
- **Protection**: Methods used
- **Practices**: Type of sexual practices (oral, anal, vaginal) and use of condoms
- **Past history of STIs**: High-risk behavior (promiscuity, prostitution) and disease risk (human immunodeficiency virus [HIV]/hepatitis)

The Centers for Disease Control and Prevention (CDC) recommends a number of specific preventive methods as part of the clinical guidelines for the prevention of sexually transmitted infections (STIs):

- Patients should be counseled in regard to abstinence/reduction in number of sex partners.
- Pre-exposure vaccination: All those evaluated for STIs should receive a hepatitis B vaccination, and men who have sex with men (MSM) and illicit drug users should receive hepatitis A vaccination.
- Male latex (or polyurethane) condoms should be used for all sexual encounters with only water-based lubricants used with latex.
- Female condoms may be used if male condom can't be used properly.
- Condoms and diaphragms should not be used with spermicides containing nonoxynol-9 (N-9) and N-9 should not be used as a lubricant for anal sex.

- Non-barrier contraceptive measures provide no protection from STIs and must not be relied on to prevent disease.
- Women should be counseled regarding emergency contraception with medication or insertion of a copper intrauterine device (IUD).

MENTAL HEALTH PROMOTION PRESENTATIONS

ORGANIZATION

Most presentations can be organized into three main sections. These sections include an introduction, body, and conclusion.

- The **introduction** should include the main purpose of the presentation and can include important statistics or facts.
- The **body** should include the main ideas.
- The **conclusion** should summarize all the information presented and can allow for questions and answers.

Determine a format for the presentation by deciding upon a **sequence**. This section can be organized by simply stating a sequence of events, placing information into categories, stating problems and solutions, or providing contrasts and comparisons. Then decide if **visual aids** should be utilized and what type will most effectively present the information. Examples of visual aids include a flip chart, transparencies, and more commonly the use of an LCD projector. Visual aids can include words, pictures, graphs, or charts.

PREPARATION

When preparing a presentation for peers, interdisciplinary members of the health care team, accreditation agencies, or anytime an individual will be speaking publicly, **preparation** is the most important part of a successful presentation. For many people, the most difficult part of preparing a presentation is getting started. First, all the facts and information on the subject should be gathered and reviewed. Determine which information is the most important along with how much and what parts of the content should be presented. Try not to read the presentation. Visual aids with topic headings and subheadings can be a very effective tool to help guide the speaker. When utilizing visual aids within a presentation, always practice using the equipment before the presentation begins.

Mental Health Screening

NURSING ASSESSMENT AND PATIENT HISTORY

Nursing assessment is defined as the gathering of patient information in a comprehensive, accurate, and systematic manner. A history is taken from patients and others (such as family members) to complete the assessment. Information relevant to a psychiatric nursing assessment includes the **biopsychosocial assessment** and the **mental status exam**.

A thorough biopsychosocial history includes:

- Identifying data
- Chief complaint
- History of present illness
- Psychiatric history
- Medical history
- Medication history
- Developmental history
- Family history
- Social history
- History of alcohol and substance abuse
- Occupational and educational history
- Culture, spirituality, and values
- Coping skills

The mental status exam assesses:

- Appearance
- Behavior
- Cognition
- Speech and language
- Thought process
- Thought content
- Mood
- Affect
- Memory
- Insight and judgment
- Intellectual functioning

EVALUATION AND DECISION MAKING IN THE ASSESSMENT PROCESS

Evaluation is the process of accumulating data in order to improve a person's ability to make a decision based on reliable standards. The accumulated data is given careful consideration and appraisal by the evaluator to ensure that it is complete and accurate. The evaluator must make some kind of interpretation or inference about the data that has been collected. This inference is known as a value judgment and is a common task for the mental health care provider who uses a methodical and well-organized system to help make these value judgments. Decision making is a process in which the collected data have been weighed against possible consequences and test results. Decisions are made every day. Some lead to mistakes that need to be corrected, but it is still best to make decisions with confidence.

Decision making is a process in which the collected data have been weighed against possible consequences and test results. Decision-making is applied in both actuarial and clinical predictions.

- **Actuarial (statistical) predictions** are those based on empirically validated data. They may incorporate regression or multiple-regression equations.
- **Clinical predictions** are based on the intuition and experience of the observing clinician.

LEVELS OF OBSERVATION

One type of assessment involves nonstandard procedures that are used to provide individualized assessments. **Nonstandard procedures** include observations of client behaviors and performance. There are three **levels of observation** techniques that can be applied:

- The **first level** is casual informational observation, where the provider gleans information from watching the client in unstructured activities throughout the day.
- The **second level** is guided observation, an intentional style of direct observation accomplished with a checklist or rating scale to evaluate the performance or behavior seen.
- The **third level** is the clinical level, where observation is done in a controlled setting for a lengthy period of time. This is most often accomplished on the doctoral level with applied instrumentation.

INSTRUMENTS USED DURING THE OBSERVATION PROCESS

The following **instruments** can be used in an observation:

- The **checklist** is used to check off behaviors or performance levels with a plus or minus sign to indicate that the behavior was observed or absent. The observer can converse with the client as they mark the checklist.
- The **rating scale** is a more complex checklist that notes the strength, frequency, or degree of an exhibited behavior. The evaluator of the behavior makes a judgment about whatever question has been asked on the rating scale.
- The **anecdotal report** is used to record subjective notes describing the client's behavior during a specified time or in a specified setting, and is often applied to evaluate a suspected pattern.

Structured interviews, questionnaires, and personal essays or journals are additional instruments that may be used during the observation process.

ACTUARIAL AND CLINICAL PREDICTIONS AND ASSESSING CHILDREN

In order to obtain a useful interview from a child, the clinician must establish a good rapport and maintain the cooperation of the child. Establish rapport by:

- Using **descriptive** statements to encourage the child (e.g., "You're doing well.")
- Using **reflective** statements that encourage the child to think about what he or she has said (e.g., "You sound very angry about that.")
- **Praising** the child specifically for those things that contribute to a good interview
- **Avoiding criticism**

Some clinicians use anatomically correct dolls to help children discuss issues of sexual function and abuse.

THEMATIC ASSESSMENT AND METHODOLOGICAL INNOVATIONS

Thematic assessment appraises major themes that have happened over the lifetime of a patient. As the patient verbalizes his or her life events, the provider makes notes of the themes or predominant topics that create a pattern. The predominant themes are then related to the assessment, which attempts to bring into focus a better understanding of what these themes mean. The assessment can be a pencil-and-paper test, a behavioral assessment, or a clinical interview.

- One type of **paper-and-pencil test** is the Minnesota Multiphasic Personality Inventory (MMPI), with the most recent version updated in 2008, the MMPI-2-RF (Restructured Form). This test is now also available online via telepractice.
- **Behavioral chart** assessments can be used to document a person's habitual, explosive angry episodes.
- **Clinical interviews** are used for cognitive imagery assessments.

Methodological innovations are concerned with processes, strategies, and techniques, which can be used to help a client change his or her behavior.

ASSESSING MEMBERS OF CULTURALLY DIVERSE POPULATIONS

Guidelines mental health care providers should remember when assessing members of culturally diverse populations are:

- Clarify the purpose of the evaluation for the examinee.
- Be sensitive to any test material that unfairly discriminates against individuals of a particular culture.
- Use an alternate method of assessment that is more appropriate to the individual, if necessary.
- Before beginning an assessment, become familiar with the norms and values of the examinee's culture.
- Recognize that the job is to establish a good rapport with the examinee, and call a replacement provider if good rapport is not possible.

SEXUALITY

Sexuality is an integral part of each individual's personality and refers to all aspects of being a sexual human. It is more than just the act of physical intercourse. A person's sexuality is often apparent in everything they do, their appearance, and how they interact with other people. There are four main aspects of sexuality and they include the following: **genetic identity** or chromosomal gender, **gender identification** or how they perceive themselves with regards to male or female, **gender role** or the attributes of their cultural role, and **sexual orientation** or the gender to which they are attracted. By assessing and attempting to conceptualize a person's sexuality, the health care provider can gain a broader understanding of the patient's beliefs and will be able to provide a more holistic approach to providing care.

PSYCHIATRIC ILLNESS AND SEXUALITY

Many times, psychiatric illness can affect a person's sexuality. **Mental illness**, such as depression, can often decrease the patient's sexual desire, while the manic patient will often become hypersexual. **Bipolar patients** can experience a lack of sexual inhibition and may have many sexual affairs or act very seductively or overtly sexual. **Psychotic patients** may experience hallucinations or delusions of a sexual nature, and the **schizophrenic patient** may exhibit inappropriate sexual behaviors such as masturbation in public. Long-term care facilities will need to keep their residents safe from sexually transmitted infections, unwanted pregnancies, and unwanted sexual advances or assaults from others.

BARRIERS TO PATIENT ASSESSMENT

LANGUAGE OR CULTURAL BARRIERS

Language or cultural barriers to performing the patient assessment should be evaluated by the staff member performing the assessment. If there is a **language barrier**, the staff member should be able to obtain an interpreter to assist with communication. Most facilities provide access to an interpreter at all times to facilitate patient-provider communication. The staff member should also be aware of any **cultural beliefs or practices** that may influence the assessment. Staff members should always strive to work within the cultural context of the patient. They should work to develop a sense of cultural awareness and knowledge. Each patient should be viewed as an individual with individual influences and beliefs and be treated with respect and consideration.

PHYSICAL AND COGNITIVE BARRIERS

There may be certain physical or cognitive barriers to performing the patient assessment.

- An example of certain **physical barriers** could be if the patient has decreased hearing or speaking abilities or other diminished motor abilities. The patient may simply be physically unable to participate in certain portions of the examination. This information and an exact description of the patient's deficits should be documented in the record.
- Certain **cognitive barriers** may also be present. Some patients may not be able to understand certain questions or be able to effectively communicate their answers.

Tool Selection and Interpretation

PSYCHOLOGICAL ASSESSMENT TERMINOLOGY

A **standardized test** is one in which the questions and potential responses from all tests can be compared with one another. Every aspect of the test must remain consistent.

A **behavioral assessment** assumes that an individual can only be evaluated in relation to his or her environment. Behavioral assessments must include a stimulus, organism, response, and consequences (SORC).

A **dynamic assessment** involves systematic deviation from the standardized test to determine whether the individual benefits from aid. This includes the process called "testing the limits," in which an examinee is provided with a sequence of extra clues.

Domain-referenced testing breaks evaluation into specific domains of ability—for instance, reading or math ability.

MEASUREMENT AND TESTS IN THE ASSESSMENT PROCESS

The mental health care provider develops a representation of the client through the collection of facts. Psychometric instruments are used to collect pertinent data on the client. **Measurement** is a numerical value that has been allocated to a mannerism, attribute, or characteristic on the instrument. The measurement used must be one that is commonly understood by the general population.

A **test** is a task or series of tasks used to examine a psychomotor behavior or action that is indicative of a state of being. The state of being can be cognitively based or affective in nature. Answering written questions is a typical test scenario. The student goes through the task of answering academically based questions to indicate that cognitive learning has been accomplished in an academic class. The teacher grades the test and makes the inference that the student has learned on a cognitive or affective level.

TEST SELECTION AND ADMINISTRATION

The primary concern in test selection should be the client's needs and wants. Out of this consideration, the mental health care provider makes an informed decision about which **tests and psychometric techniques** to apply. A provider should suggest testing if there is a need to gain further information, but testing is not necessarily required. The client may perceive the testing to be some kind of threat or manipulative tool. In that case, the client should be reassured and educated about the real purpose of the test. **Competency level** should also be considered when selecting, administering, measuring, and evaluating the test results, including legal issues involving a particular assessment, and any **ethical issues** that may be associated with an assessment. The mental health care provider may require additional training in test procedures before giving and assessing a particular test.

USING THE INTERNET FOR TEST SELECTION

The internet provides an excellent search tool for the mental health provider. The internet can be used to locate specific tests that are applicable to the client's needs and wants. The **decision-making model** presented by Drummond in 1996 can be used to help select the most appropriate test. Any tests being considered should be evaluated for dimension, traits, and attributes. The decision should be based on what kind of information is anticipated to be the most useful. This involves a thorough perusal of the information already available at hand. The internet can also be used to search through objective evaluations given by others. Prospective tests should also be appraised for validity and reliability. The test and its results must provide the mental health care provider and the client with a practical use.

ISSUES IMPACTING TEST SELECTION

The test-related issues that may impact the selection of a test include validity, reliability, and norm standards.

- The issue of **validity** in a test involves an effective examination that gives the desired results. Tests used within the mental health profession should have well founded, criterion-based content that measures what it is supposed to measure.
- Before using a test, make sure it has received an independent appraisal from established sources, and is considered **reliable**, meaning that the test results should be able to stand up over a period of time. The test should give a precise and accurate score. The entire test should be evaluated for its *reliability coefficient* and *standard of error measurement*. The test may present a split-half reliability that measures internal consistency among other assessment instruments.
- The test should follow the **norm-referenced criteria** for the client's age, sex, ethnic origin, culture, and socioeconomic status.

PAPER-AND-PENCIL TESTS VS. PERFORMANCE TESTS

Another choice in test selection is that between administering a paper-and-pencil test vs. a performance test.

- **Paper-and-pencil tests** are used by a variety of test takers. One drawback is found when the client cannot read at the same level at which the test is written.
- **Performance tests** are given with a verbal request. The verbal request elicits a response that measures whether the client can follow the instruction given.

Paper-and-pencil and performance tests can either be applied in group settings or in individual treatments. Group-administered tests may be given by untrained proctors in a variety of settings. Typically, the group completes a paper-and-pencil test. Individuals may take the test under the supervision of an administrator. The administrator understands the complexities involved in giving the test, scoring the test, and interpreting the test results. Paper-and-pencil tests or performance tests are used to collect data about an exhibited behavior. The data is then evaluated. Paper-and-pencil tests are used to provide a fast, inexpensive, and objective grade. Test publishers develop most of the commercial grade paper-and-pencil assessment tests available. The administrator or proctor of the paper-and-pencil test will distribute materials, read the directions to the group, time the test, and collect the test.

USING COMPUTERS IN PSYCHOLOGICAL ASSESSMENTS

The computer has gained popularity over paper-and-pencil tests and has changed the field of assessment through a wide range of mechanically based scoring mechanisms. The analog computer has been incorporated in tallying the score of the Strong Vocational Interest Blank, now called the Strong Interest Inventory, developed by Edward Kellog Strong in 1946. Computer software capabilities have given way to school-based vocational preference instruments. National testing organizations like the Educational Testing Service (ETS) uses computers to administer multiple college-admissions tests like the GRE and to score them. The computer is also used to administer and interpret some psychological instruments like the Rorschach and the MMPI tests.

NORM-REFERENCED VS. CRITERION-REFERENCED TESTS

Tests can be **norm-referenced** or **criterion-referenced**. Both require that the test is graded with a raw score. The raw score indicates the number of right answers or a pattern found. The client's raw score is then compared to a group score. The raw score in a criterion-related test is compared to a criterion that can determine mastery or minimum competency levels within a subject.

STRUCTURED VS. UNSTRUCTURED TESTS

The difference found between a **structured** and an **unstructured test** is the range or degree of structure applied. For instance, the Strong Interest Inventory is a structured vocational preference test that only allows the client to give one of six possible answers. The Rorschach inkblot test allows the client to answer with any response that comes to mind.

STANDARDIZED ASSESSMENT TOOLS USED IN EVALUATION PROCESS

The five standardized assessment tools or tests are the achievement test, the aptitude test, the intelligence test, the vocational preference instrument, and the personality test:

- The **achievement test** is used to measure what has been learned in academics, vocation, or other life experience.
- The **aptitude test** is used to make a prediction on the subject's future performance in a given field of study.
- The **intelligence test** predicts a person's academic performance in the future by determining the person's mental potential.
- The **vocational preference instrument** is used to discover a pattern of characteristics that describe the individual's preferences or inclination to do something in leisure, work, and educational settings.
- The **personality test** describes the person's behavior, attitudes, beliefs, and values, and is used to diagnose psychopathology or in relationship counseling.

ASSESSING TRAITS, STRENGTHS, AND WEAKNESSES

An assortment of tests is available to **delineate capabilities, tendencies, and personalities**:

- The selection category can include tests like the Graduate Record Exam (GRE) or the Law School Admissions Tests (LSAT). **Selection tests** may also include vocational preference tests or personality tests used in educational and occupational counseling.
- **Placement tests** are used to determine where a client belongs in a program. Colleges may use these tests to determine in which class a student should start a program of study.
- **Diagnostic tests** use a combination of psychometric techniques and tests to evaluate human performance levels, and incorporate the DSM diagnostic labels to determine a remediation program for a client. Many insurance carriers also require this DSM label before payment is released for services rendered. Individual progress is also typically measured using psychometric instruments to help evaluate progress toward a goal.

INTELLIGENCE TESTS
STANFORD-BINET INTELLIGENCE SCALES

The Stanford-Binet intelligence scales (SB5) measure cognitive ability, assist in psychoeducational evaluation, diagnose developmental disabilities, and perform various assessments for individuals 2 to 85+. The SB5 test measures five **categories of intelligence**:

- Fluid reasoning
- Knowledge
- Quantitative reasoning
- Visual-spatial processing
- Working memory

SB5 measures each of these domains through both verbal and nonverbal activities. Subtests indicate which components of the SB5 are appropriate for the examinee. These subtest scores are combined to give four kinds of **composite score**:

- Factor index
- Domain
- Abbreviated battery
- Full-scale IQ

The standardization sample of the SB5 was based on 4,800 participants of various ages, socioeconomic statuses, geographic regions, and races.

WAIS-IV
MAIN INDEX SCORES OF WAIS-IV

The fourth edition of the **Wechsler Adult Intelligence Scale (WAIS-IV, 2008)** is used to measure the intellectual ability of late-adolescents and adults. The newest edition, WAIS-V, is currently under the clinical validation phase and has not yet been released. Wechsler considered intelligence to be a global ability made up of a number of interrelated functions. This interrelationship between the various types of intelligence is described in the current test in terms of four index scores:

- Verbal Comprehension Index (VCI)
- Perceptual Reasoning Index (PRI)
- Working Memory Index (WMI)
- Processing Speed Index (PSI)

CORE SUBTESTS OF WAIS-IV

There are **ten core subtests** on the WAIS-IV:

- VCI: Similarities (abstract reasoning)
- VCI: Vocabulary (semantic knowledge)
- VCI: Information (general knowledge)
- PRI: Block Design (spatial processing)
- PRI: Matrix Reasoning (inductive reasoning)
- PRI: Visual Puzzles (spatial reasoning)
- WMI: Digit Span (working memory)
- WMI: Arithmetic (quantitative reasoning)
- PSI: Symbol Search (processing speed)
- PSI: Coding (associative memory)

ADMINISTRATION AND SCORING OF WAIS-IV

There are 2 **broad scores** in the WAIS-IV.

- **Full Scale IQ (FSIQ)**: Based on the combined scores for the ten VCI, PRI, WMI and PSI subtests
- **General Ability Index (GAI)**: Based only on the six subtests that test VCI and PRI

The **administration** of the test begins with picture completion and then a series of alternating verbal and nonverbal subtests. The only exception to this is that the digit span and information subtests are administered together. Some tests will be timed, while others will be allowed to go on until the examinee has finished. The raw **scores** for each subtest are converted into scaled scores with a standard conversion table. In the subtests, the mean score is 10 and the standard deviation is 3. For the full-scale performance and verbal IQs and factor indices, the mean is 100 and the standard deviation is 15.

SUPPLEMENTAL SUBTESTS OF THE INTELLIGENCE SCALES OF THE REVISED WAIS-IV

Additional supplemental subtests are included with each intelligence scale in the WAIS-IV:

- Verbal Comprehension (VCI) Supplemental Subtest: Comprehension
- Perceptual Reasoning (PRI) Supplemental Subtests: Picture Completion and Figure Weights
- Working Memory (WMI) Supplemental Subtest: Letter-Number Sequencing
- Processing Speed (PSI) Supplemental Subtest: Cancellation

GROUP INTELLIGENCE TESTS

Many different organizations, from schools to the armed forces, administer **group intelligence tests**:

- The **Kuhlman-Anderson Test (KA)** is for children in grades K-12; it measures verbal and quantitative intelligence. This test is unique in that it relies less on language than do other individual and group tests.
- The **Woodcock Johnson IV** consists of a test of cognitive abilities and a test of achievement; the latter of which measures oral language and academic achievement.
- The **Wonderlic Personnel Test (WPT-R)** takes about 12 minutes to fill out with paper and pencil; it purports to measure the mental ability of adults. The Wonderlic is a good predictor of performance, but some critics maintain that it unfairly discriminates against some cultural groups in certain jobs.

TESTS FOR COGNITIVE AND INTELLECTUAL DEVELOPMENT IN CHILDREN
WISC-V AND WPPSI-IV

The **WISC-V** is a variation of the WAIS made especially for children between the ages of 6 and 17. WISC-V is closely based on neurocognitive models of information processing, and gives scores through five indexes:

- Verbal comprehension
- Visual-spatial
- Fluid reasoning
- Working memory
- Processing speed

Highly asymmetrical scores on the subtests are used to diagnose autism, ADHD, and other learning disorders.

The **WPPSI-IV** (released in 2012) is made for children between the ages of 2.5 and 7.25. For children that are either 2 or 3 years old, the test can measure verbal comprehension, and perceptual organization; for older children, processing speed can also be measured.

INFANT AND PRESCHOOL TESTS

Tests administered to children aged 2 or younger are good at screening for developmental delays and disabilities, but have poor predictive validity. **The Denver II** screens for developmental delays by observing a child's performance in four developmental domains:

- Personal-social
- Fine motor adaptive
- Language
- Gross motor

If a child fails an item that 90% of younger children pass, he or she is scored as having a **developmental delay**.

The **Bayley Scales of Infant Development (BSID-III)** assess the development of children 1 to 42 months old on mental, motor, and behavior rating scales.

The **Fagan Test of Intelligence** tries to gauge the information processing speed of an infant, in order to predict childhood IQ. It does this by introducing novel stimuli and observing the reaction time of the child.

KAUFMAN TEST OF EDUCATIONAL ACHIEVEMENT, COGNITIVE ASSESSMENT SYSTEM, AND SLOSSON TESTS

The **Kaufman Test of Educational Achievement (KTEA-3)** measures academic ability in children grades 1-12. It provides scores in three core areas:

- Reading
- Math
- Written Language

Verbal instructions and responses should be minimized on these tests to make them fair for all cultures.

The **Cognitive Assessment System (CAS2)** is based on the *PASS* (planning, attention, simultaneous processing, and sequential processing) model of intelligence, and is appropriate for children between the ages of 5 and 18 of all cultures and ethnicities.

The **Slosson tests** were designed to be fast ways of estimating intelligence in order to identify children at risk of educational failure.

ASSESSMENT OF INTELLECTUAL DISABILITY

Intellectual disability is defined as limitations in mental functioning mirrored by significant limitations in everyday functioning that are present early in life and before the age of 18.

- The **Individuals with Disabilities Act** states that all disabled individuals under the age of 25 need to be evaluated, and an *individualized educational plan (IEP)* needs to be developed for each child in order to provide education in the least restrictive environment.
- The case **Larry P. v. Riles** established that IQ tests can be *racially discriminatory* and should not be used to place African-Americans in special education classrooms.
- The **Vineland Behavior Scales** measure communication, daily living skills, and socialization, for the purpose of developing *special education programs*.
- The **AAIDD Adaptive Behavior Scales** assess personal self-sufficiency, community self-sufficiency, personal-social responsibility, social adjustment, and personal adjustment for individuals ages 4-21.

VANDERBILT ADHD

Vanderbilt ADHD is used to assess whether a child has attention deficit hyperactivity disorder. The tool has 3 parts:

- Assessment by a parent
- Assessment by a teacher
- Follow-up assessment by a parent

The parental assessment evaluates 47 symptoms that may be associated with ADHD and 8 performance measures. The teacher assessment evaluates 35 symptoms, 3 academic performances (reading, math, written expression), and 5 classroom performance behaviors. The follow-up parental assessment evaluates 18 symptoms, 8 performance measures, and 12 possible side effects.

ACADEMIC ABILITY TESTING

Ability tests measure current status and predict future academic achievement. Types of **ability testing** include:

- **Curriculum-based measurement** is any form of assessment that focuses on the student's ability to perform the work of the school curriculum. Usually, a teacher will set a minimum standard for performance and provide remedial attention for any student who performs below this level.

- **Performance-based assessment** evaluates students on their execution of a task or creation of a product. It is meant to be egalitarian and culture-fair.
- The **SAT** measures verbal and mathematical reasoning skills; it is used to predict the college success of high school students. Studies show that the SAT is more effective as a predictor when it is combined with grade-point average.
- The **Graduate Record Exam (GRE)** measures general scholastic abilities and may be taken in lieu of a normal secondary course of study.

PERSONALITY TESTS

STRUCTURED PERSONALITY TESTS

A structured personality test (as opposed to a projective test) measures emotional, social, and personal traits and behaviors through a series of multiple-choice questions or other unambiguous stimuli. There are four common strategies for structured personality tests:

- **Logical content method** bases its questions on deductive logic and a systematic theory of personality.
- **Theoretical method** measures the prevalence of the personality structures identified by a particular theory of personality.
- **Empirical criterion keying** has questions that are administered to different criterion groups; there are items that distinguish between the groups in the test.
- **Factor analysis tests** administer a large number of items to a large group of examinees, and then analyze their answers for any correlations.

MMPI-3

VALIDITY SCALES

The **Minnesota Multiphasic Personality Inventory-3 (MMPI-3)** was originally developed to diagnose psychiatric patients. The attitude of the examinee towards the test is indicated by his or her scores on various validity measures. In general, the validity scales can be grouped into three measurements: those that detect inconsistent response or non-response, those that detect the exaggerated self-reporting of the prevalence/severity of psychological symptoms, and those meant to detect those under-reporting psychological symptoms. Validity scales include:

- **Inconsistent/non-response**: CNS ("cannot say"), VRIN (Variable response inconsistency, TRIN (True response inconsistency).
- **Exaggerated response**: F (Infrequency, or "faking bad" in the first half of the test); Fb (F Back; "faking bad" in the second half of the test); Fp (F-Psychopathology (frequency of presentation).
- **Downplayed response:** L (Lie; "faking good"); K (Defensiveness, denial); S (Superlative Self-Presentation).

SCORING, INTERPRETATION, AND PROFILE ANALYSIS

The MMPI-3 takes raw scores and converts them into T-scores with a mean of 50 and a standard deviation of 10. If a person scores above a 65, it is considered to be clinically significant. The most common use of the MMPI-3 is as an assessment of personality and behavior through profile analysis. Most of the time, the code is simply the two highest scores on the various subtests. The validity scales are then used to ensure that the profile is the result of an honest attempt at the test. The standardization sample approximated the 2020 US census in age, gender, race, and social class.

Rorschach Inkblot and TAT Projective Personality Tests

Projective personality tests assume that unstructured and ambiguous stimuli can elicit meaningful responses from individuals, particularly about personality and underlying conflicts. Projective tests are typically open-ended and therefore less susceptible to faking. The most famous projective test is the **Rorschach Inkblot Test**, in which a person is presented with ten cards containing bilaterally symmetrical inkblots and asked to free associate on the design. Scoring the Rorschach is very complex, but relies on the following dimensions of the individual's response:

- Location (as in where the subject sees whatever he or she describes)
- Determinants (why the subjects saw what they saw)
- Form quality (resemblance of the response to the inkblot)
- Content
- Frequency of occurrence

The Rorschach may provide interesting results, but its use in clinical work is dubious.

Another projective test is the **Thematic Apperception Test (TAT)**, in which the examinee is asked to make up a story based on a random presentation of picture cards.

EPPS, 16 PF-5, NEO-3

The **Edwards Personal Preference Schedule**, based on the personality theory of Murray, contains 225 items that present an either-or choice to the examinee. This test strives to prevent examinees from responding in ways that they know are socially desirable. The test provides ipsative scores, meaning that the strengths of the candidate are given comparative, rather than absolute, value.

The **Sixteen Personality Factor Questionnaire (16PF 5th Ed)** is a factor analysis-based exam that identifies 16 primary personality traits and 5 secondary traits.

The **NEO-Personality Inventory (NEO-PI-3)** attempts to gauge an individual's level of the Big Five personality traits (extraversion, agreeableness, conscientiousness, neuroticism, and openness to experience). These traits are then broken down into facets, for example, neuroticism contains anxiety and depression.

Tests for Dementia, Attention, and Delirium
MMSE

The mini-mental state exam (MMSE), also known as the **Folstein test**, is a commonly used assessment tool for evaluating cognition. It is typically used to evaluate for the presence and severity of **dementia**. The MMSE consists of a 30-point questionnaire that evaluates immediate and short-term memory recall, orientation, arithmetic, the ability to follow simple commands, language, and other functional abilities such as copying a drawing. In clinical settings, it is very useful to detect initial impairment or follow responses over the course of an illness and/or treatment. This tool establishes a score based on education level and age. This score can be placed on a scale to determine **functionality** of the individual. A total possible score of 30 can be achieved. A score of 24 or greater is considered a normal functioning level. The lower the score, the greater the degree of dementia or mental dysfunction. It is possible that simple physical limitations such as the inability to read or hear or decreased motor function may negatively affect the total score.

Trail Making Test

The Trail Making Test (Parts A and B) assesses brain function and indicates increasing dementia. It is useful for detecting early Alzheimer's disease, and those who do poorly on part B often need assistance with activities of daily living (ADLs). The individual is given a demonstration of each part before beginning:

- **Part A** has 25 sequentially-numbered scattered circles across the page, and the individual is advised to use a pencil/pen to draw a continuous line to connect in ascending order the circles (starting with 1 and ending with 25).
- **Part B** is slightly more complex and has circles with numbers (1-12) and circles with letters (A-L) scattered about the page. The individual is advised to draw a continuous line alternating between numbers and letters in ascending order (1-A-2-B....).

The test is scored according to the number of seconds required for completion:

- **A**: 29 seconds is average, and >78 indicates deficiency.
- **B**: 75 seconds is average, and >273 seconds indicates deficiency.

Time and Change Test

The Time and Change Test assesses **dementia** in adults and is effective in diverse populations. First, the individual is shown a clock face set at 11:10 and has one minute to make two attempts at stating the correct time. Next, the individual is given change (7 dimes, 7 nickels, and 3 quarters) and asked to give the clinician $1.00 from the coins. The individual has two minutes and two attempts to make the correct change. Failing either or both tests is indicative of dementia.

Digit Repetition Test

The Digit Repetition Test is used to assess **attention**. The individual is told to listen to numbers and then repeat them. The clinician starts with two random single-digit numbers. If the individual gets this sequence correct, the clinician then states three numbers and continues to add one number each time until the individual is unable to repeat the numbers correctly. People with normal intelligence (without intellectual disability or expressive aphasia) can usually repeat 5-7 numbers, so scores <5 indicate impaired attention.

Confusion Assessment Method

The Confusion Assessment Method is used to assess the **development of delirium** and is intended for those without psychiatric training. The tool covers 9 factors. Some factors have a range of possibilities and others are rated only as to whether the characteristic is present, not present, uncertain, or not applicable. The tool provides room to describe abnormal behavior. Factors indicative of delirium include:

- **Onset**: Acute change in mental status
- **Attention**: Inattentive, stable, or fluctuating
- **Thinking**: Disorganized, rambling conversation, switching topics, or illogical
- **Level of consciousness**: Altered, ranging from alert to coma
- **Orientation**: Disoriented (person, place, time)
- **Memory**: Impaired
- **Perceptual disturbances**: Hallucinations, illusions
- **Psychomotor abnormalities**: Agitation (tapping, picking, moving) or retardation (staring, not moving)
- **Sleep-wake cycle**: Awake at night and sleepy in the daytime

The tool indicates delirium if there is an acute onset with fluctuating inattention and disorganized thinking or altered level of consciousness.

TESTS FOR ANXIETY AND DEPRESSION

HAMILTON ANXIETY SCALE

The Hamilton Anxiety Scale (HAS or HAMA) is utilized to evaluate the anxiety related symptomatology that may present in adults as well as children. It provides an evaluation of overall **anxiety** and its degree of severity. This includes **somatic anxiety** (physical complaints) and **psychic anxiety** (mental agitation and distress). This scale consists of 14 items based on anxiety produced symptoms. Each item is ranked 0-4 with 0 indicating no symptoms present and 4 indicating severe symptoms present. This scale is frequently utilized in psychotropic drug evaluations. If performed before a particular medication has been started and then again at later visits, the HAS can be helpful in adjusting medication dosages based in part on the individual's score. It is often utilized as an outcome measure in clinical trials.

GAD-7

General Anxiety Disorder-7 (GAD-7) is used to assess the severity of an individual's anxiety and focuses on the previous 2 weeks. The questions are as follows:

1. Feeling nervous, anxious, on edge?
2. Unable to stop/control worrying?
3. Worrying excessively about different things?
4. Having trouble relaxing?
5. Being excessively restless?
6. Easily annoyed/irritated?
7. Fearful something terrible will occur?

Responses are scored as 0 (not at all), 1 (several days), 2 (more than half of days), or 3 (nearly every day). Scores and assessment:

- **5-9 mild anxiety**, requires monitoring.
- **10-14 moderate anxiety**, requires further diagnostic tests, including MMSE and referral to a professional.
- **15+ severe anxiety**, requires active treatment.

BECK DEPRESSION INVENTORY

The Beck Depression Inventory (BDI) is a widely utilized, self-reported, multiple-choice questionnaire consisting of 21 items, which measures the **degree of depression**. This tool is designed for use in adults between the ages of 17 and 80 years of age. It evaluates physical symptoms such as weight loss, loss of sleep, loss of interest in sex, and fatigue, along with attitudinal symptoms such as irritability, guilt, and hopelessness. The items rank in four possible answer choices based on an increasing severity of symptoms. The test is scored with the answers ranging in value from 0 to 3. The total score is utilized to determine the degree of depression. The usual ranges include: 0-9 no signs of depression, 10-18 mild depression, 19-29 moderate depression, and 30-63 severe depression.

GERIATRIC DEPRESSION SCALE

The Geriatric Depression Scale (GDS) is a self-assessment tool to identify older adults with depression. The test can be used with those with normal cognition and those with mild to moderate impairment. The test poses 15 questions to which individuals answer "yes" or "no" and a point is assigned for each answer that indicates depression. A score of >5 points is indicative of depression:

1. Are you basically satisfied with your life?
2. Have you dropped many of your activities and interests?
3. Do you feel your life is empty?
4. Do you often get bored?
5. Are you in good spirits most of the time?

6. Are you afraid that something bad is going to happen to you?
7. Do you feel happy most of the time?
8. Do you often feel helpless?
9. Do you prefer to stay at home rather than going out and doing new things?
10. Do you feel you have more problems with memory than most?
11. Do you think it is wonderful to be alive now?
12. Do you feel pretty worthless the way you are now?
13. Do you feel full of energy?
14. Do you feel that your situation is hopeless?
15. Do you think that most people are better off than you are?

CHILDREN'S DEPRESSION RATING SCALE-REVISED

The Children's Depression Rating Scale-Revised (CDRS-R) evaluates a child for depressive disorders and monitors treatment response. CDRS-R includes 17 items, 14 of which are assessed during an interview, and 3 of which are assessed by the clinician's interpretation of the individual's nonverbal cues. The CDRS-R is designed specifically for individuals aged 6-12 but may also be used during an interview with the individual's parents, caregivers, and teachers. The items included in the interview include the following: schoolwork, capacity to have fun, social withdrawal, sleep, appetite or eating patterns, excessive fatigue, physical complaints, irritability, guilt, self-esteem, depressed feelings, morbid ideation, suicidal ideation, weeping, depressed affect, tempo of speech, and hypoactivity.

PHQ-9

Patient Health Questionaire-9 (PHQ-9) is used to determine the severity of depression and focuses on answers to questions related to the previous 2 weeks. The questions are as follows:

1. Little interest/pleasure in activities?
2. Feelings of depression or hopelessness?
3. Sleeping difficulties?
4. Tiredness of lack of energy?
5. Poor appetite or excessive eating?
6. Feelings of being a failure or letting down self/others?
7. Difficulty concentrating?
8. Speaking/moving slowly or fidgeting?
9. Suicidal ideation?

Responses are scored as 0 (not at all), 1 (several days), 2 (more than half of days), or 3 (nearly every day). Scores and assessment:

- **0-4: minimal or no depression**—monitor but likely does not need treatment
- **5-9: mild depression**—may need treatment
- **10-15: moderate depression**—may need treatment
- **15-19: moderately severe depression**—treatment required
- **20-27: severe depression**—treatment required

Suicide risk assessment should be carried out for any individuals indicating suicidal ideation.

MULTIPLE APTITUDE TEST BATTERIES AND SPECIAL BATTERIES

Multiple aptitude test batteries measure ability in a number of different areas; one of their weaknesses is that they often lack adequate differential validity, meaning that the various parts of the test do not have different validities for different categories.

- **Differential aptitude tests (DAT)** identify job-related abilities and are used for career counseling and employee selection.
- The **general aptitude test battery (GATB)** was developed by the US Employment Service for vocational counseling and job placement. There are other tests used to measure special aptitudes.
- **Psychomotor tests** are used to assess speed, coordination, and general movement responses. These typically have low validity coefficients because they are highly specific and susceptible to practice effects.
- **Mechanical aptitude tests** are used to assess dexterity, perceptual and spatial skills, and mechanical reasoning. The different skills that fall within this category are relatively independent.

ASSESSMENT OF INDIVIDUALS WITH PHYSICAL DISABILITIES

The **Americans with Disabilities Act of 1990** declares that any test administered to a disabled job applicant or employee should reflect only the person's ability on the test, and not his or her disability. Employers are also required to make reasonable accommodations for disabled employees.

- The **Columbia Mental Maturity Scale (CMMS)** is a test of general reasoning ability that does not require fine motor skills or verbal responses. It is useful for assessing students with cerebral palsy, brain damage, intellectual disability, and speech impediments.
- The **Peabody Picture Vocabulary Test (PPVT-5)** measures receptive vocabulary without requiring verbal responses.
- The **Haptic Intelligence Scale (HIS)** uses tactile stimuli, so it is good for assessing blind and partially-sighted individuals.
- The **Hiskey-Nebraska Test of Learning Aptitude (H-NTLA)** contains twelve nonverbal subtests which can be administered verbally or in pantomime; it is good for assessing children with hearing impairments.

WORLD HEALTH ORGANIZATION DISABILITY ASSESSMENT SCHEDULE 2.0

The World Health Organization Disability Assessment Schedule 2.0 (WHODAS 2.0), is the DSM-5-TR recommended tool for assessing **global impairment and functioning**. It is based on ICD and ICF classifications. In previous versions of the DSM, global disability was assessed by the Global Assessment of Functioning (GAF) scale. WHODAS comes as a self-report tool with either 12 or 36 questions, taking around 7-15 minutes to administer. These questions help to assess the individual's performance in 6 domains over the last 30 days. The **six domains** are: cognition, participation, mobility, self-care, life activities, and interacting with other people. Using the questionnaire, the tool produces a score that represents the individual's global disability. Pros of the tool include that it is reliable and valid, even across cultures. Cons include that due to the self-report nature of the tool, there is no way to check the validity of the individual's responses to the questions.

NEUROPSYCHOLOGICAL ASSESSMENTS

The **Benton Visual Retention Test (BVRT)** assesses visual memory, spatial perception, and visual-motor skills in order to diagnose brain damage. The subject is asked to reproduce from memory the geometric patterns on a series of ten cards.

The **Beery Developmental Test of Visual-Motor Integration (Beery-VMI-6)** assesses visual-motor skills in children; like the BVRT, it involves the reproduction of geometric shapes.

The **Wisconsin Card Sorting Test (WSCT)** is a screening test that assesses the ability to form abstract concepts and shift cognitive strategies; the subject is required to sort a group of cards in an order that is not disclosed to him or her.

The **Stroop Color-Word Association Test (SCWT)** is a measure of cognitive flexibility; it tests an individual's ability to suppress a habitual reaction to stimulus.

The **Halstead-Reitan Neuropsychological Battery (HRNB)** is a group of tests that are effective at differentiating between normal people and those with brain damage. The clinician has control over which exams to administer, though he or she is likely to assess sensorimotor, perceptual, and language functioning. A score higher than 0.60 indicates brain pathology.

The **Luria-Nebraska Neuropsychological Battery (LNNB)** contains 11 subtests that assess areas like rhythm, visual function, and writing. The examinee is given a score between 0 and 2, with 0 indicating normal function and 2 indicating brain damage.

The **Bender Visual-Motor Gestalt Test (Bender-Gestalt II)** is a brief examination that involves responding to 16 stimulus cards containing geometric figures, which the examinee must either copy or recall.

AIMS

The abnormal involuntary movement scale (AIMS) is an assessment tool that can be utilized to assess **abnormal physical movements**. These movements can often be the resulting side-effects of certain antipsychotic medications and can be associated with tardive dyskinesia or chronic akathisia. These motor abnormalities can also be associated with particular illnesses. Based on a five-point scale, the movements of three specific physical areas are evaluated to determine a total score. These areas are the face and mouth, trunk area, and the extremities. The AIMS has been established as a reliable assessment tool and also has a very simple design that provides a short assessment time. This allows it to be easily utilized in an inpatient or outpatient setting to provide an objective record of any abnormal physical movements that can change over the course of time.

BRIEF PSYCHIATRIC RATING SCALE FOR CHILDREN

The Brief Psychiatric Rating Scale for Children (BPRS-C) is designed to identify presenting symptoms and annotate the severity of each symptom, on a scale ranging from "not present" to "extremely severe." BPRS-C is used to diagnose psychiatric disorders for both children and adolescents through an interview with the child and parent(s).

Symptoms evaluated on the scale include:

- **Behavioral symptoms**, such as uncooperativeness and hostility
- **Mood symptoms**, such as depressive mood and anxiety
- **Sensory symptoms**, such as hallucinations, delusions, and speech characteristics
- **Symptoms of awareness and alertness**, such as disorientation, hyperactivity, distractibility, and others
- **Symptoms of affect**, such as emotional withdrawal and blunted affect

The BPRS-C assessment tool is a cursory look at many symptoms typically displayed with mental disorders.

YALE-BROWN OBSESSIVE-COMPULSIVE SCALE

The Yale-Brown Obsessive-Compulsive Scale (Y-BOCS) is a useful tool for identifying and diagnosing obsessive-compulsive disorders. Y-BOCS aims to identify obsessions, including: aggressive, contamination, sexual, hoarding/saving, religious, need for symmetry, somatic, and miscellaneous compulsions such as cleaning/washing, checking, repeating, and counting. Y-BOCS asks the individual to rate the time he or she spends on obsessions and compulsions during the week prior to the clinician's interview. It asks the individual how much control he or she has over the compulsion/obsession, and how much distress it causes him or her. Y-BOCS has questions about resistance and interference. The clinician can ask for clarification and if the individual volunteers information, it is included in the assessment. The final rating is based on the clinician's judgment.

COMMUNICATING TEST RESULTS

Test results must be communicated to the client in an ethical manner that will be of benefit to the client. This information should not add to the client's sense of bewilderment, embarrassment, unworthiness, or be perceived as critical in nature. The mental health care provider should provide significant results to the client out of a sincere desire to help. The client should understand the reason for giving the test and what information will be gleaned from its results. Then, the results and the scores should be discussed in relation to the questions asked on the test. The client should be encouraged to make his or her own interpretation of the results discussed. This can alleviate an attitude of passive acceptance or a more defensive rejection concerning the outcome of the test. The client should be affirmed by the communication efforts of the provider.

ETHICAL ISSUES ASSOCIATED WITH CLIENT TESTING

Mental health providers should be thoroughly familiar with their **Code of Ethics**. The American Nurses Association (ANA) has issued *The Code of Ethics for Nurses with Interpretive Statements* and also created the Center for Ethics and Human Rights Annual Report to "help nurses navigate ethical and value conflicts... common to everyday practice." Revisions have been made in recent years to cover computer applications. The computer has changed the construction, administration, scoring, and interpretation of tests used in the mental health field. The revisions also address validity in measuring ability levels of the client. **Ethical issues** address professional competence, qualifications, and confidentiality of the client. The ethical consideration given to professional competency involves graduate level training in the use of tests. Most tests require administration under the supervision of a licensed practitioner. Test publishers can only sell their tests to those who are legally qualified to administer it.

The client's information is handled with strict confidentiality throughout the entire process. **Confidentiality** can be compromised with the use of computers, so apply every protective precaution. Seek permission from the client before performing the test. Inform the client about how the information obtained will be stored and about what happens to the information after counseling has been completed. Keep in mind the potential for misuse of information and make sure that any test performed is absolutely necessary. Remain diligent in protecting the client's right to privacy. The client must sign a release before any information can be shared with other organizations or other professionals. Refer to the Code of Ethics whenever there is any question of how to proceed.

Family Assessment

FAMILY TYPES

A **family** consists of a group of people that are connected by marriage, blood relationship, or emotions. There are many different variations when referring to the concept of family.

- The **nuclear family** is one in which two or more people are related by blood, marriage, or adoption. This type of family is typically parents and their children.
- The **extended family** is one in which several nuclear families related by blood or marriage function as one group.
- In a **single-parent structure**, there is only one parent caring for the children in the household.
- In a **blended family** a parent marries or remarries after he or she has already had children. Blended families are often referred to as stepfamilies because they consist of a parent, a stepparent, and one or more children.

A **household** consists of an individual or group of people residing together under one roof. The nurse will often interact with families on many different levels. This may involve meeting the family once during treatment or establishing a long-term relationship with the family over the course of long-term treatment.

FAMILY LIFE CYCLE

The family life cycle is a process in which the family undergoes changes to allow for the introduction of new family members, exiting of existing family members, and the development of present family members in a positive functional manner. This cycle is described in **stages** and includes times of **transition**. Many times, stress and dysfunction can occur during these times of transition and the family may seek assistance to be able to successfully navigate this period of time. The stages of the family life cycle include leaving home as a young adult, joining of families though marriage or establishment of an emotional relationship, having young children, having adolescent children, launching young adult children and moving forward, and finally the family later in life.

FAMILY FUNCTION AND DYSFUNCTION

FUNCTIONAL FAMILY

A functional family will be able to change roles, responsibilities, and interactions during a stressful event. This type of family can experience nonfunctional behaviors if placed in an acute stressful event; however, they should be able to reestablish their family balance over a period of time. The functional family will have the ability to deal with **conflict and change** in order to deal with negative situations without causing long-term dysfunction or dissolution of the family. They will have completed vital life cycle tasks, keep emotional contact between family members and across generations, avoid over-closeness, and use distance to resolve issues. When two members of the family have a conflict, they are expected to **resolve** this conflict between themselves and there is **open communication** between all family members. Children of a functional family are expected to achieve age-appropriate functioning and are given age-appropriate privileges.

HOW A FAMILY AIDS THE DEVELOPMENT, EDUCATION, AND FUNCTION OF ITS MEMBERS

A family can aid the development, education, and function of its members in two major ways. First, parents and grandparents typically pass their heritage down to their children and teach them what is considered acceptable through their actions, customs, and traditions. In other words, a person typically acquires culture through his or her family, and that culture helps the person function in society and interact socially with other people. Second, a person's family can act as an effective support network in many situations. A family may be able to provide some of the emotional, financial, or other types of support a person needs.

INCONGRUOUS HIERARCHY

An incongruous hierarchy is a family relationship in which a minor figure controls the family dynamic. The control engine may be the exhibition of inappropriate behavior at crucial times. It is a "tail wags the dog" type of scenario. A child throws an entire family into turmoil by ranting and throwing a fit each evening at bedtime. The child's father reacts by attempting to soothe her, offering her candy and letting her stay up late. The child's mother is angry with the father for doing so, and begins shouting at him and withholding affection. An older brother loses sleep because of the daily hysterics, and subsequently performs poorly in school. This type of family dysfunction is called incongruous hierarchy.

FAMILY ASSESSMENT

When performing a family assessment, the health care provider will collect many different types of data relevant to the family's health and wellbeing. They will evaluate the **psychological and social functioning of the family** and utilize this information to help identify nursing diagnoses. Information gathered may include the creation of a **genogram**, which is a graphical depiction of generations that identifies family members and their relationships. It includes their geographic relationship, age, date of death, and marriages. This picture should also include any known psychiatric disorders. By using the genogram, patterns can be identified. A **family APGAR** can also be used to help identify the family structure. It assesses adult satisfaction with social support from the family in the domains of adaptation, partnership, growth, affection, and resolve.

CULTURAL AND ETHNIC DIFFERENCES WITHIN THE FAMILY

Different cultural and ethnic backgrounds can affect the **definition of family**. They may have different beliefs about the functions of family members. Conflict may be resolved differently within families, and adaptive and maladaptive responses may vary. Outside events may be viewed differently and interventions within the family may differ between cultural groups. Many times, African American and Latino families often look to other family members instead of health care professionals for support early in the problem. These families also have higher rates of attrition and termination of family therapy than Caucasian families.

CHANGE IN FAMILY ROLES OF MEN AND WOMEN IN UNITED STATES

The family roles of men and women in the United States have changed drastically over the past several decades. Women were traditionally the primary caretakers of children, so they were expected to maintain the household while the men worked to provide for the family. However, this is no longer the case, as there has been a drastic increase in the number of women entering the work force in the recent years. This change is partially due to the fact that it has become more difficult for families to live off of one income. It can be extremely difficult for a family to find the time and money to care for a child, especially if that child has a disability, because both parents are typically required to work.

REASONS WHY WOMEN COMPRISE ONE-HALF OF U.S. JOB MARKET

The high divorce rate may have contributed to an **increase in working women,** as more women are required to support themselves and their children. Economic and material motivations have driven more women into the workforce and created the phenomenon of dual-career households. Research shows that two-earner families enjoy higher income than families in which only one person is working outside the home. Parts of the Civil Rights Act of 1964 and its amendments in 1972 were meant to secure equal opportunities for women and equal pay for the same work. These efforts at eliminating gender bias have been a major factor in the increased presence of women in all career fields.

EFFECTS OF MENTAL ILLNESS ON FAMILY

Families with a member that has a chronic mental illness will provide several functions that those without mentally ill members may not need. These functions can include providing support and information for care and treatment options. They will also monitor the services provided the family member and address concerns with these services. Many times, the family is the biggest **advocate** for additional availability of services for those with mental health problems. There can often be disagreements between the health care providers and the family members concerning the dependence of the patient within the family. Parents can often be viewed as overprotective when the nurse attempts to encourage patient independence and self-reliant functioning. The parents will need support and reassurance if the patient leaves home. On the other hand, many parents will provide for their child for as long as they live. Once the primary care provider dies, the patient may be left with no one to care for them, and they may experience traumatic disruptions.

FAMILY VIOLENCE

Family violence can include physical, emotional, sexual, or verbal behaviors that occur between members of the same family or others living within the home. This behavior can include both abuse and neglect and involve the elderly, spouses, and children. Family violence is often kept a secret and may be the main issue with many family problems. Many times, actions that would be considered unacceptable to strangers or friends are often the norm between family members. Violence and abuse occur due to the unique interactions between the family members based upon personality differences, situational variations, and sociocultural influences.

CHARACTERISTICS OF VIOLENT FAMILIES

Violent families will often share many of the same characteristics. Many times, the abusive family member will have suffered abuse from their family while growing up. This type of abuse is a **multigenerational transmission** and is a cycle of violence. These abusers have learned to believe that violent behavior is a way to solve problems. Violent families are also usually socially isolated so that others such as friends, teachers, neighbors, or law enforcement officials do not become aware that the abuse is occurring. The abuser will also use and abuse power to **control** the victim. They may be considered a person of authority, such as a parent would be to a child. Power is a very important factor with abuse of an intimate partner. The abuser is often very controlling of their partner and will attempt to dominate every aspect of their life. Another commonality among abusers is **substance abuse**; however, one is not dependent upon the other. Many times, the use of alcohol or drugs may escalate violent behaviors by decreasing inhibitions.

Risk Assessment

COMPONENTS OF A RISK ASSESSMENT

A risk assessment evaluates the patient's condition and their particular situation for the presence of certain risk factors. These risks can be influenced by age, ethnicity, spiritual beliefs, or social beliefs. They can include risk for suicide, harming others, exacerbation of symptoms, development of new mental health issues, falls, seizures, allergic reactions, or elopement. This assessment should occur within the first hour of their arrival and then continue to be an ongoing process. The patient's specific risks should be prioritized and documented, and then nursing interventions should be put into place to protect this patient from these risks.

EVALUATION FOR SUICIDAL OR HOMICIDAL THOUGHTS

During a risk assessment two of the most important areas to evaluate are the patient's **risk for self-harm or harm to others**. The staff member performing the assessment should very closely evaluate for any descriptions or thoughts the patient may have concerning these risks. Direct questioning on these subjects should be performed and documented. Close evaluation of any delusional thoughts the patient may be having should be carefully evaluated. Does the patient believe he or she is being instructed by others to perform either of these acts? Safety of the patient and others needs to be a top priority and carefully documented. If the patient indicates that they are having these thoughts or ideas, they must be placed in either suicidal or assault precautions with close monitoring per facility protocol.

SUICIDE RISK ASSESSMENT

A suicide risk assessment should be completed and documented upon admission, with each shift change, at discharge, or any time suicidal ideations are suggested by the patient. This risk assessment should evaluate some of the following criteria: would the patient sign a contract for safety, is there a suicide plan, how lethal is the plan, what is the elopement risk, how often are the suicidal thoughts, and has the patient attempted suicide before. Any associated symptoms of hopelessness, guilt, anger, helplessness, impulsive behaviors, nightmares, obsessions with death, or altered judgment should also be assessed and documented. The higher the score the higher the risk for suicide.

GUIDELINES FOR SUICIDE PREVENTION

The initial step in decreasing suicide rates is to identify the **patterns** of suicidal behaviors and the **risk factors**. Educating the public on some of the behavior changes seen in those who are at increased risk for suicide can help to better identify those individuals. There can be a stigma associated with seeking mental health services and this negativity needs to be reversed so that those who need the help of a mental health professional will seek out that help. An increase in **access to mental health and counseling services** needs to occur so that those services are available to those who exhibit or express behaviors and feelings of suicidal ideation. Efforts have been made in gun control and the pharmaceutical industry to decrease access to the lethal means in which someone could carry out a suicide attempt. The overall goal is to **increase awareness** across the larger population to help decrease the risk within the smaller group of those who are at greatest risk.

ASSESSMENT OF VETERANS

Assessment of **veterans** must include not only the standard assessments appropriate for the patient's age and gender but also assessment of combat-associated injuries and illnesses:

- Shrapnel or gunshot injuries: Associated physical limitations, pain
- Amputations: Mobility and prosthesis issues; body image issues
- PTSD: Extent, frequency of attacks, limiting factors, triggers
- Depression, suicidal ideation
- Substance abuse: Type and extent

Because a large number of veterans are among the homeless population, the veteran's living arrangements should be explored and appropriate referrals made if the patient is in need of housing. Veterans may be unaware of programs offered through the U.S. Department of Veterans Affairs and should be provided information about these programs as appropriate for the patient's needs.

COLLECTING A TRAUMA HISTORY

According to the Joint Commission National Quality Measures, a trauma history should be collected within the first three days of admission in a hospital setting. Additionally, a trauma history should be collected from any patient with a known history of physical or emotional abuse, accident involvement, or signs and symptoms of PTSD from known or unknown events. There are several methods of trauma history collection:

- **Trauma History Screen (THS)**: The patient self-reports (via questionnaire) by responding with *yes* or *no* to 14 event types, and includes the number of times the event occurred. These events include abuse, accidents, natural disasters, military service, loss of loved ones, life crises, and life transitions. Next, the patient is prompted to respond to the question, "Did any of these things really bother you emotionally?" If the patient responds with *yes*, they are then asked to provide details about every event that bothered them.
- **Trauma History Questionnaire (THQ)**: Similar to the THS, this questionnaire requires the patient to self-report experiences with 24 potentially traumatic events, and then to provide the frequency and details of each experience.

DOCUMENTATION OF OCCURRENCE REPORTS

Occurrence reports are utilized for facilities to track **negative or averted negative events** that occur within the facility. These reports are usually forwarded to the manager of the department who then forwards them on to risk management for review. They can be utilized to document occurrences such as patient injury due to a fall or any other cause; medication errors or averted errors; and inadvertent removal of IV's, feeding tubes, or other invasive patient lines by a staff member or the patient themselves. Any negative event or averted event should be documented on this form. Only the facts of what occurred are documented. No opinions or judgments about what the staff member thought might have happened are included. Witness names, patient identification, and an exact explanation of what occurred are documented on this report.

Substance Use Screening

SUBSTANCE ABUSE DISORDERS

Substance abuse disorders are behaviors related to taking an abusive substance such as alcohol, amphetamines, marijuana, cocaine, hallucinogens, sedatives, or other unidentified substances. This group of disorders is classified into four different categories that include substance dependence, substance abuse, substance intoxication, and substance withdrawal. The United States has one of the highest rates of substance abuse when compared to other countries. It is a chronic disease process with many relapses. It is a huge cost to the US, with substance abusers utilizing a large amount of health care dollars. These individuals will have long-term serious medical sequelae associated with abuse, along with frequent hospitalizations and emergency department visits. Note: Substance-related and addictive disorders now include **gambling disorder**, as evidence shows that the behaviors of gambling trigger similar reward systems as drugs.

STAGES OF PROGRESSION IN DRUG AND ALCOHOL USE

Not everyone who has used drugs or alcohol has a problem with addiction. The mental health provider must determine if the patient has a pathological addiction or just engages in experimental use. Grade the patient on the continuum of drug use, based on a five-stage progression.

Stage 1 is the patient who is abstinent or involved in self-denial of use. **Abstinence** may allow for an occasional glass of wine. However, the person who chooses this route probably was heavily addicted to alcohol in the past, and completely abstains now to keep from falling back into old, addictive ways. Twelve step programs such as Alcoholics Anonymous (AA) advocate complete abstinence. Self-help groups like these are complementary reinforcement for formal therapy because meetings are held daily in most metropolitan areas, and peer pressure can prevent a relapse. The therapeutic role in cases of past addictions is to help them stay "on the wagon" of abstinence. Even one drink can be detrimental to an alcoholic because it can trigger a drinking binge.

Stage 2 of progression on the continuum of drug use involves **experimental use**. Teens and young adults partake of a chemical to find out what it feels like. It is an expected rite of passage for many segments of our culture. Problems with experimentation include drunk driving and date rape. GHB is dissolved in alcohol at raves because it enhances the libido and lowers inhibitions. Victims enter a dream state and act drunk. They relax, sometimes to the point of unconsciousness, have problems seeing clearly, are confused, and have no recall of events or the passage of time while drugged.

Stage 3 of the progression involves **social use** of drugs or alcohol. The test to determine if a person is a social user or addicted is whether or not the person can stop the drug use. Social users do not get outside help without coercion from either a parent or an authority figure. Counseling involves an educational group to develop coping skills and relationship skills with peers.

Stage 4 of progression on the continuum of drug use involves **abuse**. The patient's problem can be physiological or psychological in nature, or both. The addiction is detrimental to personal safety, family relationships, academic life, and work functions. Spousal and child abuse often coincide with drug abuse. Drunk driving and theft to support a habit are societal problems resulting from addictive behavior. Friends and associates are probably uncomfortable around the abuser by the time the addiction is visibly evident. At this point, the employer can insist the abuser get help on a professional level through Employee Assistance or public programs as a condition of continued employment. Abusers benefit from psychological counseling on a weekly basis and an intervention program to stop the alcohol or drug abuse. Antabuse (disulfiram), methadone, LAAM, buprenorphine, ibogaine, and naltrexone are useful adjuncts to counseling/therapy to wean the abuser off the drug. Intensive out-patient programs may be sufficient for recovery.

Stage 5 of progression involves **chemical dependency** or addictions that must be relieved. The addict experiences withdrawal symptoms when the drug or alcohol is not available for consumption. The addict builds up a tolerance to the drug to the point that more and more is needed just to keep from experiencing physical withdrawal. The high is harder and harder to reach. The addict is now at increased risk for **unintentional overdose**, because street drugs have inconsistent strengths. The addict is also now on the verge of failing in marriage, academics, and work. The addict experiences serious medical issues like ventricular tachycardia and atrial fibrillation and more powerful drugs like Clonidine (Catapres patches or tablets) are used to prevent death. Permanent damage from Korsakoff's syndrome or Wernicke's encephalopathy may result from a poor diet lacking in vitamins. Long-term, in-patient rehabilitation programs are crucial in most cases. Intensive out-patient programs may be sufficient for the minority.

PATHOPHYSIOLOGY OF ADDICTION

Genetic, social, and personality factors may all play a role in the development of **addictive tendencies**. However, the main factor of the development of substance addiction is the pharmacological activation of the **reward system** located in the central nervous system (CNS). This reward systems pathway involves **dopaminergic neurons**. Dopamine is found in the CNS and is one of many neurotransmitters that play a role in an individual's mood. The mesolimbic pathway seems to play a primary role in the reward and motivational process involved with addiction. This pathway begins in the ventral tegmental area of the brain (VTA) and then moves forward into the nucleus accumbens located in the middle forebrain bundle (MFB). Some drugs enhance mesolimbic dopamine activity, therefore producing very potent effects on mood and behavior.

> **Review Video: Addictions**
> Visit mometrix.com/academy and enter code: 460412

INDICATORS OF SUBSTANCE USE DISORDER

Many people with substance use disorders (alcohol or drugs) are reluctant to disclose this information, but there are a number of **indicators** that are suggestive of substance use disorder:

- Physical signs
  - Needle tracks on arms or legs
  - Burns on fingers or lips
  - Pupils abnormally dilated or constricted, watery eyes
  - Slurring of speech, slow speech
  - Lack of coordination, instability of gait
  - Tremors
  - Sniffing repeatedly, nasal irritation
  - Persistent cough
  - Weight loss
  - Dysrhythmias
  - Pallor, puffiness of face
- Other signs
  - Odor of alcohol/marijuana on clothing or breath
  - Labile emotions, including mood swings, agitation, and anger
  - Inappropriate, impulsive, and/or risky behavior
  - Lying
  - Missing appointments
  - Difficulty concentrating/short term memory loss, disoriented/confused
  - Blackouts
  - Insomnia or excessive sleeping
  - Lack of personal hygiene

INITIAL INTERVIEW WITH A PATIENT WHO ABUSES SUBSTANCES

Issues to discuss with a patient who abuses substances during an initial interview include:

- Drug(s) and/or drink of choice: amount, frequency and duration of use, route of administration, and when last used
- The use of any other substances
- Any history of and response to withdrawal
- Any history of DTs, seizures, blackouts, alcoholic amnesia, or past events of injury to self or others
- Changes in mood and/or behavior
- Sleep pattern changes, eating habits and any changes
- Problems with: relationships, finances, legal system, occupation, school, family, medical disorders, psychiatric disorders
- Any family history of drug or alcohol use
- Any family history of mental health disorders
- Access to substances of abuse
- Previous substance abuse treatments
- Longest period of being substance-free
- Interviews with family members and/or significant others may be warranted if denial or rationalization is suspected

QUESTIONS ASKED IN A CLINICAL INTERVIEW OF A PATIENT WITH SUBSTANCE ABUSE

There are the 12 questions to ask a patient with substance abuse in a clinical interview:

- **Question 1**: Find out the client's motivation for getting a mental health referral.
- **Question 2**: Obtain historical background about the beginning and severity of the client's drug and alcohol use. Discuss changes or deterioration in the client's behavior from the alcohol and drug use.
- **Question 3**: Determine the longest length of time that the client has stayed sober. Delve into the reasons why this period of sobriety ended.
- **Question 4**: Ask about the intoxication level that the client reaches when drinking or drugging. Are there blackouts? Violent incidents? Is it harder to get a high now than when the client first started using drugs?
- **Question 5**: Find out the arrest record of the client. Pay particular attention to impaired driving (DUI) and domestic violence charges resulting from chemical abuse.
- **Question 6**: Find out about military service where drug or alcohol use was part of the client's service time.
- **Question 7**: Discuss addictive cycles of abuse found in the client's family. Note psychological disorders in family members and dysfunctional family relationships.
- **Question 8**: Find out the psychiatric history of the client.
- **Question 9**: Ask the client about his or her educational and work experience, including any drug or alcohol activities at school or in the workplace.
- **Question 10**: Get the medical and substance use history of the client. Note chronic pain treated with OxyContin or other pain relievers, which subsequently led to addiction.
- **Question 11**: Ask about prior drug and alcohol abuse treatment programs in which the client participated. Is the client a recidivist? If so, use a different treatment technique.
- **Question 12**: Discuss drug and/or alcohol levels revealed by the client's latest toxicology screen.

The answers gleaned in the clinical interview should correspond with other data collected from various sources. If there is a discrepancy, determine the truth of the situation.

ABUSE OF ALCOHOL

Alcohol is a **CNS depressant**, or sedative-hypnotic, which depresses tissues within the brain. These drugs decrease anxiety and/or induce sleep. Even though alcohol is a sedative, it also causes a sense of euphoria. Its effects also include decreased inhibitions, relaxation, impaired coordination, slurred speech, and nausea. In cases of toxicity and overdose it can cause respiratory depression leading to respiratory or cardiac arrest. Withdrawal symptoms can include shaking, seizures, hyperthermia, tachycardia, hypertension, and delirium. Long-term complications can affect all body systems and lead to death.

ASSESSMENT TECHNIQUES FOR ALCOHOL USE

All patients should be assessed for alcohol use as part of the initial history and physical exam as well as at subsequent visits, especially if there are health indications (abnormal liver function tests, falls, insomnia) or social indications (family problems, divorce, job loss). There are numerous **self-assessment screening tools** that ask the patient a number of questions about the frequency and amount of drinking as well as questions such as if he or she drinks in the morning or alone; has been arrested, lost a job, or missed work because of drinking; feels depressed; or if he or she drinks to gain confidence. The assessment tools have a **scale indicator** that suggests a problem with certain scores. The nurse should discuss the assessment and score with the patient and provide information about resources (such as Alcoholics Anonymous and alcohol rehabilitation programs) and health consequences of drinking to the patient.

CAGE TOOL

The CAGE acronym is used as a quick assessment tool to determine if people are drinking excessively or are problem drinkers. Moderate drinking, (1-2 drinks daily or 1 drink a day for older adults), unless contraindicated by health concerns, is usually not harmful to people, but drinking more than that can lead to serious psychosocial and physical problems. One drink is defined as 12 ounces of beer/wine cooler, 5 ounces of wine, or 1.5 ounces of liquor.

C	Cutting down	Do you think about trying to cut down on drinking?
A	Annoyed at criticism	Are people starting to criticize your drinking?
G	Guilty feeling	Do you feel guilty or try to hide your drinking?
E	Eye opener	Do you increasingly need a drink earlier in the day?

A "yes" answer on 1 question suggests the possibility of a drinking problem while a "yes" answer on 2 or more questions indicates a drinking problem. The patient should be provided with information about reducing drinking and appropriate referrals made.

ALCOHOL INTOXICATION AND ALCOHOL WITHDRAWAL

Symptoms of **alcohol intoxication** include:

- Maladaptive behavior and psychological changes
- Slurred speech
- Poor coordination
- Unsteady gait
- Nystagmus (uncontrolled eye movements)
- Impaired attention and memory
- Stupor or coma

Maladaptive behaviors and **psychological changes** associated with alcohol intoxication include inappropriate sexual or aggressive behaviors, impaired judgment, and emotional lability.

Symptoms of **alcohol withdrawal** are:

- Autonomic hyperactivity (diaphoresis and tachycardia)
- Hand tremors
- Insomnia
- Nausea and vomiting
- Transient illusions or hallucinations
- Anxiety
- Psychomotor agitation
- Tonic/clonic seizures if use was heavy or prolonged

ALCOHOL USE IN CHILDREN AND ADOLESCENTS

Alcohol is a significant problem in adolescents and even in younger children. It is the **most-commonly abused substance**. Studies have shown that about 32% of young people drink and 20% are binge drinkers. While alcohol can impair development of almost all body systems in a growing child, it is of particular concern for the effects on the neurological system and liver. Additionally, because it interferes with impulse control, adolescents who drink are often involved in violence, abuse, and risky sexual behavior. Drinking should be suspected if a child has memory problems, changes in behavior, poor academic progress, emotional lability, and physical changes, such as slurring of speech, general lethargy, or lack of coordination. Intervention includes teaching children from about age 9 about the dangers of drinking, identifying those who are drinking, identifying underlying problems, and providing programs to help teenagers stop drinking, such as counseling or Alcoholics Anonymous.

KORSAKOFF SYNDROME

Korsakoff syndrome is characterized by retrograde and anterograde amnesia and confabulation due to **thiamine deficiency.** It is a late sign of **Wernicke's syndrome**, which is characterized by ataxia, abnormal eye movements, and confusion. In Korsakoff syndrome, the anterograde amnesia is more severe, especially for declarative memories. The retrograde amnesia seems to affect recent long-term memories more than those formed long ago. **Confabulation** occurs when an individual unconsciously attempts to compensate for memory loss by making up memories. It is associated with damage to the frontal lobe and basal forebrain.

ALCOHOL WITHDRAWAL DELIRIUM AND ALCOHOL-INDUCED SLEEP DISORDER

Symptoms associated with **alcohol withdrawal delirium** are:

- Disturbances in consciousness and other cognitive functions
- Autonomic hyperactivity
- Vivid hallucinations
- Delusions
- Agitation following periods of prolonged or heavy use of alcohol

Alcohol-induced sleep disorders may be caused by either intoxication or withdrawal, and usually manifest as insomnia. Intoxicative sleep disorder entails a period of drowsiness followed by excessive wakefulness, restlessness, and vivid, anxious dreams. **Withdrawal sleep disorder** manifests as a severe disruption in sleep continuity, accompanied by vivid dreams.

DISEASE MODEL OF ALCOHOLISM

The disease model is accepted by self-help organizations such as Alcoholics Anonymous (AA). The disease model contends that alcoholism is chronic (an unremitting, gradual disease that becomes more severe over time) and requires treatment. Alcoholism likely has a genetic root. Persons predisposed to the disease of alcoholism have **genetic markers** for lowered levels of platelet MAO activity, serotonin function, prolactin, adenylate cyclase, and ALDH2. Other theorists believe alcoholism is a **learned behavior**, rather than genetic. Research in this area is inconclusive. In 1956, E. M. Jellinek endorsed the American Medical Association's adoption of alcoholism as a disease. He described alcoholism as an infirmity with four stages of progression: Pre-alcoholic; prodromal, crucial, and chronic. Jellinek believed that alcoholics suffered from chemical dependencies that became relentless cravings for alcohol.

ALCOHOLICS ANONYMOUS

Alcoholics Anonymous is a 12-step self-help plan with many locations throughout the U.S. that encourages sobriety. Meetings are held in church halls, libraries, and clubs. AA should be offered along with appropriate counseling by a therapist, because the meetings are not considered psychological therapy. The benefit of an AA meeting to the client is the reinforcement of the coping skills taught in counseling sessions, and access to a peer group that is supportive. The group provides a same-sex sponsor to help the client see a good role model who has enjoyed a long period of sobriety. The alcoholic develops a more positive outlook of self and a sense of unity with the group, so feelings of isolation are removed. The client gains a sense of hope about his or her future, and comes to recognize that the substance use is out of control. Alcoholics are encouraged to seek God or a higher power of authority for outside help.

AA RELAPSE PREVENTION CARD AND OTHER COPING STRATEGIES

The alcoholic carries an AA relapse prevention card. The client is given this card to help him or her find alternative activities that do not include drugs or alcohol. The card contains instructions to communicate his or her feelings to a trusted AA member, and phone numbers for the sponsor and the client's spouse, or parents. The card may also instruct the client in relaxation techniques or imagery to get through the cravings. A client may find it beneficial to write down his or her feelings in a journal and bring it to the counseling sessions. Teach the client assertiveness techniques to stand up to his or her AA peers if they make inappropriate suggestions.

ABUSE OF BARBITURATES AND BENZODIAZEPINES

Barbiturates and benzodiazepines are classified as **CNS depressants** or **sedative-hypnotics**. These drugs can be taken orally or injected. Their effects include depression of the major brain functions such as mood, cognition, memory, insight, or judgment and can cause feelings of euphoria and emotional lability. They can also lead to sedation and decreased sexual desire.

- **Overdose** can lead to unresponsiveness, coma, respiratory arrest, and cardiac arrest.
- **Withdrawal** symptoms can include anxiety and agitation, hypertension, tachycardia, diaphoresis, increased temperature, excitability, insomnia, seizures, delirium, or hallucinations.
- **Long-term complications** can include those acquired from shared needle use as well as medical conditions associated with other dependencies.

ABUSE OF AMPHETAMINES AND COCAINE

Amphetamines and cocaine are both classified as **CNS stimulants**. They can both be taken orally or injected. Cocaine can also be smoked or used topically. These drugs cause a sudden sensation of euphoria, energy, wakefulness, diminished appetite, and insomnia. They can also cause paranoia, aggressiveness, dilated pupils, shaking, hyperactivity, pressured speech, constipation, dry mouth, tachycardia, and chest pain.

- An **overdose** can lead to sudden cardiac death or myocardial infarction due to coronary artery spasm, cardiac dysrhythmias, hyper or hypotension, respiratory depression or arrest, seizures, psychosis, dyskinesias, dystonias, coma, or death.

- **Withdrawal** symptoms can include feelings of depression and fatigue with suicidal ideations, agitation, insomnia, anxiety, nightmares, and increased appetite.
- These drugs are often alternated with depressants and can result in **malnutrition** or a **schizophrenia-like syndrome**.

PHYSIOLOGIC RESPONSE

Stimulants such as cocaine and amphetamines increase levels of **dopamine, serotonin, and norepinephrine** in the synapse. However, the mechanisms between the two differ somewhat. Cocaine inhibits the monoamine reuptake mechanism. The inhibition of reuptake increases dopamine levels and leads to a rewarding sense of euphoria. Cocaine's effect is usually short lived and the abuser will repeat the abuse to achieve the desired effect. Amphetamines both increase the release of norepinephrine and dopamine and also inhibit their reuptake.

INTOXICATION AND WITHDRAWAL

Characteristics of amphetamine and cocaine **intoxication** are:

- Maladaptive behavioral and psychological changes, including euphoria, hyperactivity, grandiosity, confusion, anger, paranoid ideation, and auditory hallucinations
- Tachycardia
- Hypertension or hypotension
- Dilated pupils
- Perspiration or chills
- Nausea or vomiting
- Weight loss
- Psychomotor agitation
- Muscular weakness
- Confusion
- Seizures

Symptoms of amphetamine and cocaine **withdrawal** are:

- Dysphoric mood
- Fatigue
- Vivid and unpleasant dreams
- Insomnia or hypersomnia
- Increased appetite
- Psychomotor agitation or retardation
- Intense depression after prolonged or heavy use

ABUSE OF OPIATES

Opiates include heroine, morphine, meperidine, codeine, opium, and methadone. All of the drugs can be given orally except meperidine, which can only be given by injection. Opium can also be smoked. Heroine, morphine, codeine, and meperidine can also be given by injection. These drugs cause a sense of euphoria, relaxation, pain relief, sedation, decreased sexual desire, impaired judgment, constricted pupils, nausea, slurred speech, and memory and concentration impairment.

- **Overdose** can lead to unresponsiveness, coma, or respiratory and cardiovascular depression leading to arrest and death.
- **Withdrawal** symptoms include watery eyes, runny nose, yawning, dilated pupils, goose bumps, diaphoresis, GI upset, insomnia, anorexia, flushing, hypertension, paresthesias, headaches, and fatigue.
- **Chronic use** can lead to malnutrition and dehydration along with medical problems caused by use of dirty needles.

PHYSIOLOGIC RESPONSE TO OPIATES

Opiates are powerful **pain relievers** and many are utilized medically for pain control. There are three types of opiate related drugs: **agonists** that increase the central nervous system effects, **antagonists** that block these effects, and **mixed agonist-antagonists**. Opiates act by elevating the production of **dopamine** by increasing the neuronal firing rate of dopamine producing cells. The opiate abuser's mood is elevated resulting in a sense of euphoria brought on by the increased dopamine activity. Opiate receptors are located throughout the brain and body and are activated by endorphins.

CLINICAL OPIATE WITHDRAWAL SCALE (COWS)

The Clinical Opiate Withdrawal Scale (COWS) is used to evaluate the severity of opiate withdrawal and the patient's level of drug dependence. Eleven items are assessed by the clinician based on observations of the patient and include:

- Resting pulse rate
- Sweating, chills, or flushing
- Restlessness
- Pupil size (normal, pinpoint, dilated)
- Bone, joint, or muscle aches
- Runny nose or tearing
- GI upset
- Tremors (on outstretched hands)
- Yawning
- Anxiety or irritability
- Gooseflesh

Each item is scored from 0 (normal) to 4 or 5, with the score higher with increased symptoms. The severity level of the withdrawal is based on the score:

- 5-12: Mild opiate withdrawal
- 13-24: Moderate opiate withdrawal
- 25-36: Moderately severe opiate withdrawal
- 36+: Severe opiate withdrawal

ABUSE OF CANNABIS

Cannabis includes hashish, THC, and marijuana (also known as grass, dope, joint, weed, or J). They can be smoked or taken orally. These drugs alter the user's state of awareness and can cause euphoria or dysphoria, sleepiness, heightened color and sound perceptions, red eyes, decreased inhibitions, dry mouth, increased appetite, or tingling sensations.

- **Overdose** can lead to tachycardia, disorientation, or toxic psychosis.
- There are usually no associated **withdrawal** symptoms; however, users can become irritable and may have insomnia for a few days.
- Usually, there are **no long-term medical complications**; however, the individual may experience an inability to concentrate and experience some memory disturbances.

No pharmacologic treatment has been evidenced to promote the reduction of cannabis abuse. First line treatment recommendation includes psychotherapy such as CBT and motivational enhancement therapy.

ABUSE OF PCP

Phencyclidine (PCP) can be taken orally or smoked to achieve the desired effects. This drug causes the user to feel as if they are **superhuman**. They have enhanced strength and endurance and will often experience intense rage. They may become agitated and hyperactive, acting out violently, or they may become catatonic and withdrawn or move back and forth between the two states. They may also have an increased pain threshold and stimulation of the cardiovascular and respiratory systems.

- In **overdose**, they may experience hallucinations, paranoia, psychosis, adrenergic crisis, cardiac arrest, stroke, malignant hyperthermia, seizures, or death.
- There are usually no associated **withdrawal** side effects.
- **Long-term problems** can include mild flashbacks or organic brain syndromes with psychosis lasting up to 6 months after drug use was discontinued. These individuals commonly have frequent police arrests.

ABUSE OF HALLUCINOGENS

Hallucinogens include LSD, DMT, mescaline, and MDMA, also known as ecstasy. These drugs can be taken orally or smoked. Effects can include distorted or sharpened visual and hearing perceptions, hallucinations, distortions of space and time, depersonalization, mystical experiences, mood lability, euphoria or dysphoria, altered body image, bizarre behaviors, confusion, impaired judgment and memory, dilated pupils, diaphoresis, palpitations, or panic reactions.

- **Overdose** symptoms can include paranoia, seizures, hyperthermia, hallucinations, or death.
- There are usually **no withdrawal** side effects and **long-term problems** may include flashbacks that may last for many months or the user may develop a chronic state of psychosis.

ABUSE OF INHALANTS

Abuse of inhalants can include use of glue, aerosol sprays, paint thinners, or lighter fluid. Using inhalants can cause the user to feel a sense of euphoria and giddiness. It can also cause impaired judgment, apathy, and assaultive behaviors.

- **Overdose** of these drugs causes CNS depression, dizziness, slurred speech, nystagmus, unsteady gait, dysarthria, shaking, depressed reflexes, and decreased appetite. In overdose, these drugs can lead to coma, seizures, respiratory or cardiac arrest, and death.
- **Withdrawal** symptoms are very similar to those seen with alcohol withdrawal; however, they are usually milder.
- **Long-term use** can lead to liver and kidney disease, blood disorders, interstitial lung disease, CNS damage, or permanent cognitive impairment that could require placement in a long-term care facility.

RELAPSE AND REMISSION

While many individuals are able to temporarily abstain from a substance on which they were formerly dependent, few of them will be able to avoid **relapse**. When an individual relapses into substance abuse behavior, he or she develops an **abstinence violation effect** that is manifested as self-blame, shame, and an increased susceptibility to relapse. The type of **remission** is based on whether any of the criteria for abuse/dependence have been met and over what time frame:

- **Early Remission**: After the criteria for a substance use disorder have been met, none of those criteria are fulfilled (except for the criteria for craving) for at least three months but not more than 1 year.
- **Sustained Remission**: After the criteria for a substance use disorder have been met, none of those criteria are fulfilled (except for the criteria for craving) for 1 year or longer.
- **Maintenance Therapy**: A replacement medication that can be taken to avoid withdrawal symptoms. The client could still be considered in remission from a substance use disorder if while using maintenance therapy, they do not meet any criteria for that substance use disorder except for craving. For tobacco use disorder this would include using nicotine replacement systems. For opioid use disorder this could include medications such as methadone. If the client is in remission in a controlled environment, this should be specified.

STAGES OF RELAPSE AND THE CREATION OF A RELAPSE PREVENTION PLAN

Patients suffering from substance abuse and addiction should be educated on the **stages of relapse** so that they can seek help.

- The first stage of relapse is **emotional relapse**. During this stage, the individual experiences emotions that signify the beginning of a possible relapse, such as anxiety, anger, isolation, and defensiveness. They may also become withdrawn, stop going to meetings, or develop poor eating and sleeping habits.
- The next stage of relapse is **mental relapse**, during which the patient starts to think about using the substance or reminisces on using in the past. The patient may begin to plan relapse at this stage.
- The third and final stage of relapse is **physical relapse** in which actions are taken to use the substance again. The earlier that relapse is addressed, the less likely the individual will reach the stage of physical relapse.

Patients must be empowered with a **relapse prevention plan** so that they are prepared in the face of early signs of relapse. This plan should identify triggers for use/abuse, detail a list of tools and coping mechanisms to use should the early stages of relapse occur, identify support systems (family, mentors, sponsors, etc.) to call in the case of triggers/cravings, and identify the support group(s) that will provide consistent reinforcement and encouragement in the path to recovery.

IDENTIFYING AND DELINEATING BETWEEN SUBSTANCES BEING ABUSED

To diagnose substance use disorder correctly, find a clear connection relating the patient's **symptoms** to the **substance**. There are a number of different ways to ascertain substance abuse:

- Direct physical evidence
- Time of substance use and subsequent onset of symptoms
- Cessation of symptoms after a period of abstinence
- Presence of symptoms not associated with any other mental disorder
- Direct empirical evidence of a relationship between the substance and the observed symptoms

The most **common substances of abuse** are nicotine, caffeine, alcohol, marijuana, amphetamines, phencyclidine, opiates, cocaine, sedative-hypnotics, anabolic steroids, hallucinogens, inhalants, and laxatives. Assess for these substances first.

TREATMENT OPTIONS FOR SUBSTANCE USE DISORDER

Treatments for substance use disorder include:

- **Aversion therapy** techniques like covert sensitization or Antabuse (disulfiram) for alcoholism
- **Multicomponent interventions** involving social skills training, stress management, moderation training, and contingency management
- Learning strategies for **self-control**
- **12-step peer group treatment programs** like AA
- **Rapid Opiate Detoxification** (ROD or Waismann Method) with general anesthesia
- Cold turkey withdrawal in **detox facilities**

TREATMENTS FOR NICOTINE USE DISORDER

Because of the major health risks associated with smoking, there have been numerous attempts to devise successful **programs for smoking cessation**. Unfortunately, nicotine addiction is very difficult to break; one study indicated that only 2.5% of all those who tried to quit were successful. This is especially tragic considering that the health risks associated with smoking are almost entirely negated after five years of cessation. At present, research suggests that the most successful programs for smoking cessation include nicotine replacement therapy (patches and gum); a multicomponent behavioral therapy including skills training, relapse prevention, stimulus control, or rapid smoking; and support and assistance from a clinician.

Abuse and Domestic Violence

INDICATORS OF ABUSE THAT MAY BE IDENTIFIED IN THE PATIENT HISTORY

The healthcare provider should always be aware of the presence of any **indicators** that may present a potential for or an actual situation that involves **abuse**. These indicators may present in the **patient's history**. Some examples of indicators concerning their primary complaint may include the following: vague description about the cause of the problem, inconsistencies between physical findings and explanations, minimizing injuries, long period of time between injury and treatment, and over-reactions or under-reactions of family members to injuries. Other important information may be revealed in the family genome, such as family history of violence, time spent in jail or prison, and family history of violent deaths or substance abuse. The patient's health history may include previous injuries, spontaneous abortions, or history of pervious inpatient psychiatric treatment or substance abuse.

During the collection of the patient history, the financial history, the patient's family values, and the patient's relationships with family members can also reveal actual or potential **abuse indicators**.

- The **financial history** may indicate that the patient has little or no money or that they are not given access to money by a controlling family member. They may also be unemployed or utilizing an elderly family member's income for their own personal expenses.
- **Family values** may indicate strong beliefs in physical punishment, dictatorship within the home, inability to allow different opinions within the home, or lack of trust for anyone outside the family.
- **Relationships** within the family may be dysfunctional. Problems such as lack of affection between family members, co-dependency, frequent arguments, extramarital affairs, or extremely rigid beliefs about roles within the family may be present.

During the collection of the patient history, the sexual, social, and psychological history of the patient should be evaluated for any signs of actual or potential abuse.

- The **sexual history** may reveal problems such as previous sexual abuse, forced sexual acts, sexually transmitted infections (STIs), sexual knowledge beyond normal age-appropriate knowledge, or promiscuity.
- The **social history** may reveal unplanned pregnancies, social isolation as evidenced by lack of friends available to help the patient, unreasonable jealousy of significant other, verbal aggression, belief in physical punishment, or problems in school.
- During the **psychological assessment** the patient may express feelings of helplessness and being trapped. The patient may be unable to describe their future, become tearful, perform self-mutilation, have low self-esteem, and have had previous suicide attempts.

OBSERVATIONS THAT MAY INDICATE ABUSE

During the initial assessment, observations may also be made by the provider that can provide vital information about actual or potential abuse. **General observations** may include finding that the patient history is far different from what is objectively viewed by the provider or that there is a lack of proper clothing or lack of physical care provided. The home environment may include lack of heat, water, or food. It may also reveal inappropriate sleeping arrangements or lack of an environmentally safe housing situation. Observations concerning **family communications** may reveal that the abuser answers all the questions for the whole family or that others look to the controlling member for approval or seem fearful of others. Family members may frequently argue, interrupt each other, or act out negative nonverbal behaviors while others are speaking. They may avoid talking about certain subjects that they feel are secretive.

INDICATORS OF ABUSE THAT MAY BE EVIDENT DURING THE PHYSICAL ASSESSMENT

During the **physical assessment** the provider should always be aware of any **indicators of abuse**. These indicators may include increased anxiety about being examined or in the presence of the abuser; poor hygiene; looks to abuser to answer questions for them; flinching; over or underweight; presence of bruises, welts, scars or cigarette burns; bald patches on scalp for pulling out of hair; intracranial bleeding; subconjunctival hemorrhages; black eye(s); hearing loss from untreated infection or injury; poor dental hygiene; abdominal injuries; fractures; developmental delays; hyperactive reflexes; genital lacerations or ecchymosis; and presence of STIs, rectal bruising, bleeding, edema, or poor sphincter tone.

DOMESTIC VIOLENCE

Men, women, elderly, children, and the disabled may all be victims of **domestic violence**. The violent person harms physically or sexually and uses threats and fear to maintain control of the victim. The violence does not improve unless the abuser gets intensive counseling. The abuser may promise not to do it again, but the violence usually gets more frequent and worsens over time. The provider should ask all patients in private about abuse, neglect, and fear of a caretaker. If abuse is suspected or there are signs present, the state may require **reporting**:

- Give victims information about community hotlines, shelters, and resources.
- Urge them to set up a plan for escape for themselves and any children, complete with supplies in a location away from the home.
- Assure victims that they are not at fault and do not deserve the abuse.
- Try to empower them by helping them to realize that they do not have to take abuse and can find support to change the situation.

> **Review Video: Domestic Violence**
> Visit mometrix.com/academy and enter code: 530581

ASSESSMENT OF DOMESTIC VIOLENCE

According to the guidelines of the Family Violence Prevention Fund, **assessment** for domestic violence should be done for all adolescent and adult patients, regardless of background or signs of abuse. While females are the most common victims, there are increasing reports of male victims of domestic violence, both in heterosexual and homosexual relationships. The person doing the assessment should be informed about domestic violence and be aware of risk factors and danger signs. The interview should be conducted in private (special accommodations may need to be made for children <3 years old). The manager's office, bathrooms, and examining rooms should have information about domestic violence posted prominently. Brochures and information should be available to give to patients. Patients may present with a variety of physical complaints, such as headache, pain, palpitations, numbness, or pelvic pain. They are often depressed and may appear suicidal and may be isolated from friends and family. Victims of domestic violence often exhibit fear of spouse/partner, and may report injury inconsistent with symptoms.

STEPS TO IDENTIFYING VICTIMS OF DOMESTIC VIOLENCE

The **Family Violence Prevention Fund** has issued guidelines for identifying and assisting victims of domestic violence. There are 7 steps:

1. **Inquiry**: Non-judgmental questioning should begin with asking if the person has ever been abused—physically, sexually, or psychologically.
2. **Interview**: The person may exhibit signs of anxiety or fear and may blame himself or report that others believe he is abused. The person should be questioned if she is afraid for her life or for her children.

3. **Question**: If the person reports abuse, it's critical to ask if the person is in immediate danger or if the abuser is on the premises. The interviewer should ask if the person has been threatened. The history and pattern of abuse should be questioned, and if children are involved, whether the children are abused. Note: State laws vary, and in some states, it is mandatory to report if a child was present during an act of domestic violence as this is considered child abuse. The provider must be aware of state laws regarding domestic and child abuse, and all healthcare providers are mandatory reporters.
4. **Validate**: The interviewer should offer support and reassurance in a non-judgmental manner, telling the patient the abuse is not his or her fault.
5. **Give information**: While discussing facts about domestic violence and the tendency to escalate, the interviewer should provide brochures and information about safety planning. If the patient wants to file a complaint with the police, the interviewer should assist the person to place the call.
6. **Make referrals**: Information about state, local, and national organizations should be provided along with telephone numbers and contact numbers for domestic violence shelters.
7. **Document**: Record keeping should be legal, legible, and lengthy with a complete report and description of any traumatic injuries resulting from domestic violence. A body map may be used to indicate sites of injury, especially if there are multiple bruises or injuries.

INJURIES CONSISTENT WITH DOMESTIC VIOLENCE

There are a number of characteristic **injuries** that may indicate domestic violence, including ruptured eardrum; rectal/genital injury (burns, bites, or trauma); scrapes and bruises about the neck, face, head, trunk, arms; and cuts, bruises, and fractures of the face. The pattern of injuries associated with domestic violence is also often distinctive. The bathing-suit pattern involves injuries on parts of body that are usually covered with clothing as the perpetrator inflicts damage but hides evidence of abuse. Head and neck injuries (50%) are also common. Abusive injuries (rarely attributable to accidents) are common and include bites, bruises, rope and cigarette burns, and welts in the outline of weapons (belt marks). Bilateral injuries of arms/legs are often seen with domestic abuse. Defensive injuries are indicative of abuse.

Defensive injuries to the back of the body are often incurred as the victim crouches on the floor face down while being attacked. The soles of the feet may be injured from kicking at perpetrator. The ulnar aspect of hand or palm may be injured from blocking blows.

ABUSIVE BEHAVIORS ASSOCIATED WITH DOMESTIC VIOLENCE

Abusive behaviors often occur in a series of escalating degrees.

1. The series begins with **verbal abuse** in the form of mocking comments, put-downs, name-calling, or abusive language.
2. The next degree is **emotional abuse** in the form of rejecting, degrading, terrorizing, isolating, corrupting, financially exploiting, and denying emotional responsiveness.
3. **Physical abuse** is next on the continuum in the form of restraining, slapping, beating, biting, burning, striking with an object, strangulation, and the use of weapons with the intent of wounding or causing death.

According to the CDC, 1 in 4 women and 1 in 10 men have experienced some form of intimate partner violence.

> **Review Video: Domestic Abuse**
> Visit mometrix.com/academy and enter code: 530581

SOCIETAL COST OF ABUSE

Abuse costs Americans over $4 billion dollars per year for:

- Physical injuries treated by medical practitioners
- Psychological injuries treated by mental health professionals
- Violence prevention campaigns
- Police and judiciary costs
- Emergency housing
- Social services costs

There are also hidden costs from **eroded social capital** like:

- Increased morbidity from stress
- Lost pay from work absences
- Low productivity from worry at work and painful movement
- Lower earnings and savings
- Increased mortality from suicide through depression
- Poor school performance by traumatized children
- Increased mortality from murder

Victims can be either a member of an intimate relationship, or children in violent homes, which are often neglected or abused. Victims of childhood abuse often become the perpetrators of violence in later life. Many suffer from poor self-esteem that undermines their job choices and social interactions.

VIOLENCE AGAINST WOMEN ACT OF 1994

President Bill Clinton signed the Violence Against Women Act of 1994, a law based on zero tolerance for violence. **Zero tolerance** means no reported abuse will be ignored; the perpetrator always faces stiff penalties. The Violence Against Women Act was not a productive deterrent from abuse because the stiff penalties caused women to withdraw from legal protection. Abused women feared:

- Police would take their children away from the violence
- Their husbands or significant others would retaliate after release from jail
- They would be unable to cope financially without their husband's or significant other's income to help support the family
- Taking on the fees charged by lawyers, bondsmen, and the courts

Women are frequent targets for abuse because they are often:

- Untrained in self-defense
- Small enough to wound and intimidate easily
- Socialized not to leave a relationship except under extreme duress

WOMEN IN ABUSIVE RELATIONSHIPS

Women tend to stay in abusive relationships for many reasons, including:

- Abuse being normalized from watching their parents participate in similarly dysfunctional relationships
- Being concerned that their children will have no traditional nurturer if they leave
- Feeling a social responsibility to keep up the facade of a happy home
- Early training from childhood that they are inferior and deserve abuse

Abuse screening tools have been implemented in doctors' and mental health providers' offices in an effort to identify abused women who do not spontaneously disclose. The woman is asked:

- Whether or not she has been physically struck over the last year
- About the safety of her present relationship
- About past relationships that may threaten her present safety

COMMON PROBLEMS THAT CHILDREN OF ABUSE MAY DEVELOP

Physical and mental issues often develop in a **child from an abusive home** that follows him or her into adulthood. Some common behavior and social problems include:

- Deficient social skills
- Inadequate problem-solving skills; aggressiveness
- Delinquency
- Oppositional behaviors
- Attention deficit/hyperactivity disorder (ADHD)
- Obsessive-compulsive disorders (OCD)
- Suicidal tendencies
- Drug and alcohol abuse
- Social disengagement
- Denial
- Anxiety and depression
- Social withdrawal
- Avoidance of problems
- Excessive self-criticism

These social, behavioral, and intimacy problems are very prevalent and costly to our society, and degrade the children's quality of life.

CHARACTERISTICS OF ABUSERS

Abusers of either sex have various unmet psychological needs or motivations. These **types of abusers** are common:

- A person who assaults his or her victims in the **home setting** and has a strong need to dominate relationships with his or her intimate partners.
- The abuser who is suffering from significant **psychological issues**, like antisocial personality disorder; who is a convicted criminal; or has past assault and battery charges (often dropped by intimidated victims).
- The person who works through a **continuum of abusive behaviors**. These often begin with verbal and emotional abuses, which lead to throwing objects at the victim, intimidation, and an effort to dominate the relationship by withholding money or restraining movement and social access. Violence can escalate, followed by feelings of remorse. The pattern can become part of a never-ending cycle of behavior. This type of abuser often victimizes seniors or the disabled.

MALE ABUSERS

Male abusers were usually abused as children, watched their mothers being abused, or saw abuse perpetrated by male friends (e.g., gang rapes as initiation rites). The **male abuser** often displays one or several of the following qualities:

- He has a **disproportionate sense of entitlement** that he has the right to hurt others, especially females. He truly believes he has the right to hit a woman if she is unfaithful or withholding sex from him.
- He usually **does not have a good opinion of women** because that is the way he has been socialized.
- He often justifies his behavior by stating he was **drunk or high on drugs** at the time of an attack.
- He may have a **psychological problem** such as post-traumatic stress disorder (PTSD), a delayed reaction caused by trauma or witnessing an event that caused him a great deal of suffering. Other psychological problems common to abusers are depression, poor self-esteem, personality disorders, and psychopathy.

Male abusers may have been abandoned as children. **Abandonment** leads to a state of rage in the adult male. Be alert to three states of child abuse that commonly have detrimental effects on the future adult male:

- The father or an adult male authority figure inflicts physical abuse on a male child.
- The father inflicts emotional abuse by rejecting and humiliating his son.
- The mother does not form a maternal bond with her son.

Anger is part of the attachment process. The attachment object may be the victim of the violence as the male abuser takes out his feelings of jealousy or rejection. The male's veneer of icy indifference conceals a strong emotional dependency on the significant other or wife.

RECOMMENDED TREATMENT APPROPRIATE FOR ABUSERS

The first step is to determine if abuse actually exists and to diagnose the type of abuser. Rule out addiction to drugs or alcohol. If the abuser is an addict, refer the abuser to a separate drug or alcohol intervention program, in conjunction with treatment. Next, determine the severity of past abuse perpetrated on the abuser when he or she was a child. The abuse need not have been directed at the child. It is sufficient that he or she witnessed violence being perpetrated on other family members. Evaluate the abuser for borderline personality disorder and post-traumatic stress disorder. Provide the abuser with anger management training in a group setting. Anger management involves discussions of dominant and controlling behaviors, and the development of personal responsibility. The abuser needs to control his own or her own behavior.

The male abuser should be **counseled** regarding the abuse that was perpetrated on him as a child. The male adult should understand that he was a victim himself, and is not to be blamed for the past abuse perpetrated upon him as a child. He is not the one that caused others to hurt him. Bring to light his wrong assumptions. Try to develop his understanding of the root of his self-esteem issues. The male needs to develop a healthier self-view and learn thought patterns that lead to appropriate behavior. Encourage him to discuss and deal with internal conflicts and the internalized pain of his past. Use a motivational approach to help the male client gain a healthy perspective on his behavior. Base the approach on cognitive, emotional, and behavioral conflicts in the client's life.

Avoid **jointly counseling** a couple in an abusive relationship, as this can lead to further abuse. Assess the clients individually, followed by group therapy. The small group of 6-8 members should be led either by a sole male counselor, or male and female co-counselors to help the clients see positive interaction between a male and female. The co-leader relationship must be evenly balanced in power and control of the group. The focus of the group is self-improvement. Each individual in the group examines his or her emotional responses that are reflected in angry behaviors. The **emotions** behind the anger are usually sadness, pain, rejection, and humiliation. Turn angry behavior to the appropriate expression of emotion. Discuss families and relationships. Relate childhood experiences to present attitudes and behaviors.

COMPONENTS OF A 20-WEEK ANGER MANAGEMENT GROUP OUTLINE

Anger management group therapy can be accomplished in 20 weeks with one session per week. The anger management treatment group should consist of 6-8 members. Here is a suggested outline for discussion topics:

- **Week 1**: The group makes a participation agreement. Each individual shares their personal violence statement.
- **Week 2**: Clients learn to take a time-out from anger. Discuss other anger management principles. Provide some stress management skill instructions.
- **Week 3**: Each client participates in a discussion on issues they face in their daily life that they can or cannot control. Follow this discussion with another discussion on conflict, emotions, and actions. Encourage clients to practice the use of "I" messages to communicate their feelings. Help clients to gain insight into assertive requests and refusals.
- **Week 4**: Involve clients in an examination of values and discuss the clients' reactions.
- **Week 5**: Discuss the continuum of abuse and the power wheel.
- **Week 6**: Discuss childhood experiences, especially the parental relationship that the child witnessed, and parenting styles.
- **Week 7**: Discuss how abuse of the child is reflected in the life of the adult. The resulting conversation will deal with emotions that this discussion conjures up.
- **Week 8**: Clients discuss the difference between punishment and discipline.
- **Week 9**: Clients discuss praise and respect.
- **Week 10**: Discuss self-talk and its impact, and examine scripts.
- **Week 11**: Discuss the abuse cycle along with a conversation regarding communication.
- **Week 12**: Incorporate empathy, listening, and reflection.
- **Week 13**: Discuss assertiveness.
- **Week 14**: Summarize and consolidate the communication skills taught in the first 13 weeks.
- **Week 15**: Review the power wheel and include a practice exercise.
- **Week 16**: Discuss intimacy.
- **Week 17**: Give empathy exercises.
- **Week 18**: Follow-up on the empathy exercises.
- **Week 19**: Outline a relapse prevention plan.
- **Week 20**: Summarize and reinforce what was learned in the previous 19 weeks. In ending conversation, discuss ways to implement the relapse prevention plan in case a problem develops.

POSSIBLE ISSUES RESULTING FROM TREATMENT

Treatment that involves discussing the client's abusive relationship with others may unearth feelings that are uncomfortable for both the client and the counselor. The client may want to place the blame for his or her violent actions on the client's spouse or significant other. Help the client to understand the motivations behind those actions and the desire to place the blame elsewhere. Understanding helps the client to establish a closer relationship with his or her spouse. Do not force the client to take responsibility for his or her behavior, or criticize the client, as this will likely cause the client to become defensive. Do not force a confrontation that could turn into an aggressive act. Confrontations increase the sense of humiliation the client is feeling. Humiliation will lead the client to express feelings of blame and anger.

ELDER ABUSE

Active abuse is intentional (such as hitting) while passive abuse occurs without intention. **Elder abuse** may be difficult to diagnose, especially if the person is cognitively impaired, but symptoms can include fearfulness, disparities in reports of injuries between patient and caregiver, evidence of old or repeated injuries, poor hygiene and dental care, decubiti, malnutrition, undue concern with costs on caregiver's part, unsupportive attitude of caregiver, and caregiver's reluctance or refusal to allow patient to communicate privately with the nurse. Diagnosis includes a careful history and physical exam, including direct questioning of the patient about abuse. Treatment includes attending to injuries or physical needs, (this can vary widely) and referral to adult protective services as indicated. Reporting laws regarding elder abuse vary somewhat from one state to another, but all states have laws regarding elder abuse and most states require mandatory reporting to adult protective services by health workers.

ELDER NEGLECT

Neglect of basic needs is a common problem of older adults who live alone or with reluctant or incapable caregivers. In some cases, passive neglect may occur because an elderly spouse is trying to take care of a patient and is unable to provide the care needed, but in other cases, active neglect reflects a lack of caring and may border on negligence and abuse. **Indications** of neglect include the following:

- Lack of assistive devices, such as cane or walker, needed for mobility
- Misplaced or missing glasses or hearing aids
- Poor dental hygiene and dental care and/or missing dentures
- Patient left unattended for extended periods of time, sometimes confined to a bed or chair
- Patient left in soiled or urine/feces-stained clothing
- Inadequate food/fluid/nutrition resulting in weight loss
- Inappropriate and unkempt clothing, such as lack of sweater or coat during the winter and dirty or torn clothing
- Dirty, messy environment

RISK OF ELDER ABUSE

Age and disability increase the **risks of elder abuse**. People over the age of 80 are more than twice as likely to suffer abuse as younger adults. Patients with dementia, such as Alzheimer's disease, are at risk of abuse in both the home environment, where they are often cared for by adult children, and in institutions. Caregivers often lose patience and become frustrated, especially if the patient's behavior is belligerent, combative, or disruptive. This type of abuse can be very difficult to diagnose, as the patient is usually unable to corroborate abuse. In fact, even older adults who are not cognitively impaired may be afraid to report abuse because they depend on the abusers to care for them. Older adults who are dependent on others for assistance with ADLs, such as dressing, bathing, and food preparation are also particularly at risk for outright abuse and neglect. Abusers often suffer from depression and or substance abuse and may be financially dependent on the victim.

PHYSICAL AND EMOTIONAL ABUSE

There are a number of different types of elder abuse. **Physical abuse** is an active form of abuse and is almost always associated with **psychological abuse** as well. Older adults, particularly those cared for by family members (often an adult child) or other caregivers, may suffer various types of assaults related to hitting, kicking, pulling hair, shoving, and pushing. Caregivers may make frequent threats to hit the older adult, sometimes brandishing a weapon, if the person doesn't cooperate and may tell the person to commit suicide. Ongoing intimidation may make the patient terrified and anxious. Sometimes, caregivers threaten to injure pets or family members, increasing patient's fear. Patients may be forcibly confined, forced into seclusion, and/or force-fed to the point that they choke on food.

Physical symptoms include the following:

- Ruptured eardrum
- Rectal/genital injury—burns, bites, trauma
- Scrapes and bruises about the neck, face, head, trunk, arms
- Cuts, bruises, and fractures of the face

The **pattern of injuries** is also often distinctive:

- Bathing suit pattern—injuries on parts of body that are usually covered with clothing as the perpetrator abuses but hides evidence of abuse
- Head and neck injuries (50%)

Abusive injuries (rarely attributable to accidents) are common:

- Bites, bruises, rope and cigarette burns, welts in the outline of weapons (belt marks)
- Bilateral injuries of arms/legs

Defensive injuries are indicative of abuse:

- Back of the body injury from being attacked while crouched on the floor face down
- Soles of the feet from kicking at perpetrator
- Ulnar aspect of hand or palm from blocking blows

Psychological symptoms include anxiety, paranoia, insomnia, low self-esteem, avoidance of eye contact, and obvious nervousness in the presence of the caregiver, who is often reluctant to leave the patient alone.

SEXUAL ABUSE

Sexual abuse of older adults occurs when the person receiving sexual attention is unwilling to participate or unable (because of cognizant impairment or other illness) to consent to sexual intimacy. Types of **sexual abuse** include:

- **Physical**: Fondling, kissing, and rape
- **Emotional**: Exhibitionism
- **Verbal**: Sexual harassment, using obscene language, threatening

Sexual abuse of older adults occurs most commonly to women in their 70s or 80s confined to nursing homes. Sexual abuse may also occur in home environments, but it is harder to detect. Most abusers are fellow nursing home residents (males over the age of 60), and the most common form of abuse is sexualized kissing and fondling of genitals. Because older adults have a right to sexual intimacy, in some cases what may appear to be abuse between residents may, in fact, be consensual. Caregivers may have raped or otherwise sexually abused patients, and this exercise of power over another person is always illegal abuse.

FINANCIAL ABUSE

Elder abuse often occurs when an older adult is unable to care for or protect himself. In many situations, another person takes advantage of an older adult and uses threats or manipulation to justify the activity. As older adults become unable to manage their own financial affairs, they become increasingly vulnerable to **financial abuse**, especially if they have cognitive impairment or physical impairments that impair their mobility. This kind of abuse often occurs when an older adult trusts another person for help with finances and is taken advantage of. Financial abuse includes the following:

- Outright stealing of property or persuading patients to give away possessions
- Forcing patients to sign away property
- Emptying bank and savings accounts
- Using stolen credit cards
- Convincing the person to invest money in fraudulent schemes
- Taking money for home renovations that are not done

Indications of financial abuse may be unpaid bills, unusual activity at ATMs or with credit cards, inadequate funds to meet needs, disappearance of items in the home, change in the provision of a will, and deferring to caregivers regarding financial affairs. Family or caregivers may move permanently into the patient's home and take over without sharing costs.

Some examples of financial abuse of an elderly client include when another person steals money or other valuable items, forges the patient's signature on checks or signs over Social Security income, uses the adult's name and identifying information to gain access to other accounts or to spend money, advises an older adult to invest money into accounts or schemes that are not legitimate, or commits fraud by telling an older adult that she has won money or is contributing to fraudulent organizations.

SOCIOECONOMIC FACTORS THAT MAY CONTRIBUTE TO ELDER ABUSE

Elder abuse is a problem that remains largely underreported. Elder abuse may be more prevalent when abusers see older adults as helpless victims who have no control over their environment or who have no access to reporting to authorities. Some older adults and their abusers may downplay the abuse or neglect, while others may be unsure of what their options are for help and safety. There are some **socioeconomic factors** that contribute to elder abuse and neglect, allowing these situations to continue. Some examples include a stressful environment, such as a long-term-care facility that houses many high-need residents, family or caregivers that are burdened by stress or who have emotional instability, the prevalence of ageism and the idea that the elderly are incompetent or frail, the increase in diagnosed cases of chronic disease, and advances in medicine and technology that allow older persons to live longer.

SCREENING QUESTIONS TO ASSESS FOR ELDER ABUSE

The nurse who cares for older adults is in a position to detect cases of abuse or neglect that may otherwise go unreported. The nurse serves as the patient's advocate to protect him from abuse taking place that he may be powerless to control. The nurse may need to ask questions when the potential abuser is not in the room. Some questions that the nurse may ask to assess for underlying abuse or neglect include:

- Has anyone been hurting you?
- Do you feel safe where you live?
- Is there someone in your family/neighborhood that you are afraid of?
- Have you ever been threatened?
- Has anyone ever touched you in a manner that made you uncomfortable?
- Do you feel that your caregiver/family/friend is there for you when you need him or her?

UNDERREPORTING OF ABUSE IN LONG-TERM-CARE FACILITIES

Abusive and neglectful situations that occur in nursing homes may go **underreported** for various reasons. Many longterm-care facilities care for a large number of residents, caregivers may be stressed, and units may be understaffed. These facilities provide care for high-need patients, potentially causing difficulties with time management and fully meeting the needs of every resident, which further contributes to abuse. Some residents may be in situations where they are unable to report any abuse because of speech or hearing difficulties, physical disabilities, or cognitive changes. Abuse or neglect may also occur and remain underreported in residents who do not have regular visits from families or friends. These residents may go for long periods without an outside person visiting to evaluate or notice any changes in behavior or appearance that may occur with abuse.

IDENTIFYING AND REPORTING NEGLECT OF THE BASIC NEEDS OF ADULTS

Neglect of the basic needs of adults is a common problem, especially among the elderly, adults with psychiatric or mental health problems, or those who live alone or with reluctant or incapable caregivers. In some cases, **passive neglect** may occur because an elderly or impaired spouse or partner is trying to take care of a patient and is unable to provide the care needed, but in other cases, **active neglect** reflects a lack of caring which may be considered negligence or abuse. Cases of neglect should be reported to the appropriate governmental agency, such as adult protective services. Indications of neglect include the following:

- Lack of assistive devices, such as a cane or walker, needed for mobility
- Misplaced or missing glasses or hearing aids
- Poor dental hygiene and dental care or missing dentures
- Patient left unattended for extended periods of time, sometimes confined to a bed or chair
- Patient left in soiled or urine- and feces-stained clothing
- Inadequate food, fluid, or nutrition, resulting in weight loss
- Inappropriate and unkempt clothing, such as no sweater or coat during the winter and dirty or torn clothing
- A dirty, messy environment

IDENTIFYING AND REPORTING NEGLECT OR LACK OF SUPERVISION IN CHILDREN

While some children may not be physically or sexually abused, they may suffer from profound **neglect** or **lack of supervision** that places them at risk. Indicators include the following:

- Appearing dirty and unkempt, sometimes with infestations of lice, and wearing ill-fitting or torn clothes and shoes
- Being tired and sleepy during the daytime
- Having untended medical or dental problems, such as dental caries
- Missing appointments and not receiving proper immunizations
- Being underweight for stage of development

Neglect can be difficult to assess, especially if the nurse is serving a homeless or very poor population. Home visits may be needed to ascertain if adequate food, clothing, or supervision is being provided; this may be beyond the care provided by the nurse, so suspicions should be reported to appropriate authorities, such as child protective services, so that social workers can assess the home environment.

Emergency Situations and Crisis Management

CRISIS

CHARACTERISTICS

A **crisis** occurs when a person is faced with a highly stressful event and their usual problem solving and coping skills fail to be effective in resolving the situation. This event usually leads to increased levels of **anxiety** and can bring about a **physical and psychological response**. The problem is usually an **acute event** that can be identified. It may have occurred a few weeks or even months before or immediately prior to the crisis and can be an actual event or a potential event. The crisis state usually lasts less than six weeks with the individual then becoming able to utilize problem-solving skills to cope effectively. A person in crisis does not always have a mental disorder. However, during the acute crisis, their social functioning and decision-making abilities may be impaired.

DEVELOPMENTAL TYPE

There are basically two different **types of crises**. These types include developmental or maturational crises and situational crises. A **developmental crisis** can occur during **maturation** when an individual must take on a new life role. This crisis can be a normal part of the developmental process. A youth may need to face crisis and resolve this crisis to be able to move on to the next developmental stage. This may occur during the process of moving from adolescence to adulthood. Examples of situations that could lead to this type of crisis include graduating from school, going away to college, or moving out on their own. These situations would cause the individual to face a maturing event that requires the development of new coping skills.

SITUATIONAL TYPE

The second type of crisis is the **situational crisis**. This type of crisis can occur at any time in life. There is usually an event or problem that occurs, which leads to a **disruption in normal psychological functioning**. These types of events are often unplanned and can occur with or without warning. Some examples that may lead to a situational crisis include the death of a loved one, divorce, unplanned or unwanted pregnancy, onset or change in a physical disease process, job loss, or being the victim of a violent act. Events that affect an entire community can also cause individual and community situation crisis. Terrorist attacks or weather-related disasters are examples of events that can affect an entire community.

CRISIS INTERVENTION

Crisis intervention occurs when the goal of treatment is to return the individual to their **pre-crisis state**. This treatment course usually lasts six weeks or less and is geared toward assisting the individual to create new **coping mechanisms** and **adaptive behaviors**. Social and cultural influences can greatly affect the ability and ways in which individuals deal with and work through a crisis. There may be preconceived ideas and beliefs about asking for and accepting assistance from others. It is very important to consider the age of the individual when assessing the need for particular crisis interventions. The needs of an elderly adult will be different than the needs of a child.

Initial focus should be based on managing the current situation at hand to prevent complications and further feelings of helplessness from the patient. In this manner, the focus becomes solving the current problem and supporting the client emotionally, rather than trying to assess or manage underlying or long-term problems. Work should focus on helping the patient to feel secure and identifying negative or irrational thoughts that could be leading the patient into the crisis situation. By focusing on negative causes, the provider can work with the patient to identify solutions to the current situation. This averts the crisis from escalating into other areas, such as violence or suicide, and diminishes the patient's feelings of helplessness. If available, family members of the patient or other members of the health care team should be called in for support, as crisis interventions can be intense and overwhelming for those involved.

The patient who is having a crisis that includes hallucinations, such as hearing voices or seeing objects or people who are not truly there, may be exhibiting behaviors or hallucinating about subjects that are related to a particular theme for the patient. When managing hallucinations during an early or initial assessment, the actual theme or underlying subject may be assessed during this time. Once this topic is uncovered, management of hallucinations may focus more on dealing with the topic at hand, rather than the specific hallucination. The provider can redirect the patient to discuss the underlying feelings rather than the specific vision, voice, or thoughts the patient is experiencing. The provider may respond by saying, "I don't hear what you are hearing, but I think we should discuss your feelings of grief." If the patient is having hallucinations that are telling him to hurt himself or others, however, the provider may need to manage the situation with a crisis intervention rather than redirecting the patient to discuss underlying issues.

BRIEF CRISIS INTERVENTION THERAPIES

Brief crisis intervention therapies help the client come to terms with a life event or societal change, for example:

- Debriefing after violence in the workplace
- Natural disasters (earthquake, tornado, flood)
- Sexual assault
- Criminal victimization
- Suicidal or homicidal ideation (telephone hot lines)
- Catastrophic illness or injury
- Drastic relationship changes, like divorce

Limited therapy sessions may be conducted because of:

- Insurance limitations
- The client's reluctance to engage in prolonged treatment
- A shortage of qualified mental health workers versus heightened public demand for mental health treatment

SIX-STEP MODEL

Brief crisis intervention therapies often follow a six-step model developed by Gilliland in 1982. The end result of these steps should be that the client feels that the therapist helped and provided a positive experience:

- **Step 1**: Identify and concentrate on the problem at hand.
- **Step 2**: Assess the patient's personal history.
- **Step 3**: Develop a therapeutic bond with the patient.
- **Step 4**: Create a plan that uses an eclectic approach in selecting a wide range of intervention strategies.
- **Step 5**: Work out a solution to the problem at hand.
- **Step 6**: End therapy with an understanding between therapist and patient that the client can return whenever necessary.

USING SOLUTION FOCUSED THERAPY FOR BRIEF CRISIS INTERVENTIONS

Solution Focused Therapy is another alternative that provides a productive atmosphere for the client, where the problem can be solved in a non-judgmental environment. The provider in this situation discusses the pros and cons of that solution.

SHORT-TERM CRISIS INTERVENTION METHODS

Short crisis intervention therapies promoted by Health Management Organizations (HMOs) emphasize the heavy cost of mental health services to the insurance system. HMOs affect how mental health care is delivered because they require traditional long-term treatment models to change. Many **short crisis intervention therapies** incorporate:

- Short meeting times of 25 minutes or less, rather than traditional 60-minute sessions
- Restricted goal setting targeted at reaching short-term objectives, rather than consistent emotional insights
- Focused interviewing regarding the problem at hand
- Concentration on the here and now, rather than a detailed history
- Practical instruction about actions to be taken
- Diagnostic care that pinpoints the problem
- Flexible and varied choices of therapeutic tools to be utilized
- Prompt intervention strategies
- Inclusion of a ventilation practice
- Positive transfer of a therapeutic bond
- Selection of clients appropriate for short term crisis intervention therapies, rather than accepting all clients

EMERGENCY MENTAL HEALTH SERVICES

Psychiatric emergency services are designed to quickly assess and make arrangements for patients suffering acute crises; in many situations, patients may be a danger to themselves or others. Emergency services can provide **long-term benefits** to psychiatric clients by preventing potential complications associated with the emergency, which will keep the client safe in the short term and may prevent future complications that would have otherwise not have been addressed. Additionally, this prevention of future complications may keep the patient from ultimately entering long-term rehabilitation facilities, correctional centers, or inpatient hospitalization for significant periods of time, because of the sufficient treatment. Emergency services may also be a faster method of gaining treatment for the mentally ill client and, while not to be used only to gain faster access to care, they typically require immediate consultation with other disciplines and a fast turnaround when devising a plan of care and treatment. This benefits the client by providing rapid assessment and treatment.

COMPONENTS OF TRIAGE IN PSYCHIATRIC EMERGENCY SITUATIONS

Triage in emergency situations focuses on helping the client in acute mental health crisis to gain access to care and treatment and to prevent further complications or harm. The components of triage in these situations include:

- Assessing the client for immediate danger, whether to himself or to others
- Determining if the client has a previous psychiatric diagnosis and what current symptoms, thoughts, or behaviors he is now experiencing
- Assessing his overall level of cognitive functioning through orientation to self and place, assessing his reasoning abilities, and assessing his capacities for self-care
- Measuring the client's abilities to follow directions and adhere to a treatment regimen
- The presence of other diagnoses or disorders, both psychiatric or physical, in conjunction with the current set of behaviors
- Reviewing the client's access to community resources, financial abilities for immediate treatment, and time constraints that may permit or prohibit immediate treatment
- Determining the presence of family or others who can provide support for the client during the crisis and the treatment period following examination

CRITICAL INCIDENT STRESS MANAGEMENT

Critical incident stress management (CISM) is a procedure to help people cope with stressful events, such as disasters, to reduce the incidence of post-traumatic stress disorder.

- **Defusing sessions** usually occur very early, sometimes during or immediately after a stressful event. These sessions are used to educate actively involved personnel about what to expect over the next few days and to provide guidance about how to handle stress reactions.
- **Debriefing sessions** usually follow in 1–3 days and may be repeated periodically as needed. These sessions may include personnel who were either directly involved or indirectly involved. People are encouraged to express their feelings and emotions about the event. The six phases of debriefing include introduction, fact sharing, discussion of feelings, describing symptoms, teaching, and reentry. Critiquing the event or attempting to place blame is not part of the CISM process.
- **Follow-up** is done at the end of the process, often after only a week, but this time period varies.

RESTRICTIVE MEASURES

IMPORTANT DOCUMENTATION

The use of **restrictive measures** is a last resort in most patient settings. When utilized, these measures are to promote **patient safety**. The most common types of restrictive measures include physical restraints and seclusion. Every patient is entitled to being treated with the greatest personal respect and dignity. When a patient's activity is restricted very careful monitoring is required. Specific documentation on the patient's wellbeing should be performed per the facilities policy and usually includes a description of what occurred and physical monitoring of the patient while in restraints. If restrictive measures have to be utilized, staff members should have attempted and documented any and all other attempts to de-escalate the situation. These restraint techniques should only be utilized during the time that the patient is considered dangerous.

SECLUSION

Seclusion involves separating the patient from others by placing them in an environment where they are unable to leave. The patient is usually placed in this environment against their will in order to protect the patient or others from **harm**. This particular type of restraint is viewed negatively, is associated with negative patient outcomes, and is rarely utilized. A **seclusion room** would have padded walls and no furniture. There would be nothing in this environment that the patient could utilize to injure themselves or someone else. Once a patient has been placed in seclusion, they must be observed continuously.

RESTRAINTS

Restraints are considered to be the most restrictive of all measures and should only be utilized if all other alternative measures have failed. There are two main **types of restraints**:

- **Chemical restraints** involve the use of medications to manage a patient's behavior problem. This type of restraint often inhibits their physical movements and is used only when absolutely necessary to prevent injury. This medication is not utilized on a regular basis.
- **Physical restraints** involve the use of a person physically restraining a patient or the use of a mechanical device to restrict movement. These restraints not only restrict the physical movements in an area, but can also restrict their access to other parts of their own body or nearby equipment. Physical restraints are very difficult for patients to remove on their own.

MONITORING AND OBSERVATION

Monitoring, directly watching patients in psychiatric and mental health care, varies, depending on the type of facility and the patient's condition. It is primarily used to ensure safety. **Monitoring** can include the following:

- **Routine checks** are done at prescribed times (e.g., every 15 minutes), or continuous observation may be necessary.
- **Security personnel** (e.g., in emergency departments) may monitor patients to ensure patient and staff safety.
- **Audio/video monitoring** is sometimes used, but patients and families must be aware that this kind of monitoring is in place. It must not violate privacy, and monitors and audio speakers must not be accessible to nonauthorized individuals. Regulations regarding audio/video recordings may vary from state to state.

Observation is an ongoing process that involves observing the patient's behavior and nonverbal actions (e.g., posture, eye contact, expression, clothing, tone of voice) during communication. Observation helps to determine which issues are important to the patient, the types of questions to ask, the patient's perceptions, and the interpretation of messages.

Psychoeducation

BANDURA'S THEORY OF SOCIAL LEARNING

In the 1970s, Bandura proposed the theory of social learning, in which he posited that learning develops from observing, organizing, and rehearsing behavior that has been modeled. Bandura believed that people are more likely to adopt the behavior if they value the outcomes, if the outcomes have functional value, and if the person modeling the behavior is similar to the learner and is admired because of status. Behavior is the result of observation of behavioral, environmental, and cognitive interactions. There are **four conditions** required for modeling:

- **Attention**: The degree of attention paid to modeling can depend on many variables (physical, social, and environmental).
- **Retention**: People's ability to retain models depends on symbolic coding, creating mental images, organizing thoughts, and rehearsing (mentally or physically).
- **Reproduction**: The ability to reproduce a model depends on physical and mental capabilities.
- **Motivation**: Motivation may derive from past performances, rewards, or vicarious modeling.

TRANSTHEORETICAL MODEL OF CHANGE

The transtheoretical model of change puts forth concepts applicable to the process of educating patients and their family members. The **stages** of the transtheoretical model of change include the following:

1. The first stage is **precontemplation**. At this point, the patient is not aware of any need for a change in the health behavior.
2. In the next stage, **contemplation**, the patient begins to realize why the change may be necessary after recognizing that the health behavior in question is unhealthy and weighing the consequences of continuing this behavior.
3. During the stage of **preparation**, the patient imagines making the change at a future time and starts to formulate a plan to do so.
4. The **action** stage occurs when the patient makes specific modifications in health behavior and begins to note the resulting positive changes.
5. During the **maintenance** stage, the patient is able to implement the change over time by utilizing strategies to prevent a return to previously unhealthy behaviors.
6. **Termination** is the stage at which a patient has incorporated the changed behavior into daily functioning, and the patient will not resume the previous unhealthy behavior.

KURT LEWIN

FORCE FIELD ANALYSIS

Force field analysis was designed by Kurt Lewin, a social psychologist, to analyze both the driving forces and the restraining forces for change:

- **Driving forces** instigate and promote change, such as leaders, incentives, and competition.
- **Restraining forces** resist change, such as poor attitudes, hostility, inadequate equipment, or insufficient funds.

The educator can use this force field analysis diagram to discuss variables related to a proposed change in process:

- Write the proposed change in the center column.
- Brainstorm and list driving forces and opposed restraining forces. Score the forces. (When driving and restraining forces are in balance, this is a state of equilibrium or the status quo.)

- Discuss the value of the proposed change.
- Develop a plan to diminish or eliminate restraining forces.

LEWIN'S MODEL OF CHANGE THEORY

Lewin's model of change theory may be used to help some patients make decisions for change. Patients can be educated about the need for change and can be assisted with making alterations in behavior or thoughts in order to better facilitate change; however, only the patient can truly implement the change permanently. Lewin's concept of change theory involves a three-part process:

- **Unfreezing** is the part of the model in which the patient becomes open to change, sees a need for it, and removes the boundaries inhibiting change.
- The patient then makes the **actual change** according to expected outcomes and goals.
- Finally, **refreezing** is the process of maintaining the change so that it becomes a habit, and one that the patient is likely to uphold for a long period of time.

Lewin's theory also involves either driving forces or restraining forces. Driving forces are those outside measures that support the change, while restraining forces inhibit success in implementing the change.

STYLES OF LEARNING

Every person has a very individualized way of learning and processing information. Upon admission a patient should be evaluated for their preferred **method of learning**. This information allows the health care providers to provide patient education in a manner that is best suited to each patient. Successful patient education is a vital part of the patient's recovery and continued successful coping and functioning throughout their life. Learning styles can include auditory, visual, hands-on, or verbal.

- A person that learns best through **auditory models** can process information best through the act of listening. They prefer to receive information through discussions, lectures, and by talking through and listening to information given by others.
- **Visual learners** process information best through the use of pictures, videos, written information, or diagrams. Many times, these learners need to see the body language and gestures of the person teaching.
- A person that learns best through tactile or **hands-on education** prefers to receive the information through touch and doing. They may have difficulty sitting for long periods of time and prefer to be actively involved in the education process.
- A **verbal learner** often thinks in words instead of pictures. They are often great speakers and listeners. They have the ability to understand the meanings of words and are great at remembering information.

IDENTIFYING LEARNING NEEDS PRIOR TO PATIENT EDUCATION

Identifying the specific needs of the patient prior to education is imperative in order for that education to be effective. Identifying any barriers to different types of education and the material on which the patient needs to be educated can also impact compliance with treatment. Assessing the needs of an individual or group became part of government policy in 1998 in order to ensure the appropriate education requirements were being met to address the learning needs in healthcare. There are several different **types of needs** that have been identified:

- **Felt needs**: The needs that individuals or groups believe they have
- **Expressed needs**: The needs that individuals or groups say (express) that they have
- **Normative needs**: The needs of individuals or groups relative to a predetermined norm (e.g., the federal poverty level defines a norm for minimum income)
- **Comparative needs**: Those needs identified as a result of the comparison of different groups

Needs can be further broken down into individual versus organizational/group needs, clinical versus administrative needs, and subjective versus objective needs.

ELEMENTS OF A CONDUCIVE LEARNING ENVIRONMENT FOR PSYCHIATRIC PATIENTS

The **environment** in which a psychiatric patient is taught can greatly influence their ability to completely focus on the material presented. An environment that is very loud with a lot of activity can be very distracting and stress-inducing, decreasing the patient's ability to concentrate on what is being taught and increasing their anxiety and stress levels. Teaching areas that are cluttered can be over stimulating and can produce barriers to effectively teaching a patient. The ideal environment would be **free of external distractions** such as noise, clutter, and excess people. There should be **adequate lighting** that is soft, but sufficient for the patient to see clearly. If the patient has any **hearing deficits**, the person teaching should have a quiet environment in which they can speak slowly and clearly. If a **visual magnifying aid** is necessary to read any information, this should be provided.

BARRIERS TO LEARNING

Many times, psychiatric patients may have many different **barriers to learning** that can impact patient education. Upon admission to an inpatient facility, many patients may be in **crisis** and unable to take in the simplest instructions. The patient may need **further education** on the same information after they have moved through their crisis stage. Other barriers can include visual, hearing, physical, or cognitive impairments. Patients should be individually evaluated for their preferred method of receiving information. A patient's ability to read or educational level will also affect which type of information is best suited for that specific patient. Cultural and language barriers should also be evaluated and considered when providing patient and family education.

INFLUENCE OF SENSORY IMPAIRMENT ON LEARNING

The major recognized **senses** are sight, hearing, taste, smell, and touch. Of these, any **impairment** in sight and hearing can have a major impact on the ability of the patient to learn. Without adequate **sight**, they cannot read instructions on a medication bottle to ensure they are taking it correctly. They are also not able to read any additional instructions that are necessary for specific therapies for their illness. **Hearing** can greatly affect their ability to understand instructions. When discussing a patient's illness or specific instructions regarding medications, behavior, or cognitive therapies, it is imperative that the patient can clearly hear the healthcare professional speaking to them in order to follow these directions. Impairments in these sensations are common when dealing with elderly patients. Magnifying aids can assist with seeing medication labels or instructions clearly. Referring patients for an audiologist consultation may be necessary to have them fitted for hearing aids.

INFLUENCE OF COGNITIVE DEFECT ON LEARNING

A cognitive defect can affect a patient's ability to process, understand, and follow the directions related to medical treatments and therapies. A **comprehension deficit** can affect a patient's ability to understand written or spoken instructions. This can also impair their memory to remember how something should be done. Understanding multi-step instructions may be affected which could result in an adverse outcome for the patient. Understanding the disease process, severity, and outcomes can also be affected with a cognitive defect. When educating the patient on all aspects of their disease process, along with education on treatments, it is important to teach this on a **level at which they can understand**. They may need frequent cues to remember to take their medication or written instructions that they can refer to follow specific steps that need to be taken. The education process must be tailored to suit the patient's needs and any cognitive deficits they may have.

INFLUENCE OF ENVIRONMENTAL AND CULTURAL DIFFERENCES ON LEARNING

Environmental factors that influence learning can originate with life at home and psychosocial issues that may be influencing the learning process. **Cultural differences** can also begin at home, but can be influenced by society as a whole. When formulating a teaching plan for a patient, it is important to take into account the effect that these factors will have on the learning process. For example, certain cultures may have specific preconceived ideas regarding mental health or treatment of mental health issues. These cultural elements must be identified and addressed to ensure there is an understanding by the patient of their condition and treatment. Certain cultures and ethnicities may have a hierarchy within the family structure for decision-making when it comes to medical concerns. If the patient is not going to be the primary person making any decisions in their treatment, it is important to know who that person will be within the family structure to ensure the education is provided to the appropriate person.

Diagnosis and Treatment

Diagnostic Impression

DIAGNOSTIC REASONING PROCESS

There are a number of models for the diagnostic reasoning process but all essentially involve developing a hypothesis and testing it in order to arrive at a diagnosis. When diagnosing, a healthcare provider first looks for recognizable patterns of symptoms or presentation to suggest a diagnosis. If the patient does not fit a pattern, then a list of possible hypotheses is developed along with a **consideration of probabilities**:

- Data is gathered and clustered.
- Diagnostic studies and assessment help to narrow the choice of hypotheses. Decisions are made about the type and extent of testing, including the sensitivity and specificity of different tests and the value of invasive vs non-invasive testing.
- Hypotheses are evaluated, using the gathered data and probabilities, to prioritize differential diagnoses.
- Treatment, based on the probable diagnosis, is provided and evaluated for efficacy. If treatment fails to bring improvement, then further hypothesis testing is indicated.

IMPORTANCE OF DATA GATHERING TO DIAGNOSTIC REASONING

The gathering and recording of data are of utmost importance to the diagnostic evaluation process. The history and physical section of the **patient chart** contains a wealth of information (ideally), and should always be taken into consideration when developing a care plan for the patient. Because any number of clinicians can add information to the patient chart (and because all of these clinicians will be reading this information), it is important to record all information clearly and in an organized manner. This can be a daunting task when considering the various sources of information, including the patient interview, family member interviews, previous charts, and lab results. By keeping this information clear and concise, the nurse practitioner can minimize errors, and can be sure that the **differential diagnosis** is comprehensive.

PROBLEMS ENCOUNTERED DURING DATA EVALUATION

The **data** that are available within the patient's chart are an integral part of the patient's overall care plan. However, **errors** may be present in the records, and these errors may negatively influence clinical decision making; thus, it is important to look at the information as a whole. Does it make sense? Confirm that the patient's **verbal history** agrees with what is in his or her records. Also, remember that not every **test result** in the patient's chart is necessarily accurate. If a test result doesn't make sense in the clinical picture as a whole, consider why this might be. It could simply be an error (e.g., the wrong number was recorded, the blood was drawn incorrectly), or the patient may have a result that would be considered "abnormal," though for this particular patient it is not. For example, a marathon runner may have a resting heart rate of 40 bpm; while this is a bradycardic rate, it is not pathological, but rather a result of physical conditioning.

SENSITIVITY AND SPECIFICITY IN RELATION TO DIAGNOSTIC TESTING

Some degree of error is inherent in almost all diagnostic testing. When ordering a diagnostic test for a patient, how confident should the practitioner be that the result will be accurate? The terms **sensitivity and specificity** are used to illustrate the accuracy of diagnostic tests.

- The **sensitivity** of a diagnostic test refers to its ability to correctly identify patients who *do have the disease*. If a test is administered to 1000 patients with diabetes, and all 1000 patients test positive, the test is considered to have a sensitivity of 100%. If only 850 test positive, however, that means that the test has a false-negative rate of 15%, and a sensitivity of 85%.

- The **specificity** of a diagnostic test refers to its ability to identify patients who *do not have the disease*. If 1000 nondiabetic patients are tested for diabetes, and 200 of them test positive, the test has a false-positive rate of 20% and a specificity of 80%.

PREDICTIVE VALUES IN RELATION TO DISEASE PROBABILITY

Sensitivity and specificity are useful in evaluating the efficacy of a diagnostic test, but the predictive value of a test is more immediately relevant to individual patients. The **positive predictive value (PPV)** of a test is the likelihood that a patient who has *tested positive* truly has the condition that is being tested for. Similarly, the **negative predictive value (NPV)** of a test is the likelihood that a patient who has *tested negative* truly does not have the condition being tested for.

For a given controlled trial, PPV is calculated by dividing the number of true positive results by the number of total positive results (true and false positives). NPV is calculated by dividing the number of true negative results by the number of total negative results. Calculating the PPV and NPV is straightforward, but in order for these values to be applied to an individual patient, the assumption has to be made that the patient's pre-test likelihood of having the tested condition matches that of the trial's population.

FORMULATING A PSYCHIATRIC DIAGNOSIS

The purpose of formulating a psychiatric diagnosis is to develop a plan of care to meet the needs of the patient. Steps include:

1. **History**: Include the presenting problem and any initiating factors. Explain how the symptoms are affecting the patient's life. Note any prior history of psychological/psychiatric disorders as well as any history of disorders that may be associated with mental disorders, such as lupus erythematosus.
2. **Mental status exam**: Note important or significant findings.
3. **Physical exam**: Note any abnormalities. Order diagnostic tests as indicated to rule out non-psychiatric conditions.
4. **Differential diagnosis**: List only those that are plausible and must be ruled out.
5. **Single diagnosis**: Base diagnosis on best evidence. In some cases, two diagnoses may be determined.
6. **Etiology**: Note significant factors related to the diagnosis.
7. **Management plan**: Outline the recommended treatment options to meet somatic needs (medications), psychological needs (therapy), and social needs (family intervention, support, community programs).

Diagnostic and Laboratory Tests

PET SCAN

Positron-emission tomography (PET) involves injecting the individual with a radioactive glucose tracer that is taken up by active brain cells. By analyzing images of brains that have been injected with radioactive glucose, doctors can gauge regional cerebral blood flow, glucose metabolism, and oxygen consumption, all of which correlate with the brain's level of activity. PET scans are often used by clinicians to assess the cerebral damage that has been done by cerebrovascular disease, major neurocognitive disorder (formerly dementia), schizophrenia, Alzheimer's disease, and other disorders. Researchers often use PET scans to determine which areas of the brain are active during certain functions.

CT SCAN

The procedure known as **neuroimaging** has vastly improved scientists' ability to assess the structure and function of living brains. The two most common techniques of neuroimaging are computed axial tomography (CT or CAT) and magnetic resonance imaging (MRI). In **CT scans**, an x-ray is taken of various horizontal cross-sections of the brain. CT scans are good for diagnosing pathological conditions like tumors, blood clots, and multiple sclerosis.

HEAD CT FOR AN INDIVIDUAL WITH ALTERED MENTAL STATUS

The **CT scan** is a common imaging technique used to diagnose individuals who present with altered mental status. The CT scan can identify **traumatic brain injury** and **mass lesions**, such as brain tumors or hematomas, as well as cerebral edema, so it may be invaluable for neurological disorders, but it is primarily used to **rule out differential diagnoses** rather than to diagnose mental health disorders. CT scans may also be used in addition to other tests to help confirm a possible diagnosis. For example, individuals with schizophrenia tend to have enlarged ventricles with increased CSF and a concomitant reduction in brain volume with sulci that are more widened than in a non-schizophrenic brain. Despite these findings, the CT alone cannot be used for diagnosis, and no specific pattern of abnormality has been noted with depression or bipolar disorder, although there is evidence that the frontal cortex shrinks in size with uncontrolled bipolar disease and depression and increases with treatment, so long-term monitoring may show differences.

MRI

An MRI uses magnetic fields and radio waves to produce cross-sectional images. MRIs are able to produce more detailed images than CT scans, and MRIs can produce images from any angle, not just horizontally. MRIs are able to construct three-dimensional representations of brains.

EEG TESTING IN AN INDIVIDUAL WITH ALTERED LEVEL OF CONSCIOUSNESS

The **electroencephalogram (EEG)** is sometimes used to test individuals with altered level of consciousness in order to evaluate the individuals' **electrical impulses** (brain waves). EEG is indicated for suspected seizure activity, encephalopathies, infarcts, and altered consciousness. The purpose is to identify abnormal electrical activity, which may be noted as slowing, which occurs where there has been injury or an infarct. Waves include delta (1-4 Hz), alpha (8-13 Hz), theta (4-7 Hz), beta (12-40 Hz), sleep spindles (12-14 Hz), and spikes and waves (variable frequency). Spikes and waves indicate that tissue is irritated. Findings indicate:

- **Metabolic encephalopathy:** Intermittent slowing with triphasic waves
- **Cerebral anoxic damage:** Generalized slowing in delta and theta range
- **Coma state:** Prognosis poor if EEG shows unchanging alpha waves with stimulation
- **CNS depressant overdose:** Transient periods of absence of electrical activity
- **Epilepsy:** Unusual electrical activity within the brain, partial seizures evident from only some of the electrodes while generalized seizures evident from all electrodes
- **ADHD:** A 20-minute EEG procedure FDA-approved to diagnose children with ADHD

TESTING FOR DELIRIUM

Appropriate testing for an individual presenting with delirium, transient confusion and alterations in consciousness depends on the age and circumstances. **Delirium** is most common in older adults in response to illness or surgery but can occur at any age. **Hyperactive delirium** may be associated with alcohol withdrawal or drug toxicity. **Hypoactive delirium** may result from disease processes, such as hepatic encephalopathy. Some have mixed symptoms, becoming more agitated during the evening and night. Testing includes:

- **Confusion Assessment Method (CAM) or CAM-ICU** helps to differentiate confusion from other causes of altered consciousness.
- The **CAM-S** form of the CAM test is used to determine the severity of delirium.
- A **Delirium Symptom Interview** also helps to identify delirium.
- **Laboratory tests**: If the cause of the individual's confusion is not evident, numerous tests may be done to rule out other causes, including CBC, blood glucose, renal and liver function tests, drug and alcohol screening, sed-rate, thyroid function tests, HIV, and thiamine and vitamin B_{12} levels.

LABORATORY TESTS FOR PSYCHIATRIC ILLNESSES

At the current time, diagnosis of psychiatric illnesses is based almost completely on symptoms and history, and no laboratory tests have been FDA approved for diagnosis; however, **biochemical markers** have been identified for some psychiatric disorders, including schizophrenia, bipolar disorder, and depression. Some companies have collected data and applied for FDA approval for these tests and are now marketing tests. This testing is not in common use because its use is not yet reimbursed by Medicare/Medicaid or insurance companies. Some researchers believe that genetic testing and imaging (PET, MRI) may also have larger roles in diagnosis in the future. Currently, **laboratory tests** are used for primarily two reasons:

- Rule out differential diagnoses and identify concomitant disorders. Many different tests may be used, but in many cases the results of tests don't alter the original diagnosis, so testing is done selectively, based on individual's age, history, and physical exam.
- Monitor serum levels of drugs during therapy, such as lithium levels.

LABORATORY TESTS FOR INDIVIDUALS PRESENTING WITH NEW ONSET PSYCHIATRIC ISSUE

When individuals present with a new onset psychiatric issue, a series of **laboratory tests** may be conducted to determine potential causes, rule out differential diagnoses, and identify concomitant disorders:

- **Blood alcohol level and urine drug screening** to determine if the individual is experiencing overdosing, withdrawal symptoms, or toxic reaction
- **Blood glucose level** to determine if the individual has hypoglycemia or hyperglycemia that may be affecting mental status
- **Urinalysis and urine culture** to determine if an infection is present (may result in confusion in older adults)
- **Pregnancy testing** to determine if females are pregnant before initiating treatment.
- **Liver and kidney function tests** to evaluate for hepatic and renal encephalopathy
- **CBC** to assess for anemia, infection, or other abnormalities
- **HIV antibodies** to rule out HIV/AIDS
- **Lyme antibodies** to rule out neuropsychological symptoms related to Lyme disease
- **Lumbar puncture** to examine cerebrospinal fluid for suspected infection

Psychiatric Disorders and Diagnosis

DSM-5-TR CLASSIFICATIONS

The major DSM-5-TR classifications are as follows:

- Neurodevelopmental disorders
- Schizophrenia spectrum and other psychotic disorders
- Bipolar and related disorders
- Depressive disorders
- Anxiety disorders
- Obsessive-compulsive and related disorders
- Trauma- and stressor-related disorders
- Dissociative disorders
- Somatic symptom and related disorders
- Feeding and eating disorders
- Elimination disorders
- Sleep-wake disorders
- Sexual dysfunctions
- Gender dysphoria
- Disruptive, impulse-control, and conduct disorders
- Substance-related and addictive disorders
- Neurocognitive disorders
- Personality disorders
- Paraphilic disorders
- Other mental disorders and additional codes
- Medication-induced movement disorders and other adverse effects of medications
- Other conditions that may be a focus of clinical attention

NEURODEVELOPMENTAL DISORDERS

Neurodevelopmental disorders are a group of conditions affecting the brain that occur during childhood development. These conditions cause various degrees of functional impairments in the school, work, home, and community settings. Neurodevelopmental disorders include:

- Intellectual developmental disorders
- Communication disorders
- Autism spectrum disorder
- Attention deficit hyperactivity disorder (ADHD)
- Specific learning disorders
- Motor disorders
- Other neurodevelopmental disorders

The DSM-5-TR emphasizes that the diagnosis of neurodevelopmental disorder can be determined after evaluating a child's cognitive, social, motor, behavioral, adaptive, and language skills. In many cases, a full neuropsychological assessment using standardized instruments is required. Symptoms of neurodevelopmental disorders cannot be attributed to medical or neurological conditions. Child and adolescent cross-cutting assessment measures found in Section III of the DSM-5-TR can also aid in clinical decision making. Caretakers play an integral role in determining how a child presents in multiple contexts and diagnostic domains, and their involvement is an invaluable component of a child's treatment. Neurodevelopmental disorder diagnosis occurs in the presence of functional impairment and diagnostic symptomatology.

INTELLECTUAL DEVELOPMENTAL DISORDERS (INTELLECTUAL DISABILITY)

DIAGNOSIS

Intellectual developmental disorder is characterized by deficits in mental abilities and adaptive functioning. Children with the disorder may exhibit impairments in judgment, learning, reasoning, problem solving, planning, and abstract thinking. The diagnosis is often supported by psychometrically sound intelligence testing yielding IQ scores that are two standard deviations below the mean (e.g., 65–75). However, IQ scores should not be a confirmatory, stand-alone criterion for the diagnosis of intellectual developmental disorder.

Severity levels are measured along conceptual (e.g., academic), social (e.g., empathy, social judgment), and practical (e.g., personal care, task organization) domains. Hereditary and other medical conditions, including epilepsy and cerebral palsy, may co-occur with intellectual developmental disorder and are listed separately.

There are two additional diagnoses in the category of intellectual developmental disorder. **Global developmental delay** is a diagnosis used in children **younger than age 5** who show symptoms of intellectual developmental disorder (e.g., delays in developmental milestones) but are too young for a comprehensive clinical evaluation. **Unspecified developmental disorder** is reserved for individuals **older than age 5** who cannot be assessed because of a severe sensory, physical, or mental impairment. Global developmental delay and unspecified developmental disorder require continued reassessment.

DIFFERENTIAL DIAGNOSES

The diagnosis of intellectual disability (intellectual developmental disorder) can be differentiated from other diagnoses in that there must be deficits in intellectual and adaptive functioning that begin in childhood. Differential diagnoses include neurocognitive disorder, communication disorders, specific learning disorders, and autism spectrum disorder (ASD).

COMMUNICATION DISORDERS

DIAGNOSIS

Communication disorders affect a person's ability to engage in effective discourse due to problems with sending, receiving, expressing, and understanding concepts and information. A number of disorders are included under the heading of communication disorders, including:

- Language disorders
- Speech sound disorders
- Childhood-onset fluency disorders (stuttering)
- Social communication disorders

Differential diagnoses for communication disorder include hearing or other sensory impairment, normal language variations, ADHD, autism, intellectual disability (intellectual developmental disorder), neurological disorders, traumatic brain injury (TBI), structural deficits, selective mutism, medication side effects, Tourette disorder, and social anxiety disorder.

LANGUAGE DISORDER

Language disorder involves problems with receiving and expressing language, including difficulties with syntax, grammar, sentence structure, and vocabulary. To receive a diagnosis, there must be deficits in an individual's social, academic, or occupational functioning. Symptoms of language disorder include developmental delays in a child's first words or phrases, reduced vocabulary, and issues with comprehension. A child's conversations are also impacted by difficulty recognizing and understanding new words or sound sequences.

SPEECH SOUND DISORDER

Speech sound disorder is characterized by difficulties with pronunciation and articulation. A speech-language pathologist can determine if a child has difficulty making certain sounds (e.g., "sh") or if he or she is misarticulating sibilants (i.e., lisping). It is not uncommon for young children to have difficulties with speech and sounds because this skill is acquired over time. If significant difficulties are present early on, or if difficulties persist past the age of 8, intervention and treatment may be warranted.

CHILDHOOD-ONSET FLUENCY DISORDER

Childhood-onset fluency disorder, also known as stuttering, occurs when interruptions to a person's speech manifest in repeated sounds, syllables, and broken words. Children with childhood-onset fluency disorder are identified between the ages of 2 and 7, and the disorder is more common in males than females. There are higher instances of stuttering in children than adults, with a male-to-female ratio of 4:1 in childhood and 2:1 in adulthood. Stressful situations tend to worsen stuttering, which can be complicated by anticipatory fear or performance anxiety.

Many individuals find success in management through controlled breathing exercises, positive encouragement, and stress management. Families can help by avoiding criticism or corrections. For example, saying things such as "slow down" or "take your time" can place undue pressure on the child. Instead, caregivers can help by providing a calm home environment, allowing children to complete their thoughts and sentences, and by speaking to their child purposefully and slowly. Children who receive early intervention are more likely to prevent the disorder from advancing in later developmental stages.

SOCIAL COMMUNICATION DISORDER

Social communication disorder involves problems with the social use of language and communication (i.e., pragmatics). This applies to verbal and nonverbal communication. Children with social communication disorder exhibit deficits in social contexts, including matching communication to persons or situations—for example, speaking the same way on the playground as in the classroom. There are also problems understanding the meaning behind words, including comprehension of metaphors or sarcasm. Social rules and conversations are also difficult, which can involve problems with taking turns, listening without interruption, shaking hands to greet others, and interpreting conversational tones. Social communication **disorder** shares traits with autism spectrum disorder (ASD). The difference is that ASD occurs in the presence of restricted or repetitive behavior patterns.

AUTISM SPECTRUM DISORDER (ASD)

DIAGNOSIS

There are two categories of symptoms necessary for a diagnosis of autism spectrum disorder (ASD). The first category is **deficits in social interaction and social communication**, which include:

- Absence of developmentally appropriate peer relationships
- Lack of social or emotional reciprocity
- Marked impairment in nonverbal behavior
- Delay or lack of development in spoken language
- Marked impairment in the ability to initiate or sustain conversation
- Stereotyped or repetitive use of language or idiosyncratic language
- Lack of developmentally appropriate play

The other category of symptoms necessary for diagnosis of ASD is **restricted, repetitive patterns of behavior, interests, and activities**. These include:

- Preoccupation with one or more stereotyped and restricted patterns of interest
- Inflexible adherence to nonfunctional routines or rituals
- Stereotyped and repetitive motor mannerisms
- Persistent preoccupation with the parts of objects

Both categories of symptoms will be present in the ASD diagnosis and occur across multiple contexts. The **severity levels** are as follows: **level 1** (requiring support), **level 2** (requiring substantial support), and **level 3** (requiring very substantial support). Individuals with ASD associated with other known conditions or language/intellectual impairment should have the diagnosis written as "autism spectrum disorder associated with (name of condition/impairment)." It should also be specified if catatonia is present.

Some very noticeable, specific behavior patterns that characterize ASD include:

- Lack of eye contact and disinterest in the presence of others
- Infants who rarely reach out to a caregiver
- Hand-flapping
- Rocking
- Spinning
- Echolalia (the imitating and repeating the words of others)
- Obsessive interest in a very narrow subject, such as astronomy or basketball scores
- Heavy emphasis on routine and consistency and violent reactions to changes in the usual environment

ETIOLOGY

There are a few structural abnormalities in the brain that have been linked to ASD. These include **cerebellar abnormalities** and **enlarged ventricles**. Research has also suggested that there is a link between autism and abnormal levels of **norepinephrine**, **serotonin**, and **dopamine**. Support for a genetic etiology of ASD has been increased by studies indicating that siblings of children with autism are much more likely to have autism themselves.

PROGNOSIS AND TREATMENT

Children with ASD show signs in early childhood, with the average age of onset between 12 and 24 months. More severe symptomatology is recognized in the child's first year of life, with more subtle signs appearing after 24 months. The prognosis of individuals with ASD largely depends on their **IQ, language development, and level of severity**. Individuals classified as **level 1** display impaired social interactions and a limited repertoire of behaviors, interests, and activities, but they do not have significant delays in language, self-help skills, cognitive development, or environmental curiosity. Children in this category show improvement with less intensive work and early intervention focusing on emotional growth and interpersonal communication.

Children at **levels 2 and 3** respond well to applied behavior analysis therapy. Treatment focuses on developing appropriate social skills and reducing restricted, repetitive, and often ritualized behaviors. Children with more severe ASD may exhibit hyper- or hyporeactivity to sensory input, with sensitivity to touch, sounds, sights, tastes, and textures. Occupational therapists and physiotherapists can assist with sensory integration issues. Therapists also help adults with ASD to learn practical skills required for independent living.

DIFFERENTIAL DIAGNOSIS

Symptoms of autism disorder are shared with other neurodevelopmental disorders, with language and social communication (pragmatic) disorders being the most common. Differential diagnoses also include attention deficit hyperactivity disorder (ADHD), intellectual developmental disorder (without ASD), selective mutism, stereotypic movement disorder, and Rett syndrome. Disorders commonly diagnosed in adulthood serving as differential diagnoses include symptoms of anxiety disorder, obsessive-compulsive disorder (OCD), schizophrenia, and some personality disorders (i.e., narcissistic, schizotypal, or schizoid). ASD commonly co-occurs with depression, anxiety, and ADHD. Comorbid conditions also include epilepsy and constipation.

Review Video: **Autism**
Visit mometrix.com/academy and enter code: 395410

ATTENTION DEFICIT HYPERACTIVITY DISORDER (ADHD)

DIAGNOSIS

Attention deficit hyperactivity disorder (ADHD) can be diagnosed if a child displays at least six symptoms of inattention or hyperactivity-impulsivity in more than one setting (e.g., home, school). Their onset must be before the age of 12, and the symptoms must have persisted for at least 6 months.

Inattentiveness Symptoms (must have six for diagnosis in children)	Impulsivity/Hyperactivity Symptoms (must have six for diagnosis in children)
• Forgetful in everyday activities • Easily distracted (often) • Makes careless mistakes and does not give attention to detail • Difficulty focusing attention • Does not appear to listen, even when directly spoken to • Starts tasks but does not follow through • Frequently loses essential items • Finds organizing difficult • Avoids activities that require prolonged mental exertion	• Frequently gets out of chair • Runs or climbs at inappropriate times • Frequently talks more than peers • Often moves hands and feet or shifts position in seat • Frequently interrupts others • Frequently has difficulty waiting on turn • Frequently unable to enjoy leisure activities silently • Frequently "on the go" and seen by others as restless • Often finishes other's sentences before they can

SUBTYPES

There are three subtypes of ADHD:

- **Predominantly inattentive type** is diagnosed when a child has six or more symptoms of inattention and fewer than six symptoms of hyperactivity-impulsivity.
- **Predominantly hyperactive-impulsive type** is diagnosed when there are six or more symptoms of hyperactivity-impulsivity and fewer than six symptoms of inattention.
- **Combined type** is diagnosed when there are six or more symptoms of both hyperactivity-impulsivity and inattention.

PREVALENCE

Worldwide, ADHD occurs in just more than 7% of children and 2.5% of adults. Males are more likely to receive the diagnosis than females, with a **2:1 male-to-female ratio** among children. Females are more likely to present as predominantly inattentive, and many females are underidentified and underdiagnosed. The rates of ADHD among adults appear to be about equal for males and females.

PROGNOSIS AND ETIOLOGY

The behavior of children with ADHD is likely to remain consistent until **early adolescence**, when some may experience diminished overactivity but continue to exhibit attention and concentration problems. Adolescents with ADHD are much more likely to participate in antisocial behaviors and engage in substance use. More than half of all children who are diagnosed with ADHD will carry the diagnosis through to adulthood. Adults with ADHD are more susceptible to divorce, work-related trouble, accidents, depression, substance abuse, and antisocial behavior. Children with ADHD who are co-diagnosed with conduct disorder are especially likely to have these problems later in life.

There is significant evidence suggesting that ADHD is a **genetic disorder**. ADHD occurs at a slightly higher rate among biological relatives than among the general population, and there are higher rates among identical twins, rather than fraternal twins. However, like many neurodevelopmental disorders, ADHD can be attributed to a combination of genetics, environment, and epigenetics.

ADHD is associated with structural abnormalities in the brain, such as subnormal activity in the frontal cortex and basal ganglia and a relatively small caudate nucleus, globus pallidus, and prefrontal cortex. Prenatal care also contributes to ADHD. Children exposed to alcohol and nicotine in utero have higher instances of ADHD, as well as those with viral infections and nutritional deficiencies.

TREATMENT

Treatment for ADHD is a combination of behavioral therapy and medication. Children with ADHD tend to exhibit trouble in school because executive functioning interferes with planning and organization and their impulsivity and inattention interfere with focusing and retaining information. This is compounded by low frustration tolerance, lability, and difficulty with peers. Research has consistently shown that **pharmacotherapy** works best when it is combined with **psychosocial intervention**. Many teachers use basic elements of **classroom management (e.g., behavioral modification)** to assist children with ADHD. This involves providing clear guidelines and contingencies for behavior so that students do not have to speculate on what will happen in class or what they should be doing. Treatment is most effective with **parental involvement.**

Stimulants and nonstimulant medications are the pharmacologic therapies approved for ADHD. Somewhat counterintuitively, central nervous system stimulants such as **methylphenidate (Ritalin)** and **amphetamine (Dexedrine)** control the symptoms of ADHD. Side effects include headaches, gastrointestinal upset, anorexia, sleep difficulty, anxiety, depression, blood sugar increases, blood pressure increases, tics, and seizures.

Nonstimulant medication options include antidepressants (e.g., atomoxetine, bupropion) and alpha agonists (e.g., clonidine, guanfacine). The trigeminal nerve stimulation system is a US Food and Drug Administration (FDA)-approved nonpharmacological treatment effective in children with mild to moderate symptoms and those whose primary symptoms involve executive functioning impairments.

DIFFERENTIAL DIAGNOSIS

Practitioners must distinguish between ADHD and several other disorders, including other externalized and behavioral disorders, such as oppositional defiant disorder, intermittent explosive disorder, and disruptive mood regulation disorder. The DSM-5-TR lists mood disorders as differential diagnoses, including depressive disorders, anxiety disorders, and bipolar disorder. Reactive attachment disorder, post-traumatic stress disorder (PTSD), ASD, other neurological disorders, specific learning disorders, and intellectual developmental disorders are also included, along with psychotic disorders, substance use disorders, medication-induced symptoms of ADHD, and personality disorders.

SPECIFIC LEARNING DISORDER

DIAGNOSIS

A specific learning disorder is diagnosed as learning and academic difficulty, as evidenced by at least one of the following for at least 6 months (after interventions have been tried):

- Incorrect spelling
- Problems with math reasoning
- Problems with math calculation and number sense
- Difficulty reading
- Problems understanding what is read
- Difficulty using grammar and syntax

Children with learning disorders may score substantially lower than their peers on a standardized achievement test; however, this alone does not substantiate a clinical diagnosis because information from a comprehensive clinical assessment, rating scales, and educational history must also be considered. According to the DSM-5-TR, the learning difficulties are "persistent, not transitory." Persistent difficulties are those than lack improvement for at least 6 months in the presence of targeted assistance. Roughly 5–15% of children receive the diagnosis of specific learning disorder in either reading, math, or writing.

PROGNOSIS AND ETIOLOGY

Specific learning disorders include specific learning disorder with **impairment in reading**, specific learning disorder with **impairment in mathematics**, and specific learning disorder with **impairment in written expression**. Males are more likely to develop specific learning disorders with impairment in reading than females. Although learning disorders are typically diagnosed during childhood or adolescence, they do not subside without treatment; indeed, they may become more severe with time. Children who have a learning disorder with impairment in reading are far more likely than others to display antisocial behavior as an adult. At present, many researchers believe that reading disorders derive from problems with **phonological processing**.

Proposed **causes of learning disorders** include:

- Incomplete dominance and other hemispheric abnormalities
- Cerebellar-vestibular dysfunction
- Exposure to toxins such as lead

DIFFERENTIAL DIAGNOSIS

Specific learning disorder varies from intellectual developmental disorder, normal variations in academic attainment, ADHD, psychotic disorders, neurocognitive disorders, and learning difficulties due to neurological or sensory disorders (e.g., audiovisual impairments, pediatric stroke). Children with academic deficiencies cannot be diagnosed with specific learning disorder due to poor instruction, the absence of educational opportunities, or limited English proficiency. It is important to note that specific learning disorder is often diagnosed along with other (i.e., comorbid) neurodevelopmental disorders.

TREATMENT

Treatment options can be considered once the child has completed psychological testing and evaluation. Children can obtain targeted assistance after it is determined that they qualify. Response-to-intervention (RTI) supports are also helpful for developing a specific plan to assist the child in school. Children who do not progress with RTI may be issued an individualized education plan or a 504 accommodation plan, depending on the outcome of a comprehensive evaluation and assessment.

MOTOR DISORDERS
DIAGNOSIS

Motor disorders are malfunctions of the nervous system that cause involuntary, and often excessive, movements or purposeless behavior. Motor disorders include the following:

- **Developmental coordination disorder** is diagnosed when an individual's movements are impaired while engaging in specific motor tasks. Children with developmental coordination disorder exhibit clumsy behaviors, such as running into things or dropping objects. Symptoms also include the slow or inaccurate performance of motor skills, such as difficulty using scissors, throwing a ball, grasping forks and knives, or walking up and down stairs.
- **Stereotypic movement disorder** is characterized by repetitive and purposeless motions. Motor behaviors include rocking, head banging, hand shaking, waving, or hitting oneself. The diagnoses must include a specifier indicating whether or not the behavior would cause self-harm without prevention or intervention.

- **Tic disorders** include **Tourette disorder, motor or vocal tic disorder,** and **provisional tic disorder.** The DSM-5-TR defines a tic as a "sudden, rapid, recurrent, nonrhythmic motor movement or vocalization." **Tourette disorder** is characterized by multiple motor and vocal tics, which may abate from time to time but remain consistent for 1 year. Motor or vocal tic disorder requires at least one motor or vocal tic, but not a combination of vocal or motor tics. Provisional tic disorder is most similar to Tourette disorder, with symptoms that include multiple motor or vocal tics; however, it differs in that the tics have been present for less than 1 year. All tic disorders cannot be attributed to the effects of cocaine, Huntington disease, or post viral encephalitis.

TREATMENT

Treatment for motor disorders varies. Physiotherapy, occupational therapy, and behavior therapy are used to treat developmental coordination disorder and stereotypic movement disorder. Habit reversal therapy is an evidence-based practice for tic disorder; it works by pairing situations and sensations associated with the tic or habit followed with a competing response. Symptoms of Tourette disorder can also be treated with antipsychotics, such as **haloperidol (Haldol)** and **pimozide (Orap).** In some cases, psychostimulant drugs amplify the tics displayed by the individual. In these cases, a doctor may treat the hyperactivity and inattention of Tourette with **clonidine** (which is usually used to treat hypertension) or **desipramine** (which is typically used as an antidepressant).

DIFFERENTIAL DIAGNOSIS

Differential diagnoses for developmental coordination disorder includes motor impairments due to another medical condition, specific neurological disorders (e.g., cerebral palsy), intellectual disability (intellectual developmental disorder), ADHD, ASD, and joint hypermobility syndrome.

Stereotypic movement disorder should be differentiated from normal development, ASD, tic disorders, OCD, and other neurological and medical conditions.

Differential diagnoses for tic disorder includes abnormal movements that may accompany other medical conditions and stereotypic movement disorder, substance-induced and paroxysmal dyskinesias, myoclonus, and OCD.

SCHIZOPHRENIA SPECTRUM AND OTHER PSYCHOTIC DISORDERS

Schizophrenia spectrum and other psychotic disorders include the following:

- Delusional disorder
- Brief psychotic disorder
- Schizophreniform disorder
- Schizophrenia
- Schizoaffective disorder
- Substance-/Medication-induced psychotic disorder
- Psychotic disorder due to another medical condition
- Catatonia

Schizophrenia spectrum and other psychotic disorders are a group of conditions characterized by deficits in one or more of the following five domains:

- **Delusions** are firmly held beliefs that persist despite contradictory evidence. The most common delusion is **persecutory,** in which the person believes that someone or something is out to get then. Delusions can be **referential,** in which the individual believes that someone in the public domain is targeting them. Delusions can also be **bizarre**, involving the belief that something impossible has happened, or **grandiose**, in which the person believes they have superior qualities or capabilities. **Erotomanic** delusions refer to the erroneous belief that another person is in love with them, **somatic** delusions are false beliefs that are health related, and **nihilistic** delusions are known as delusions of nonexistence.
- **Hallucinations** involve individuals seeing or hearing things that do not exist. Although hallucinations can be experienced through all of the senses, auditory hallucinations (i.e., hearing voices) is most common.
- **Disorganized thinking (speech)** manifests as incoherence (i.e., word salad), free or loose associations that make little sense, and random responses to direct questions (i.e., tangential thinking).
- **Grossly disorganized or abnormal motor behavior (including catatonia)** manifests as a shabby or unkempt appearance, inappropriate sexual behavior, unpredictable agitation, and decreased motor activity (i.e., catatonia).
- **Negative symptoms of schizophrenia** include a restricted range of emotions; reduced use of body language; lack of facial expression; lack of coherent thoughts; and avolition, which is the inability to set goals or work in a rational, programmatic manner.

DELUSIONAL DISORDER

Delusional disorder is typified by the presence of a persistent delusion, which may be of the persecutory type, jealous type, erotomanic type (that someone is in love with a delusional person), somatic type (that one has a physical defect or disease), grandiose type, or mixed. Criteria for delusional disorder include:

Criterion A	The individual experiences at least one delusion for at least 1 month or longer.
Criterion B	The individual does not meet criteria for schizophrenia.
Criterion C	Functioning is not significantly impaired, and behavior except that dealing specifically with the delusion is not bizarre.
Criterion D	Any manic or depressive episodes are brief.
Criterion E	The symptoms cannot be attributed to another medical condition or a substance.

It should be specified if the delusions are bizarre. The severity is rated by the quantitative assessment measure Clinician-Rated Dimensions of Psychosis Symptom Severity.

Differential diagnoses for delusional disorder include but are not limited to OCD, neurocognitive disorders, mood disorders, schizophrenia, and schizophreniform disorder.

BRIEF PSYCHOTIC DISORDER

Brief psychotic disorder is characterized as a delusion that has sudden onset and lasts less than 1 month. Brief psychotic disorder is a classification of the schizophrenia spectrum and other psychotic disorders. Criteria for brief psychotic disorder include:

Criterion A	At least one of the following symptoms exist: delusions, hallucinations, disorganized speech, or catatonic behavior.
Criterion B	The symptoms last more than 1 day but less than 1 month. The individual does eventually return to baseline functioning.
Criterion C	The disorder cannot be attributed to another psychotic or depressive disorder.

Differential diagnoses include mood disorders, personality disorders, medical disorders, malingering and factitious disorders, and other psychotic disorders.

SCHIZOPHRENIFORM DISORDER

The criteria for schizophreniform disorder include:

Criterion A	Diagnosis requires at least two of the following symptoms, one being a core positive symptom: • Hallucinations (known as a core positive symptom) • Delusions (known as a core positive symptom) • Disorganized speech (known as a core positive symptom) • Severely disorganized or catatonic behavior • Negative symptoms (such as avolition or diminished expression)
Criterion B	An illness of at least 1 month but less than 6 months in duration.
Criterion C	Depressive disorder, bipolar disorder, and schizoaffective disorder have been ruled out.
Criterion D	The symptoms cannot be attributed to another medical condition or a substance.

Differential diagnoses for schizophreniform disorder include other mental disorders, medical disorders, and brief psychotic disorder.

SCHIZOPHRENIA

DIAGNOSIS

Schizophrenia is a psychotic disorder. Psychotic disorders feature one or more of the following: delusions, hallucinations, disorganized speech or thought, or disorganized or catatonic behavior. Schizophrenia **diagnostic criteria** are as follows:

Criterion A	Diagnosis requires at least two of the following symptoms, one being a core positive symptom: <ul><li>Hallucinations (core positive symptom)</li><li>Delusions (core positive symptom)</li><li>Disorganized speech (core positive symptom)</li><li>Severely disorganized or catatonic behavior</li><li>Negative symptoms (such as avolition or diminished expression)</li></ul>
Criterion B	The individual's level of functioning is significantly below the level prior to onset.
Criterion C	If the individual has not had successful treatment, there are continual signs of schizophrenia for more than 6 months.
Criterion D	Depressive disorder, bipolar disorder, and schizoaffective disorder have been ruled out.
Criterion E	The symptoms cannot be attributed to another medical condition or a substance.
Criterion F	If the individual has had a communication disorder or ASD since childhood, a diagnosis of schizophrenia is only made if the individual has hallucinations or delusions.

Differential diagnoses for schizophrenia include bipolar and depressive disorders with psychotic features, schizoaffective disorder, and the effects of prolonged and large-scale use of amphetamines or cocaine.

ETIOLOGY

Twin and adoption studies have suggested that there is a **genetic component** to the etiology of schizophrenia. The rates of instance (concordance) among first-degree biological relatives of people with schizophrenia are greater than among the general population. **Structural abnormalities** in the brain linked to schizophrenia are enlarged ventricles and diminished hippocampus, amygdala, and globus pallidus. **Functional abnormalities** in the brain linked to schizophrenia are hypofrontality and diminished activity in the prefrontal cortex. An abnormally large number of the people with schizophrenia in the Northern Hemisphere were born in the late winter or early spring. There is speculation that this may be because of a link between prenatal exposure to influenza and schizophrenia.

SCHIZOPHRENIA AND DOPAMINE

For many years, the professional consensus was that schizophrenia was caused by either an excess of the neurotransmitter **dopamine** or oversensitive **dopamine receptors**. The **dopamine hypothesis** was supported by the fact that antipsychotic medications that block dopamine receptors had some success in treating schizophrenia and by the fact that dopamine-elevating amphetamines amplified the frequency of delusions. The dopamine hypothesis has been somewhat undermined, however, by research that found elevated levels of norepinephrine and serotonin, as well as low levels of gamma-aminobutyric acid and glutamate in schizophrenics. Some studies have shown that clozapine and other atypical antipsychotics are effective in treating schizophrenia, even though they block serotonin rather than dopamine receptors.

ASSOCIATED FEATURES

Features commonly associated with schizophrenia are:

- Inappropriate affect
- Anhedonia (loss of pleasure)
- Dysphoric mood
- Abnormalities in motor behavior
- Somatic complaints

Compliance rates for individuals with schizophrenia are low, with some researchers attributing a lack of insight into treatment needs. People with schizophrenia often develop substance dependencies, especially to nicotine. The onset of schizophrenia is typically during the ages of 18–25 for males and 25–35 for females. Males are slightly more likely to develop the disorder.

PROGNOSIS

Individuals typically develop schizophrenia as a **chronic condition**, with very little chance of full remission. Positive symptoms of schizophrenia tend to decrease in later life, although the negative symptoms may remain. The following factors tend to **improve prognoses**:

- Good premorbid adjustment
- Acute and late onset
- Female gender
- Presence of a precipitating event
- Brief duration of active-phase symptoms
- Insight into the illness
- Family history of mood disorder
- No family history of schizophrenia

TREATMENT

Treatment of schizophrenia begins with the administration of **antipsychotic medication**. Antipsychotics are very effective at diminishing the positive symptoms of schizophrenia, although their results vary from person to person. Antipsychotics have strong side effects, however, including tardive dyskinesia. Medication is more effective when it is taken in combination with psychosocial intervention. Many people with schizophrenia are prone to relapse if they are unsupported by family members. Depending on the symptoms, individuals with schizophrenia can benefit from **family therapy, social skills training,** and **employment support.**

SCHIZOAFFECTIVE DISORDER

The criteria for schizoaffective disorder are as follows:

Criterion A	The individual must have an uninterrupted period of time concurrent with a major depressive or manic episode, as well as symptoms matching criterion A for schizophrenia.
Criterion B	The individual experiences hallucinations or delusions for at least 2 weeks that do not occur during a significant depressive or manic mood episode.
Criterion C	The individual experiences significant depressive or manic mood symptoms for most of the length of the illness.
Criterion D	The symptoms cannot be attributed to another medical condition or a substance.

Differential diagnoses for schizoaffective disorder include bipolar, schizophrenia, depressive disorders, psychotic disorders, and other mental and medical conditions.

CATATONIA

Criteria for catatonia include at least three of the following:

- Catalepsy
- Defying or refusing to acknowledge instruction
- Echolalia
- Echopraxia
- Little to no verbal response
- Grimacing
- Agitation
- Semiconsciousness
- Waxy flexibility
- Posturing
- Mannerisms
- Stereotypy

Catatonia is not an independent diagnosis; rather, it is a potential feature associated with several mental disorders, including psychotic disorders, neurodevelopmental disorders, bipolar disorders, and depressive disorders. Certain medical conditions are also associated with catatonia (e.g., cerebral folate deficiency).

BIPOLAR AND RELATED DISORDERS

BIPOLAR I DISORDER

The criteria for bipolar I disorder are as follows:

Criterion A	The individual must meet the criteria (listed below) for at least one manic episode. The manic episode is usually either preceded or followed by an episode of major depression or hypomania.
Criterion B	At least one manic episode cannot be attributed to schizoaffective disorder, nor can the episode be superimposed on another schizophrenia spectrum disorder or psychotic disorder.

The criteria for a **manic episode** include:

Criterion A	A significant period of maladaptive and persistently increased, expansive, or irritable mood along with a distinct increase in energy or goal-directed behaviors. These symptoms are present for most of the day nearly every day and last at least 1 week.
Criterion B	During the period described in criterion A, the individual will experience three of the following symptoms (if the individual presents with only an irritable mood, four of the following symptoms need to be present for diagnosis): <ul><li>An inflated sense of self</li><li>Decreased need for sleep</li><li>Overly talkative; pressured speech</li><li>Racing thoughts; flight of ideas</li><li>Distractibility</li><li>Either increased or decreased (purposelessness) goal-directed behaviors; agitation</li><li>Excessive engagement in activities with problematic consequences</li></ul>
Criterion C	The episode causes significant social and occupational impairment.
Criterion D	The symptoms cannot be attributed to the effects of a substance.

Differential diagnoses for bipolar I disorder include major depressive disorder, other bipolar disorders, generalized anxiety disorder, schizoaffective disorder, ADHD, disruptive mood regulation disorder, PTSD, and personality disorders.

BIPOLAR II DISORDER

The criteria for bipolar II disorder are as follows:

Criterion A	The individual has had one or more major depressive episodes and one or more hypomanic episodes.
Criterion B	The individual has never experienced a manic episode.
Criterion C	A minimum of one hypomanic episode and a minumum of one major depressive episode cannot be explained by schizoaffective disorder and are not superimposed on other schizophrenia spectrum disorders or other psychotic disorder.
Criterion D	The depressive episodes or alterations between the two moods cause significant impairment socially or functionally.

The criteria for a **hypomanic episode** are as follows:

Criterion A	An episode of significantly elevated, demonstrative, or irritable mood. There are significant goal-directed behaviors, activities, and an increase in the amount of energy that the individual normally has. These symptoms are present for most of the day and last at least 4 days.
Criterion B	During the period described in criterion A, the individual experiences three of the following symptoms (if the individual presents with only an irritable mood, four of the following symptoms need to be present for diagnosis): • An inflated sense of self • Decreased need for sleep • Overly talkative; pressured speech • Racing thoughts; flight of ideas • Distractibility • Either increased or decreased (purposelessness) goal-directed behaviors; agitation • Excessive engagement in activities with problematic consequences
Criterion C	The episode causes a change in the functioning of the individual.
Criterion D	The episode causes changes noticeable by others.
Criterion E	The episode does not cause social impairments.
Criterion F	The symptoms cannot be attributed to a substance.

A **hypomanic episode** is severe enough to be a clear departure from normal mood and functioning, but not severe enough to cause a marked impairment in functioning nor to require hospitalization.

Differential diagnoses for bipolar II disorder include major depressive disorder, cyclothymic disorder, schizophrenia, schizoaffective disorder, substance- or medication-induced bipolar-related disorder, ADHD, personality disorders, and other bipolar disorders.

CYCLOTHYMIC DISORDER

Cyclothymic disorder is characterized by chronic, fluctuating mood with many hypomanic and depressive symptoms, which are not as severe as either bipolar I or bipolar II. The diagnostic **criteria** are as follows:

Criterion A	The individual experiences a considerable number of hypomania symptoms without meeting all of the criteria for hypomanic episodes and experiences depressive symptoms that do not meet the criteria for major depressive episode for 2 or more years (can be for 1 or more years in those <18 years of age).
Criterion B	During the above time period, the individual exhibits the symptoms more than half of the time and they are never symptom free for more than 2 months at a time.
Criterion C	The individual has not met the criteria for manic, hypomanic, or major depressive episodes.
Criterion D	The episodes do not meet the criteria for schizophrenia spectrum or other psychotic disorder.
Criterion E	The symptoms cannot be attributed to a substance.
Criterion F	The episodes cause significant impairment socially or functionally.

Differential diagnoses for cyclothymic disorder include bipolar and related disorders, bipolar I disorder, borderline personality disorder, and substance-/medication-induced bipolar and related disorders.

DEPRESSIVE DISORDERS

DISRUPTIVE MOOD DYSREGULATION DISORDER

The criteria for disruptive mood dysregulation disorder includes **recurrent temper outbursts** at least three times per week, with intermittent irritability for a period of 1 year or longer. The behavior must occur in more than one setting and is only diagnosed in individuals **ages 6–18**.

There are also parameters for co-occurring diagnoses. For example, the diagnosis **cannot co-occur** with any of the following:

- Oppositional defiant disorder
- Bipolar disorder
- Intermittent explosive disorder

The diagnosis **can co-occur** with any of the following:

- ADHD
- Major depressive disorder
- Conduct disorder
- Substance use disorders

The primary diagnostic feature of disruptive mood dysregulation disorder is frequent, severe, and persistent irritability as evidenced by (1) frequent verbal or physical outbursts/aggression that are inconsistent with developmental levels, with reactions grossly disproportional to the situation, and (2) frequent and chronic anger and irritability between outbursts.

Differential diagnoses include ADHD, oppositional defiant disorder, anxiety disorders, major depressive disorder, intermittent explosive disorder, bipolar disorder, oppositional defiant disorder, and ASD.

MAJOR DEPRESSIVE DISORDER

The criteria for major depressive disorder are as follows:

Criterion A	The individual experiences five or more of the following symptoms during 2 consecutive weeks. These symptoms are associated with a change in normal functioning. (Note: Of the presenting symptoms, either depressed mood or loss of ability to feel pleasure must be included to make this diagnosis.) • Depressed mood • Loss of ability to feel pleasure or have interest in normal activities • Weight loss or gain of more than 5% in 1 month • Hypersomnia or insomnia (almost daily) • Observable motor agitation or psychomotor retardation • Fatigue (daily) • Inappropriate guilt or feelings of worthlessness • Poor concentration • Suicidality
Criterion B	The episode causes distress or social or functional impairment.
Criterion C	The symptoms cannot be attributed to a substance or another condition or disease.
Criterion D	The episode does not meet the criteria for schizoaffective disorder and cannot be superimposed on additional schizophrenia spectrum disorders or another psychotic disorder.
Criterion E	The individual does not meet the criteria for a manic episode or a hypomanic episode.

Major depressive disorder is diagnosed when an individual has one or more major depressive episodes without having a history of manic, hypomanic, or mixed episodes. There are a few different specifiers (i.e., categories of associated features) for major depressive disorder issued by the DSM-5-TR:

- With anxious distress
- With melancholic features
- With peripartum onset
- With seasonal pattern
- With psychotic features (mood congruent or mood incongruent)
- With catatonia
- With atypical features
- With mixed features

Symptoms of major depressive disorder vary with age. Children may have symptoms that include somatic complaints, irritability, or social withdrawal. Symptoms in older adults can manifest as memory loss, distractibility, disorientation, and other cognitive problems.

Differential diagnoses include sadness, ADHD, adjustment disorder with depressed mood, substance-induced mood disorders, medical conditions, and bipolar disorders.

ETIOLOGY

There are multiple biopsychosocial factors implicated in the development of major depressive disorder. Early theories contend that depression is caused by neurotransmitter abnormalities, particularly dopamine, serotonin, and norepinephrine, lending support for the use of antidepressants as a common treatment modality. Recent theories support the notion that depression is caused by secondary neuroregulatory system disturbances, such as gamma-aminobutyric acid. Socioemotional stress can also cause depression due to alterations in neuroendocrine responses contributing to changes in the cerebral cortex. Increased levels of cortisol, one of the stress hormones secreted by the adrenal cortex, is also a known contributor.

TREATMENT

Cognitive-behavioral therapy (CBT), an evidence-based treatment for major depressive disorder, is based on several theories, some of which include:

- The **learned helplessness model,** proposed by Martin Seligman, stems from the belief that one does not have control over negative life events. Cognitive distortions associated with this model are internal (e.g., "it's my fault"), stable (e.g., "it's never going to change"), or global (e.g., "this will always happen to me").
- Lynn Rehm's **self-control model of depression** suggests that depression is caused by individuals ruminating over negative outcomes, setting extremely high standards for themselves, having low rates of self-reinforcement, and having high rates of self-punishment.
- Aaron Beck's **cognitive theory** suggests that depression is the result of negative and irrational thoughts and beliefs about oneself, the world, and the future (i.e., the cognitive triad).

The typical treatment for major depressive disorder combines **antidepressant drugs** and psychotherapy. The main categories of antidepressants include tricyclic antidepressants, monoamine oxidase inhibitors, selective serotonin reuptake inhibitors (SSRIs), serotonin and norepinephrine reuptake inhibitors, and atypical antidepressants.

> **Review Video: Major Depression**
> Visit mometrix.com/academy and enter code: 632694

PERSISTENT DEPRESSIVE DISORDER

The criteria for persistent depressive disorder include:

Criterion A	For adults, individuals must experience depressed mood for most of the day on more days than not for at least 2 years. For children and adolescents, the mood can be depressed or irritable for at least 1 year.
Criterion B	Depressive symptoms must be accompanied by two or more of the following: • Low self-esteem • Decreased appetite or overeating • A feeling of hopelessness • Fatigue • Difficulty concentrating • Insomnia or hypersomnia
Criterion C	During the episode, the individual has not had relief from symptoms for longer than 2 months at a time.
Criterion D	The individual may have met the criteria for a major depressive disorder.
Criterion E	The individual does not meet the criteria for cyclothymic disorder, manic episode, or hypomanic episode.
Criterion F	The episode does not meet the criteria for schizophrenia spectrum or other psychotic disorder.
Criterion G	The symptoms cannot be attributed to a substance.
Criterion H	The symptoms cause distress or impairment socially or functionally.

Differential diagnoses include major depression, psychotic disorders, bipolar disorders, personality disorders, substance-induced depression, and depression due to a medical condition.

Review Video: Persistent Depressive Disorder
Visit mometrix.com/academy and enter code: 361077

PREMENSTRUAL DYSPHORIC DISORDER

Premenstrual dysphoric disorder is a severe and chronic condition, with **symptoms** occurring during most menstrual cycles. Symptoms of premenstrual dysphoric disorder include but are not limited to mood lability, depressed mood, increased tension and anxiety, poor concentration, and anhedonia. Vegetative symptoms may also be present, including appetite changes, sleeplessness, lethargy, and muscle pain.

A depletion in serotonin is known to accompany hormonal changes during menses. As such, the pharmacological treatment for premenstrual dysphoric disorder consists of **selective serotonin reuptake inhibitors (SSRIs)**, which are effective for treating the physical and emotional symptoms of premenstrual dysphoric disorder. Treatment recommendations also include dietary changes, exercise, and smoking cessation.

Differential diagnoses of premenstrual dysphoric disorder include premenstrual syndrome, dysmenorrhea, bipolar disorders, depressive disorders, and other medication-induced conditions.

ANXIETY DISORDERS
SEPARATION ANXIETY DISORDER

Separation anxiety disorder is characterized by developmentally inappropriate and excessive anxiety that occurs when an individual is separated or threatened with separation from an attachment figure. Symptoms include recurrent distress over the attachment figure dying, being harmed, or becoming ill. Individuals with separation anxiety often avoid school or work, choosing instead to stay at home with their attachment figure. Symptoms also include repeated nightmares involving separation and somatic complaints (e.g., headaches, stomachaches).

There are many differential diagnoses for separation anxiety disorder, some of which include other anxiety disorders, PTSD, psychotic disorders, personality disorders, depressive disorders, oppositional defiant disorder, and conduct disorder.

SELECTIVE MUTISM

Individuals with selective mutism consistently fail to communicate with adults or children in social situations. Many children with selective mutism will speak at home with their immediate family but refuse to interact with extended family or close friends. To receive a diagnosis of selective mutism, the failure to engage in social conversations must interfere with educational or occupational functioning. Selective mutism can begin as early as 2 years old and, if left untreated, can carry into adulthood.

Differential diagnoses for selective mutism include communication disorders, neurodevelopmental disorders, autism, and social anxiety disorder.

SPECIFIC PHOBIA

A specific phobia is a marked and persistent fear of a particular object or situation that is out of proportion to the actual hazards associated with the object or situation. When an individual with a phobia is exposed to the feared object or event, an anxiety response is exhibited. As a result, the phobic object or situation is avoided or is endured with significant distress. To substantiate a diagnosis, symptoms must occur for at least 6 months and must cause substantial functional impairment. According to the DSM-5-TR, there are five **subtypes** of specific phobia:

- Animal
- Natural environment
- Situational
- Blood-injection-injury
- Other

The **blood-injection-injury** subtype has different physical symptoms than other subtypes. Individuals with a blood-injection-injury phobia have a brief increase in heart rate and blood pressure, followed by a drop in both, often ending in a momentary loss of consciousness (fainting). Phobic reactions to other subtypes mainly entail increased heart rate and blood pressure without loss of consciousness.

Differential diagnoses include agoraphobia, social anxiety disorder, separation anxiety disorder, panic disorder, OCD, eating disorders, PTSD, and psychotic disorders.

SOCIAL ANXIETY DISORDER

The characteristics of social anxiety disorder are a marked and persistent fear of social situations or occasions in which the individual may be called upon to perform. Typically, the individual fears criticism and evaluation by others. The response to the feared situation is an immediate panic attack. Those with social anxiety disorder either avoid the feared situation or endure it with much distress. The fear and anxiety regarding these social situations have a negative impact on the individual's life, and they are present for at least 6 months. As with other phobias, social anxiety disorder is best treated with **exposure therapy** in combination with **social skills** and **cognitive therapy**. Antidepressants and propranolol, a beta blocker, are also recommended for the treatment of social anxiety disorder.

There are several differential diagnoses for social anxiety disorder including but not limited to specific phobia, major depressive disorder, body dysmorphic disorder, delusional disorder, other anxiety disorder, and personality disorders.

PANIC DISORDER

The cardinal manifestation of panic disorder is unexpected and reoccurring panic attacks. To substantiate a diagnosis, one of the panic attacks must be followed by 1 month of either persistent concern regarding the possibility of another attack or a significant change in behavior related to the attack. **Panic attacks** are brief, defined periods of intense apprehension, fear, or terror. They develop quickly and usually reach their greatest intensity after about 10 minutes.

Attacks must include at least four characteristic **symptoms**, which include:

Palpitations or accelerated heart rate (tachycardia)	Shaking
Sweating	Shortness of breath
Chest pain	Fear of losing control
Nausea	Fear of dying
Dizziness	Chills or heat sensation
Derealization	Feeling of choking
Paresthesia (feelings of pins and needles or numbness)	

Differential diagnoses for panic disorder include social anxiety disorder and medical conditions such as hyperthyroidism, hypoglycemia, cardiac arrhythmia, and mitral valve prolapse. Panic disorder can be distinguished from social anxiety disorder by the fact that attacks will sometimes occur while the individual is alone or sleeping.

PREVALENCE AND GENDER ISSUES

It is estimated that 2–3% of individuals in the United States have panic disorder and that just over 10% have experienced a panic attack. Females are twice as likely to be diagnosed with panic disorder than males.

TREATMENT

Evidence-based treatment for panic disorder includes flooding or implosion therapy, implemented through in vivo exposure and response prevention. Flooding is typically accompanied by cognitive therapy, relaxation, breathing training, or pharmacotherapy. **Antidepressant medications** are often prescribed to relieve the symptoms of panic disorder. If stand-alone drug treatment is used, the risk of relapse is very high.

AGORAPHOBIA

Symptoms of agoraphobia include the fear of being in a situation or place from which it could be difficult or embarrassing to escape or of being in a place where help might not be available in the event of a panic attack. These symptoms must occur in two or more of the following situations: (1) while riding in public transportation, (2) in open spaces, (3) in enclosed spaces, (4) waiting in line or in a crowded area, and (5) outside of the home. Individuals with agoraphobia will typically go to great lengths to avoid problematic situations, or they only enter certain situations with a companion or while distressed. Functional impairments result from the individual's fear, severely limiting places they are willing to go.

Differential diagnoses of agoraphobia include phobias, separation anxiety disorder, panic disorder, PTSD and related disorders, and major depressive disorder.

ETIOLOGY AND TREATMENT

Orval Mowrer's **two-factor theory** asserts that phobias are the result of avoidance conditioning, which occurs when a neutral or controlled stimulus is paired with an anxiety-producing unconditioned stimulus. Avoiding the situation prevents anxiety, positively reinforcing the behavior and leading to repeated avoidance.

Another theory for the etiology of phobias is offered by **social learning theorists,** who state that phobic behaviors are learned by watching avoidance strategies used by others. As with panic disorder, **in vivo exposure** is considered the best treatment for a specific phobia. **Relaxation** and **breathing techniques** are also helpful in dispelling fear and controlling physical responses.

GENERALIZED ANXIETY DISORDER

Individuals with generalized anxiety disorder have excessive anxiety about multiple events or activities. This anxiety must have existed for at least 6 months and must be difficult for the individual to control. The anxiety must also be disproportionate to the feared event. Anxiety must include at least three of the following:

- Restlessness
- Fatigue on exertion
- Difficulty concentrating
- Irritability
- Muscle tension
- Sleep disturbances

The treatment for generalized anxiety disorder usually entails a **multicomponent cognitive-behavioral therapy (CBT)**, occasionally accompanied by pharmacotherapy. **SSRI** antidepressants and the anxiolytic buspirone have both demonstrated success in diminishing the symptoms of generalized anxiety disorder. CBT can be used to address **cognitive distortions** that accompany generalized anxiety disorder, including all-or-nothing thinking (e.g., "I'll always be destined for failure"), catastrophic thinking (e.g., "This breakup means I'll be alone forever"), and mind reading (e.g., "She didn't return my text because I am 'nobody' to her").

Different differential diagnoses for generalized anxiety disorder include but are not limited to anxiety disorder due to another medical condition, social anxiety disorder, separation anxiety disorder, panic disorder, OCD, PTSD, and depressive and bipolar disorders.

> **Review Video: Anxiety Disorders**
> Visit mometrix.com/academy and enter code: 366760

OBSESSIVE-COMPULSIVE AND RELATED DISORDERS
OBSESSIVE-COMPULSIVE DISORDER (OCD)

The criteria for obsessive-compulsive disorder (OCD) include:

Criterion A	The individual exhibits obsessions, compulsions, or both. **Obsession**: Continuous, repetitive thoughts, compulsions, or things imagined that are unwanted and cause distress. The individual will try to suppress thoughts, ignore them, or perform a compulsive behavior. **Compulsion**: A recurrent behavior or thought that the individual feels obliged to perform after an obsession to decrease anxiety; however, the compulsion is usually not connected in an understandable way to an observer.
Criterion B	The obsessions and compulsions take at least 1 hour per day and cause distress.
Criterion C	The behavior is not caused by a substance.
Criterion D	The behavior could not be better explained by a different mental disorder.

Additional criteria and diagnostic specifiers are used to indicate whether the individual has ever had a tic disorder and whether the criteria are met with good insight (i.e., the individual realizes that the OCD beliefs are not true), poor insight (i.e., the individual thinks that the OCD beliefs are true), or absent insight (i.e., the individual is delusional, truly believing that the OCD beliefs are true).

Differential diagnoses for OCDs include anxiety disorders, major depressive disorder, eating disorders, tic disorders, psychotic disorders, and obsessive-compulsive personality disorder.

GENDER ISSUES, ETIOLOGY, AND TREATMENT

OCD is slightly more common among women than men, with men experiencing earlier childhood onset and women experiencing earlier adolescent onset. **Irrational beliefs** associated with OCD manifest in irrational obsessions and cognitive biases, including overestimating the perceived threat, inflation of personal responsibility, and underestimating one's coping abilities. Cognitive distortions also include the belief that thinking about an action causes it to happen (i.e., thought–action fusion) and the notion that one cannot tolerate a specific situation or outcome.

OCD is also attributed to low levels of **serotonin**. Structurally, OCD is believed to be linked to overactivity in the **right caudate nucleus**. The most effective treatment for OCD is exposure with response prevention in tandem with medication, usually tricyclic medications, such as clomipramine or an SSRI.

> **Review Video: Obsessive-Compulsive Disorder (OCD)**
> Visit mometrix.com/academy and enter code: 499790

BODY DYSMORPHIC DISORDER

Criteria for body dysmorphic disorder include the following:

Criterion A	Preoccupation with one or more bodily flaws that are nonexistent or slight in appearance to others.
Criterion B	Engaging in repetitive grooming behaviors (e.g., mirror checking) or constantly compares their appearance with that of others.
Criterion C	The condition causes significant functional impairments across multiple domains (e.g., social, educational).
Criterion D	The preoccupation cannot be better explained by individuals who meet the criteria for eating disorder.

Individuals with body dysmorphic disorder tend to avoid social situations due to perceived **appearance-related flaws** in which they believe they are "hideous," "disgusting," or "embarrassingly unattractive." Preoccupations with perceived flaws are often limited to one or more body areas (e.g., face, nose) and commonly occur on the skin (e.g., acne, brown spots). Individuals with body dysmorphic disorder experience unwanted and excessive preoccupations and often engage in **mental acts** and **reassurance-seeking** as a way to control their obsessions.

Differential diagnoses include eating disorders, other OCDs, illness anxiety disorder, major depressive disorder, psychotic disorders, anxiety disorders, and normal appearance-related concerns.

GENDER ISSUES, ETIOLOGY, AND TREATMENT

Women with body dysmorphic disorder are more likely than men to have a comorbid **eating disorder**, whereas men are more likely than women to have **muscle dysmorphia**. Body dysmorphic disorder is likely caused by a combination of factors, including genetics and the environment. A person's risk increases when there are immediate relatives diagnosed with OCD. Body dysmorphia is associated with **early childhood trauma**, particularly child abuse. Traits such as perfectionism enhance a person's risk, and biochemical causes include an imbalance of the neurotransmitter **serotonin**. Treatment consists of pharmacology (e.g., SSRIs) and CBT using exposure and response prevention, which involves exposure to anxiety-provoking preoccupations and response prevention, and in which the person learns to reduce urges associated with criterion B. CBT can also be used alone to address cognitive distortions, including referential thinking (e.g., "They're staring at my blemishes") and other cognitive biases related to negative appearance-related thoughts.

ADDITIONAL OBSESSIVE-COMPULSIVE AND RELATED DISORDERS

Other obsessive-compulsive and related disorders include the following:

- **Hoarding disorder** involves clinically significant levels of distress associated with parting with or discarding one's possessions, resulting in the accumulation of clutter in major living areas.
- **Trichotillomania** is repeated hair pulling resulting in hair loss, with several failed attempts to discontinue the behavior.
- **Excoriation** involves the compulsion to pick at areas of the skin, resulting in skin lesions, with several failed attempts to discontinue the behavior.

TRAUMA AND STRESSOR-RELATED DISORDERS

REACTIVE ATTACHMENT DISORDER

Children with reactive attachment disorder rarely seek or respond to comfort when upset, usually due to **neglect of emotional needs** by their caregiver. The diagnosis of reactive attachment disorder is characterized by a markedly disturbed or developmentally inappropriate social relatedness in most settings. This condition typically begins before the age of 5. To definitively diagnose this disorder, there must be evidence of **pathogenic care**, which may include neglect or a constant change of caregivers (e.g., foster care placements) that make it difficult for the child to form normal attachments. Differential diagnoses include ASD, intellectual developmental disorder, and depressive disorders.

DISINHIBITED SOCIAL ENGAGEMENT DISORDER

Children with disinhibited social engagement disorder exhibit little to no hesitation when interacting with unfamiliar adults and often interact with strangers in an overly familiar fashion. This behavior can also be coupled with diminished questioning when leaving a usual caregiver to go off with a stranger. The diagnostic criterion is similar to reactive attachment disorder in that there must be evidence of pathogenic care (e.g., social neglect). ADHD is a differential diagnosis for disinhibited social engagement disorder.

PROLONGED GRIEF DISORDER

The DSM-5-TR presents new diagnostic criteria for prolonged grief disorder, which include the following:

Criterion A	Symptoms associated with prolonged grief must follow at least 12 months after the death of a close attachment figure.
Criterion B	Since the death, maladaptive grief responses are characterized by: • Intense yearning for the deceased. • Preoccupation with memories and thoughts of the deceased.
Criterion C	At least three of the following must occur after the loss: • Feeling as if a part of oneself died along with the deceased (e.g., identity disruption). • Disbelief that the person has died. • Avoidance of painful memories associated with the death. • Intense emotional distress associated with the lost person. • Problems reintegrating into relationships and pursuing former interests and activites since the loss. • Significant reduction in emotional expression (e.g., feeling numb) as a result of the death. • Consumed with the belief that life is meaningless without the deceased. • Intense loneliness as the result of the death.
Criterion D	The disturbance results in clinically significant impairment in social, occupational, or other significant domains of functioning.
Criterion E	The maladaptive grief reaction must exceed what is culturally, socially, or religiously acceptable for the individual.
Criterion F	The symptoms cannot be explained by another mental disorder, the effects of a substance, or another medical condition.

Criteria for prolonged grief disorder in children and adolescents differ from those in adults in that symptoms may occur at least 6 (rather than 12) months after the death (criterion A). Children and adolescents also differ in avoidance (criterion C3), with youth trying to avoid memories of the lost person.

To differentiate between normal bereavement and prolonged grief, criterion B specifies that the symptoms must be clinically significant and occur almost daily for at least 1 month. Clinically significant symptoms may include intense yearning, sorrow, and frequent crying spells. It is also common for individuals with prolonged grief disorder to experience resentment, bitterness, regret, decreased appetite, physical complaints, depression, anxiety, irritability, and sleep disturbances. Context and cultural beliefs surrounding loss must also be considered.

Differential diagnoses include normal grief reactions, depressive disorders, PTSD, separation anxiety disorder, and psychotic disorder.

TREATMENT

Cognitive restructuring is the recommended treatment for prolonged grief disorder because it can co-occur with depression, anxiety, and trauma. Maladaptive beliefs about oneself, survivor's guilt, and the idea that one cannot go on without the bereaved may occur. Irrational beliefs also include preoccupation with the unfairness of the death, inaccurate appraisals surrounding the cause of the death or the need to create false narratives, maladaptive rumination, and diminished life goals.

ACUTE STRESS DISORDER

Acute stress disorder has symptoms similar to those of PTSD. Acute stress disorder is distinguished by symptoms that occur for more than 3 days but less than 1 month. An individual is diagnosed with acute stress disorder when he or she has nine or more **symptoms** from any of the following five categories, which begin after the trauma:

- Intrusion
- Negative mood
- Avoidance symptoms
- Dissociative symptoms
- Increased arousal symptoms

An individual with acute stress disorder persistently relives the traumatic event, to the extent that he or she takes steps to avoid contact with stimuli that bring the event to mind and experiences severe anxiety when reminiscing about the event. Differential diagnoses for acute stress disorder include adjustment disorders, panic disorder, anxiety disorders, ADHD, depressive disorders, personality disorders, psychotic disorders, and TBI.

> **Review Video: Acute Stress Disorder**
> Visit mometrix.com/academy and enter code: 538946

POST-TRAUMATIC STRESS DISORDER (PTSD)

The criteria for PTSD include the following:

Criterion A	Exposure to severe threats or actual injury manifested by direct exposure to the event, witnessing the event, learning about the unexpected or violent death or injury of a family member or friend, or repeatedly being exposed to trauma (such as with first responders or military soldiers).
Criterion B	One or more of the following must occur: recurrent and intrusive memories, distressing dreams, flashbacks, prolonged psychological distress, or acute physiological responses.
Criterion C	Avoidance of stimuli associated with the traumatic event.
Criterion D	Cognitive alterations (e.g., "I'm permanently ruined") and negative mood (e.g., intense fear, helplessness, horror).
Criterion E	Significant alterations in arousal and reactions associated with the traumatic event (e.g., hypervigilance, sleeplessness).
Criterion F	Symptoms must occur for more than 1 month.
Criterion G	Symptoms must cause significant functional impairment.
Criterion H	The symptoms are not better explained by the psychological effects of a substance or another medical condition.

For criterion A, it is important to note that repeated exposure to the traumatic event does not include events witnessed only in television, movies, online, or in pictures unless the exposure is work related (e.g., first responders).

TREATMENT AND DIFFERENTIAL DIAGNOSES

Treatment for PTSD includes prolonged exposure therapy, trauma-focused CBT, and cognitive processing therapy. SSRIs (e.g., sertraline, paroxetine) are also used to treat symptoms of PTSD and comorbid conditions.

Differential diagnoses for PTSD include but are not limited to adjustment disorders, acute stress disorder, anxiety disorders, ADHD, depressive disorders, personality disorders, psychotic disorders, and TBI.

ADJUSTMENT DISORDERS

Adjustment disorders appear as maladaptive reactions to one or more identifiable psychosocial stressors. In order to make a diagnosis, the onset of symptoms must be within 3 months of the stressor and the condition must cause impairments in social, occupational, or academic performance. The symptoms do not align with normal grief or bereavement. Symptoms remit within 6 months after the termination of the stressor or its consequences. The adjustment disorder should be specified with at least one of the following:

- Depressed mood
- Anxiety
- Mixed anxiety and depressed mood
- Disturbance of conduct
- Mixed disturbance of emotions and conduct

Differential diagnoses for adjustment disorders include major depressive disorder, PTSD, personality disorders, and bereavement. Clinicians must also rule out normal stress reactions and exacerbated medical conditions.

DISSOCIATIVE DISORDERS

Dissociative disorders are a disruption in consciousness, identity, memory, or perception of the environment that is not due to the effects of a substance or a general medical condition. These are all characterized by a disturbance in the normally integrative functions of identity, memory, consciousness, or environmental perception.

DISSOCIATIVE IDENTITY DISORDER

The criteria for dissociative identity disorder are as follows:

Criterion A	Significant disturbances regarding a person's sense of self paired with related changes in mood, behavior, perceptions, thinking, and/or sensory motor functioning
Criterion B	Memory loss or noted gaps in time.
Criterion C	The disturbance results in clinically significant impairment in social, occupational, or other significant domains of functioning.
Criterion D	The symptoms are not better explained by cultural or religious practices used to create dissociative psychological experiences.
Criterion E	The symptoms cannot be attributed to the psychological effects of a substance or medical condition.

Differential diagnoses for dissociative identity disorder include PTSD, major depressive disorder, depersonalization/derealization disorder, bipolar disorders, psychotic disorders, personality disorders, factitious and malingering disorder, conditions related to TBI, and functional neurological symptom disorder.

DISSOCIATIVE AMNESIA

Criteria for dissociative amnesia include:

Criterion A	One or more episodes in which important personal information is forgotten and cannot be attributed to ordinary forgetfulness.
Criterion B	The disturbance results in clinically significant impairment in social, occupational, or other significant domains of functioning.
Criterion C	The symptoms cannot be attributed to the psychological effects of a substance, medical condition, or neurological pathology.
Criterion D	The amnesia cannot be attributed to dissociative identity disorder, PTSD, acute stress disorder, somatic symptom disorder, or neurocognitive disorders.

The three most common patterns of dissociative amnesia are:

- **Localized**, in which the individual is unable to remember all events around a defined time period
- **Selective**, in which the individual cannot recall some events pertaining to a circumscribed time period
- **Generalized**, in which memory loss spans the individual's entire life

It should be specified if this is with dissociative fugue, a subtype of dissociative amnesia, which includes impulsive travel that is associated with amnesia. Differential diagnoses for dissociative amnesia include but are not limited to PTSD, neurocognitive disorders, substance-related disorders, seizure disorders, catatonic stupor, factitious disorder, and malingering.

DEPERSONALIZATION/DEREALIZATION DISORDER

Criteria for depersonalization/derealization disorder include the following:

Criterion A	Experiences of depersonalization (e.g., detachment, feeling outside of one's self) and derealization (e.g., visual distortions).
Criterion B	During experiences discribed in criterion A, reality testing remains intact.
Criterion C	Symptoms must be intense enough to cause significant distress or functional impairment.
Criterion D	Symptoms cannot be attributed to the psychological effects of a substance, medical condition (e.g., ketamine, MDMA [aka ecstasy in its pill form or Molly in its powder form]), or neurological pathology (e.g., seizures).
Criterion E	Symptoms cannot be attributed to another mental disorder (e.g., schizophrenia, panic disorder, PTSD, acute stress disorder, major depressive disorder).

Differential diagnoses for depersonalization/derealization disorder include major depressive disorder, OCD, panic disorder, psychosis, and TBI.

SOMATIC SYMPTOM AND RELATED DISORDERS

SOMATIC SYMPTOM DISORDER

Somatic symptom disorder involves symptoms associated with a medical condition that are not explainable by a specific physical condition. They also cannot be explained by the effects of a substance or another medical disorder. Mood, behavior, and thoughts that accompany the disorder include clinically significant distress over the **perceived seriousness of health concerns**, which may be coupled with high anxiety regarding the etiology of the symptoms and excessive time and energy spent focusing on these concerns. The disorder involves **recurrent multiple somatic complaints**, and although no one symptom has to be continuous, some symptoms are present for at least 6 months. The diagnosis must specify whether the health conditions are associated with pain, whether they are persistent, and their level of severity.

Differential diagnoses include but are not limited to panic disorder, anxiety disorders, depressive disorders, OCD, delusional disorder, factitious disorder and malingering, and body dysmorphic disorder.

ILLNESS ANXIETY DISORDER

Individuals with illness anxiety disorder (formerly hypochondriasis) have an unrealistic preoccupation with having or getting a severe illness. Fears associated with this preoccupation are excessive and are based on a misappraisal of bodily symptoms, which are either mild or nonexistent. The symptoms of the illness are also disproportional to medical evidence. Individuals with illness anxiety disorder likely know a great deal about their condition and frequently go to several doctors searching for a professional opinion confirming their own. They likely either experience **frequent health-related checks** (either by doctors or self-checks), or they avoid doctors and healthcare facilities. The symptoms of this disorder must be present for at least 6 months; however, the specific illness that the individual fears may change.

Differential diagnoses for illness anxiety disorder include adjustment disorders, anxiety disorders, major depressive disorder, psychotic disorders, somatic symptom disorder, and OCD and related disorders. Other medical conditions must also be ruled out.

FUNCTIONAL NEUROLOGICAL SYMPTOM DISORDER (CONVERSION DISORDER)

Functional neurological symptom disorder (conversion disorder) is characterized by one or more neurological symptoms that are **incongruent with symptoms of a serious medical condition**. Individuals with functional neurological symptom disorder present with **altered voluntary motor functioning** (e.g., paralysis, tremors, movement irregularities) or **sensory symptoms** (e.g., hearing deficits, altered sight, reduced skin sensation). These symptoms do not cause substantial structural damage to the brain, and testing reveals no underlying physical disease. The sensory loss, movement loss, or repetitive physical symptoms are not intentional. The individual is not malingering to avoid work or factitiously seeking attention. Clinicians must specify whether the symptoms occur with or without a psychological stressor and the symptom type (e.g., with paralysis, with seizures).

Differential diagnoses include somatic symptom disorder, factitious disorder and malingering, body dysmorphic syndrome, dissociative disorders, depressive disorders, and panic disorder. Clinicians must also be cognizant of other substantiated neurological conditions with similar symptoms.

FACTITIOUS DISORDER

There are two sets of criteria for factitious disorder. The **first set of criteria** is categorized as factitious disorder imposed on self. Symptoms include intentionally falsifying physical or psychological symptoms created by a deceptive scheme. Individuals with factitious disorder present with exaggerated somatic symptoms and do so for no apparent reason. These individuals may undergo multiple surgeries and invasive medical procedures. They often hide insurance claims and hospital discharge forms. This disorder was previously referred to as Munchausen syndrome.

The **second set of criteria** is categorized as factitious disorder imposed on another, previously called factitious disorder by proxy. The same criteria are included, with the difference being that the falsification of symptoms is portrayed onto another person.

Differential diagnoses include other somatic symptom and related disorders and borderline personality disorder. It is also important to distinguish factitious disorder from malingering. Malingering (V65.25) involves feigning physical symptoms to avoid something specific, such as going to work or to gain a particular reward. In contrast, in factitious disorder, the individual does not feign physical symptoms for personal gain or to avoid an adverse event but does it with no apparent external rewards.

FEEDING AND EATING DISORDERS

PICA AND RUMINATION DISORDER

A detailed breakdown of all of the feeding and eating diagnoses is beyond the scope of this overview. In brief, **pica disorder** involves the persistent eating of nonfood substances such as paint, hair, sand, cloth, pebbles, etc. Those with pica do not show an aversion to food. In order to be diagnosed, the symptoms must persist for at least 1 month without the child losing an interest in regular food. Also, the behavior must be independent and not a part of any culturally acceptable process. Pica is most often manifested between the ages of 12 and 24 months. Pica has been observed in developmentally disabled children, pregnant women, and people with anemia. **Rumination disorder** is the regurgitation and rechewing of food.

Differential diagnoses for pica disorder and rumination disorder include anorexia nervosa. Differential diagnoses for pica also include factitious disorder and nonsuicidal self-injury. Rumination disorder must be differentiated from gastrointestinal conditions and bulimia nervosa.

AVOIDANT/RESTRICTIVE FOOD INTAKE DISORDER

The diagnostic **criteria for avoidant/restrictive food intake disorder** are as follows:

Criterion A	A disruption in eating evidenced by not meeting nutritional needs and failure to gain expected weight or weight loss, nutritional deficiency requiring nutritional supplementation, or interpersonal interference.
Criterion B	This disruption is not due to cultural traditions or a lack of food.
Criterion C	There does not appear to be a problem with the individual's body perception.
Criterion D	The disturbance cannot be explained by another medical condition.

Individuals with avoidant/restrictive food intake disorder differ from individuals with anorexia nervosa in that they do not have a distorted body image, and they differ from bulimia nervosa sufferers in that they are not overly concerned with body image.

Differential diagnoses include but are not limited to other feeding conditions, ASD, other anxiety disorders, OCD, schizophrenia, and major depressive disorders.

ANOREXIA NERVOSA

DIAGNOSIS

The diagnostic criteria for **anorexia nervosa** are as follows:

Criterion A	Extreme restriction of food, which is lower than nutritional requirements, leading to low body weight
Criterion B	An irrational fear of gaining weight or behaviors that prevent weight gain, despite being at a very low weight
Criterion C	Distorted body image or a lack of acknowledgement of severity of current weight

Adults with anorexia have a **body mass index** of 17.5 or lower. Individuals with restricting type anorexia lose weight through fasting, dieting, and excessive exercise. **Physiological symptoms of anorexia** include constipation, cold intolerance, lethargy, and bradycardia. Those with binging/purging type anorexia engage in self-induced vomiting and/or laxative, diuretic, or enema misuse. The **physical problems** associated with purging are anemia, impaired renal function, cardiac abnormalities, dental problems, and osteoporosis.

Differential diagnoses for anorexia nervosa are social anxiety disorder, OCD, schizophrenia, substance use disorders, major depressive disorder, and other eating disorders. Clinicians must also rule out other medical conditions with similar symptoms (e.g., hyperthyroidism, AIDS).

BULIMIA NERVOSA

The diagnostic criteria for **bulimia nervosa** are as follows:

Criterion A	Cyclical periods of binge eating characterized by discreetly consuming an amount of food that is larger than most individuals would eat in the same time period and situation. The individual feels a lack of control over eating.
Criterion B	Characterized by binge eating followed by purging via self-induced vomiting/laxatives/fasting/vigorous exercise in order to prevent weight gain.
Criterion C	At least one binge eating episode per week for 3 months.
Criterion D	It is marked by a persistent overconcern with body shape and weight.
Criterion E	The eating and compensatory behaviors do not only occur during periods of anorexia nervosa.

The **medical complications** associated with bulimia are fluid and electrolyte disturbances, metabolic alkalosis/acidosis, dental problems, and menstrual abnormalities. Also, there are links between bulimia and low levels of the endogenous opioid beta-endorphin and the neurotransmitters serotonin and norepinephrine. Treatment often involves **CBT techniques** such as self-monitoring, stimulus control, cognitive restructuring, problem solving, and self-distraction. Some antidepressants, such as imipramine, have been effective at reducing instances of binging and purging.

BINGE-EATING DISORDER

The diagnostic criteria for **binge-eating disorder** are as follows:

Criterion A	Cyclical periods of binge eating characterized by discreetly consuming an amount of food that is larger than most individuals would eat in the same time period and situation. The individual feels a lack of control over eating.
Criterion B	Episodes of binge eating occur along with eating faster than usual; eating beyond feeling comfortably full; eating large quantities of food without an appetite; hiding eating; or feeling embarrassed, guilty, depressed, or repulsive with regard to eating.
Criterion C	Significant distress around binge eating is present.
Criterion D	Binge eating must occur once a week for 3 months.
Criterion E	Binge eating is not paired with the compensatory behaviors (e.g., vomiting, laxative use) associated with bulimia nervosa.

Medical complications for binge-eating disorder are similar to those associated with bulimia nervosa. Individuals with binge-eating disorder are at risk for type 2 diabetes and the associated complications. Weight gain is also common, which may result in hypertension, heart disease, and sleep apnea. Suicidal ideation is present in approximately 25% of individuals with binge-eating disorder. CBT is useful for treating underlying feelings of depression, shame, and guilt.

Differential diagnoses for binge-eating disorder include bulimia nervosa, borderline personality disorder, depressive disorders, bipolar disorders, and obesity.

ELIMINATION DISORDERS
ENURESIS AND ENCOPRESIS

Encopresis and enuresis make up the two major categories of elimination disorders. **Enuresis** is repeated urinating during the day or night into the bed or clothes at least twice a week for 3 or more months. Most of the time this urination is involuntary. Enuresis is diagnosed only when the child has reached an age at which continence can be reasonably expected (at least age 5 for DSM-5-TR criteria) and he or she does not have some other medical condition that could be to blame, such as a urinary tract infection. Enuresis is treated with a night alarm, which makes a loud noise when the child urinates while sleeping. This is effective about 80% of the time, especially when it is combined with techniques such as behavioral reversal and overcorrection. Desmopressin acetate nasal spray, imipramine, and oxybutynin chloride (Ditropan) may help control symptoms. **Encopresis** is involuntary fecal soiling in children who have already been toilet trained. An encopresis diagnosis cannot be made until the child is at least 4 years of age per DSM-5-TR criteria.

SLEEP-WAKE DISORDERS

Sleep-wake disorders include the following:

Insomnia disorders	Difficulty falling asleep, staying asleep, or early rising without being able to go back to sleep
Hypersomnolence disorder	Sleepiness despite getting at least 7 hours of sleep with difficulty feeling awake when suddenly awoken, lapses into sleep in the day, feeling unrested after long periods of sleep
Narcolepsy	Uncontrollable lapses into sleep, occurring at least three times each week for at least 3 months. Includes narcolepsy without cataplexy and without hypocretin deficiency
Obstructive sleep apnea hypopnea	Breathing-related sleep disorder with obstructive apneas or hypopneas
Central sleep apnea	Breathing-related sleep disorder with central apnea
Sleep-related hypoventilation	Breathing-related sleep disorder with evidence of decreased respiratory rate and increased CO_2 levels
Circadian rhythm sleep-wake disorder	Sleep-wake disorder caused by a mismatch between the circadian rhythm and the amount of sleep required by a person
Non-rapid eye movement (REM) sleep arousal disorder	A parasomnia associated with the first third of the night, associated with sleepwalking or sleep terrors
Nightmare disorder	Recurring distressing dreams that are well remembered and cause distress
REM sleep behavior disorder	Arousal during REM sleep associated with motor movements and vocalizing
Restless leg syndrome	The need to move the legs due to uncomfortable sensations, usually relieved by activity

> **Review Video: Chronic Insomnia**
> Visit mometrix.com/academy and enter code: 293232

SEXUAL DYSFUNCTIONS

A sexual dysfunction is any condition in which an individual's sexual response cycle is disturbed or there is pain during sexual intercourse, which causes distress or interpersonal difficulty. Sexual dysfunctions include all of the following:

- Delayed ejaculation
- Erectile disorder
- Female orgasmic disorder
- Female sexual interest/arousal disorder
- Genitopelvic pain/penetration disorder
- Male hypoactive sexual desire disorder
- Premature ejaculation
- Substance-induced sexual dysfunction
- Unspecified sexual dysfunction

The exact **etiology of sexual dysfunctions** is complex, dynamic, and largely unknown. Clinicians must first determine conditions that would preclude a diagnosis. These conditions include the influence of cultural factors, aging, substance use, and/or nonsexual mental conditions. Thus, individuals with sexual dysfunctions should be given a medical evaluation to identify comorbid and co-occurring conditions.

Clinicians must provide a thorough assessment to understand the biopsychosocial determinants for sexual dysfunctions and related conditions. A sexual dysfunction would not be diagnosed in the presence of **inadequate sexual stimulation** that prevents an individual from obtaining an orgasm or experiencing sexual excitation.

Contributing factors for individuals reporting insufficient sexual stimulation may include:

- A partner's sexual difficulties
- A partner's sexual health
- Psychological factors (e.g., depression)
- Poor body image or a history of childhood abuse
- Religious and cultural norms surrounding sexual intercourse
- Intimate relationship factors (e.g., intimate partner violence, divergent sexual desires).
- Other psychosocial stressors

A detailed breakdown of all sexual dysfunctions is beyond the scope of this overview. To summarize, **erectile disorder** is the inability to attain or maintain an erection and is linked to diabetes; liver and kidney disease; multiple sclerosis; and the use of antipsychotic, antidepressant, and hypertensive drugs. **Female orgasmic disorder** is any delay or absence of orgasm after the normal sexual excitement phase. **Premature ejaculation** is an orgasm with minimal stimulation before the person desires it, which may be due to deficiencies in serotonin levels. **Genitopelvic pain/penetration disorder** is persistent difficulty with vaginal pain (or the anticipatory fear of vaginal pain) associated with sexual intercourse or involuntary spasms in the pubococcygeus muscle in the vagina.

The DSM-5-TR categorizes sexual dysfunctions as **lifelong** or **acquired** and **generalized** or **situational**, depending on their cause. Generalized dysfunctions occur with every sexual partner in all circumstances. Situational dysfunctions only happen under certain circumstances. The reason may be psychological, physical, or both.

GENDER DYSPHORIA

DSM-5-TR defines gender dysphoria (formerly gender identity disorder) as a marked incongruence between one's expressed gender and one's assigned gender that causes significant distress or impairment over a period of at least 6 months. Informally, gender dysphoria is used to describe a person's persistent discomfort and disagreement with their assigned gender. DSM-5-TR criteria for diagnosis in **children** include:

- Strong desire to be of the other gender or insistence that one is the other gender
- Strong preference for clothing typically associated with the other gender
- Strong preference for playing cross-gender roles
- Strong preference for activities stereotypical of the other gender and rejection of those activities stereotypical of one's assigned gender
- Strong preference for playmates of the other gender
- Strong dislike of one's own sexual anatomy
- Strong desire for the sex characteristics that match one's expressed gender

DSM-5-TR criteria for diagnosis in **adolescents and adults** include:

- Marked incongruence between one's expressed gender and one's existing primary and secondary sex characteristics
- Strong desire to rid oneself of these sex characteristics for this reason
- Strong desire for the sex characteristics of the other gender
- Strong desire to be of the other gender and to be treated as such
- Strong conviction that one's feelings and reactions are typical of the other gender

Differential diagnoses for gender dysphoria include ASD, schizophrenia, body dysmorphic disorder, and transvestic disorder. Traits must also differ from individuals who do not conform to gender roles because a substantiated diagnosis must include symptom distress and must lead to functional impairment.

DISRUPTIVE AND IMPULSE CONTROL DISORDERS
OPPOSITIONAL DEFIANT DISORDER

Oppositional defiant disorder is a pattern of behavior lasting at least 6 months, with symptoms present in categories including angry/irritable mood, argumentative/defiant behavior, and vindictiveness as evidenced by:

- Negative or hostile behavior toward authority
- Spitefulness
- Easily annoyed
- Frequent temper outbursts
- Deliberately annoying people
- Blaming others
- Vindictiveness

This pattern of negative, hostile, defiant behavior, and vindictiveness is mild, moderate, or severe. Mild specifiers are assigned to behaviors in one setting, moderate in two settings, and severe in three or more settings.

Differential diagnoses for oppositional defiant disorder include but are not limited to other disruptive and impulse control disorders, adjustment disorder, PTSD, ADHD, depressive disorders, anxiety disorders, and bipolar disorders.

INTERMITTENT EXPLOSIVE DISORDER

Intermittent explosive disorder is a pattern of behavior occurring twice weekly and lasting at least 3 months, with recurrent temper outbursts as evidenced by:

- Physical assault
- Injury to animals
- Verbal altercations
- Property destruction
- Teasing/bullying

The temper outburst may or may not result in injury to animals or others, and it is **significantly disproportional** to the activating event. Intermittent explosive disorder differs from other disruptive disorders in that episodes are not planned or premeditated. Individuals with intermittent explosive disorder experience **impulsive reactions**, often leaving the person feeling distressed and/or experiencing functional impairment or negative consequences. Children must be at least 6 years of age to receive this diagnosis.

Differential diagnoses include other disruptive and impulse control disorders, other child-onset disorders (e.g., ASD, ADHD), delirium, antisocial personality disorder, and borderline personality disorder.

CONDUCT DISORDER

DIAGNOSIS

The diagnostic criteria for conduct disorder are as follows:

Criterion A	Persistent pattern of behavior in which significant age-appropriate rules or societal norms are ignored, and others' rights and property are violated (theft, deceitfulness); aggression to people and animals and destruction of property are common. To meet the diagnosis criteria, individuals will display 3 of the 15 possible symptoms over the course of 1 year. All of the symptoms can be sorted into one of the following four categories: • Aggression to people or animals • Destruction of property • Deceitfulness or theft • Serious violations of rules
Criterion B	The patterns of behavior cause academic, social, or other impairments.
Criterion C	The behaviors would not be better classified as antisocial personality disorder.

Individuals with conduct disorder persistently violate either the rights of others or age-appropriate rules. They have little remorse about their behavior, and in ambiguous situations, they are likely to interpret the behavior of other people as hostile or threatening.

The DSM-5-TR includes specifiers for conduct disorder, which are childhood-onset type (before age 10), adolescent-onset type, and unspecified onset. There are two basic types of conduct disorder:

- **Life-course-persistent type** begins early in life and gets progressively worse over time. This kind of conduct disorder may be a result of neurological impairments, a difficult temperament, or adverse circumstances.
- **Adolescence-limited type** is usually the result of a temporary disparity between the adolescent's biological maturity and freedom. Adolescents with this form of conduct disorder may commit antisocial acts with friends. It is quite common for children with adolescence-limited conduct disorder to display antisocial behavior persistently in one area of life and not at all in others.

Differential diagnoses for conduct disorder include other disruptive and impulse control disorders, antisocial personality disorder, bipolar and depressive disorders, and adjustment disorder.

TREATMENT

Evidence-based practices for oppositional defiant disorder, intermittent explosive disorder, and conduct disorder include multisystemic family therapy, behavior modification, anger management, and structured environments designed to reduce disruptive behavior. Research suggests that interventions are most successful when they are administered to preadolescents and include the immediate family members. This is especially true for individuals with oppositional defiant disorder and conduct disorder. Trauma-focused CBT is also useful for individuals with co-occurring trauma.

Parenting programs emphasizing behavior modification have also proven to be effective. Most programs advise positive reinforcement for prosocial behavior, clear guidelines, and consistently reinforced, preestablished consequences. There are currently no approved medications available. Instead, pharmacotherapy consists of the use of off-label medications to treat any accompanying symptoms. Examples include mood stabilizers, second-generation antipsychotics, and stimulant medications for impulsivity.

PYROMANIA AND KLEPTOMANIA

Pyromania is characterized by deliberate and purposeful fire setting. The cycle of pyromania involves excitement, arousal, or tension before setting a fire; fixation on fire-setting paraphernalia or other situational contexts; and gratification upon setting a fire and/or pleasure and excitement with the aftermath. As such, fire-setting is purposeful and deliberate. It is essential to differentiate pyromania from fire-setting that is completed in the context of protests or to obtain attention, acknowledgment, recognition, or retaliation.

Kleptomania is the failure to control the impulse to steal. The cycle of kleptomania is similar to pyromania, with initial tension and arousal before stealing and gratification and pleasure obtained after completing the act. Individuals with kleptomania do not seek items for personal use, nor do they seek to possess objects with significant monetary value. Additionally, items are not stolen to seek revenge or respond to hallucinations or delusions. Kleptomania must also be differentiated from shoplifting, malingering, or antisocial personality disorder.

SUBSTANCE-RELATED AND ADDICTIVE DISORDERS
SUBSTANCE-RELATED DISORDERS

The DSM-5-TR categorizes substance-related disorders for the following substances:

- Alcohol
- Caffeine (excludes severity level)
- Cannabis
- Hallucinogens
- Inhalants
- Opioids
- Sedatives
- Hypnotics or anxiolytics
- Stimulants (including amphetamine-type substances, cocaine, and other stimulants)
- Tobacco

Individuals with substance use disorder display a persistent pattern of behavior within a **12-month** period **along 11 criteria**, which are subdivided into the following **four categories:**

Category	Criteria
Impaired control	The substance is taken in larger amounts or for longer periods than intended. There is a desire to control substance use and an inability to do so. Significant periods of time are spent engaging in substance-related behaviors (e.g., seeking the substance, recovering from using the substance). There is a strong urge to use the substance (i.e., cravings) and an inability to think of anything else.
Social impairment	Repeated substance use leads to impairment in work, school, or home. Continued substance use despite causing or exacerbating relationship problems. The relinquishment of important social, job, or recreational activities due to substance use.
Risky use	Continued substance use in physically dangerous situations (e.g., driving a car). Failure to abstain from use despite adverse physical or psychological consequences.

Category	Criteria
Pharmacological criteria	Tolerance, as evidenced by one of the following: • the need to substantially increase substance use to obtain the desired effect. • experiencing a markedly reduced effect when the same amount of the substance is used. Withdrawal, as evidenced by one of the following: • substance-specific symptoms of withdrawal. • use of a similar substance to prevent or arrest withdrawal symptoms.

To substantiate a substance use disorder diagnosis, individuals must experience between 2 and 3 criteria. Substance use disorders include the following specifiers: **mild** (2–3 criteria), **moderate** (4–5 criteria), or **severe** (6 or more criteria).

Differential diagnoses vary according to the presenting symptoms and include but are not limited to ADHD, anxiety, sleep disorders, depression, trauma- and stressor-related disorders, mood disorders with psychotic features, delirium, eating disorders, medical conditions, and other substance use disorders.

GAMBLING DISORDER

Gambling disorder is recognized as a non-substance-related disorder. The criteria for gambling disorder include at least 12 months of ongoing and maladaptive gambling-related behavior resulting in significant functional impairment.

Individuals with gambling disorder must display four or more of the following criteria:

- Using more money to gamble to attain the same level of desired excitement
- Exhibiting distress when unable to reduce or stop gambling
- Finding it difficult to cut down or discontinue gambling
- Engaging in persistent thoughts or preoccupation with gambling, including planning and securing money for the next endeavor
- Gambling to alleviate feelings of sadness, anxiety, or related distress
- Returning to gambling to "chase" or recoup one's losses
- Telling lies about gambling or minimizing the extent of one's gambling
- Risking or losing significant relationships and opportunities due to gambling
- Relying on others to lend money to continue gambling or recoup losses

The diagnosis of gambling disorder cannot be made if the gambling-related behaviors are better explained by a manic episode. Differential diagnoses include nonproblematic gambling behavior, bipolar disorder with manic episodes, impulse control disorders, medical conditions (e.g., Parkinson's disease), and antisocial personality disorder.

ETIOLOGY

Individuals who engage in gambling from an early age have higher instances of gambling disorder as the condition worsens over time. Gambling disorder tends to co-occur with alcohol use disorder, with similar genetic and environmental causes. Researchers indicate that 96% of individuals with gambling disorder have one or more co-occurring mental disorders. Co-occurring diagnoses include mood disorders, substance use disorders, and antisocial personality disorders. Impulsivity is a predominant risk factor, as are difficulties with decision making and self-directedness.

TREATMENT

Much like other substance use disorders, a **motivational interviewing** approach has proven to be effective in generating change among individuals with gambling disorder. **Cognitive behavioral therapy (CBT)** (e.g., cognitive restructuring) is also recommended because individuals with gambling disorder tend to experience

cognitive distortions, including illusions of control, magical thinking, and gambling expectancy. Illusions of control describe the belief that the probability of gambling success is unrealistically high. The negative recency effect (aka the gambler's fallacy or the Monte Carlo fallacy) involves the erroneous belief that a specific outcome will occur more or less frequently based on the frequency of preceding occurrences—for example, believing a roulette wheel will land on red after previously landing on black for several consecutive turns.

Although there are currently no FDA-approved gambling disorder treatments, pharmacology can treat underlying symptoms. The primary drug therapies include antidepressants, mood stabilizers, and opioid antagonists, targeting neurotransmitter pathways that produce dopamine, serotonin, and glutamate.

NEUROCOGNITIVE DISORDERS

DELIRIUM

Delirium is characterized by a clinically significant deficit in cognition or memory compared to previous functioning. To diagnose delirium, the individual must have disturbances in consciousness and either a **change in personality** or the development of **perceptual abnormalities**. These cognitive changes may appear as memory loss, disorientation in space and time, and impaired language. The perceptual abnormalities associated with delirium include **hallucinations** and **delusions**. Delirium usually develops over a few hours or days, and it may vary in intensity over a couple of days or weeks. If the cause of the delirium is alleviated, it may disappear for an extended period.

The **criteria** for delirium are as follows:

Criterion A	A disturbance in consciousness or attention
Criterion B	Develops over a short period of time and fluctuates throughout the day
Criterion C	Accompanied by changes in cognition
Criterion D	Not better explained by another condition
Criterion E	Caused by a medical condition or is substance related

Risk factors for delirium include but are not limited to older age, diabetes, underlying brain conditions (e.g., stroke), human immunodeficiency virus (HIV), renal impairment, and substance or medication withdrawal. Delirium may be caused by systemic infection or toxins, metabolic disorders, postoperative states, head trauma, and immobility.

There are **three types** of delirium:

- **Hyperactive**—increased psychomotor activity (e.g., agitation, restlessness)
- **Hypoactive**—decreased psychomotor activity (e.g., stupor, slowness, extreme fatigue)
- **Mixed**—normal or rapidly changing psychomotor activity

Differential diagnoses for delirium include malingering or factitious disorder, other neurocognitive disorders, acute stress disorder, psychotic disorder, bipolar disorders, and major depressive disorder.

MAJOR NEUROCOGNITIVE DISORDER

Individuals with major neurocognitive disorder find it difficult to independently manage activities of daily living due to a **substantial decline** in cognitive functioning. Clinicians can better understand a client's cognitive functioning from informant reports, such as those received from significant others, family members, or caretakers. The impairment can also be determined by a comprehensive clinical assessment, such as the Mini-Mental State Examination, or standardized testing, including the Montreal Cognitive Assessment. This diagnosis cannot occur in the presence of delirium or must not be better explained by another mental disorder.

Individuals with major neurocognitive disorder exhibit **cognitive deficits**, including memory impairment, aphasia, apraxia, agnosia, or impaired executive functioning. Depending on the etiology of the neurocognitive disorders, these deficits may remain stable or may become progressively worse. There may be a decrease in

language skills, specifically manifested in an inability to recall the names of people or things. Individuals may also need help performing routine motor programs, and they may be unable to recognize familiar people and places. Abstract thinking, planning, and initiating complex behaviors may also be challenging.

MILD NEUROCOGNITIVE DISORDER

The diagnosis of mild neurocognitive disorder is marked by a **modest decline** in cognitive functioning. Individuals with mild neurocognitive disorder exhibit moderate difficulty with memory, planning, organization, attention, learning, or processing social cues. However, these difficulties are often managed with the use of **compensatory strategies,** such as keeping a written schedule, the use of mnemonics, assistance with organization, and related accommodations. Much like the diagnostic criteria for major neurocognitive disorder, the decline can be measured by an informant's report, a comprehensive clinical assessment, or standardized testing. The deficits cannot occur in the context of delirium, nor can they be better explained by another mental disorder.

Individuals with neurocognitive disorders, such as those caused by Alzheimer's disease, could have **anterograde** and **retrograde amnesia,** meaning that they find it difficult to learn new information and recall previously learned information. Clinicians must be careful when differentiating between other forms of amnesia, such as those caused by trauma, transient global amnesia, and dissociative amnesia. Other forms of amnesia will generally improve over time or when underlying causes are addressed. Delirium, major depressive disorder, and learning disorders also serve as differential diagnoses.

NEUROCOGNITIVE DISORDERS DUE TO ALZHEIMER'S DISEASE

The diagnosis of neurocognitive disorder due to Alzheimer's disease can be made in the presence of either:

- Evidence obtained through genetic testing, family history, or
- Evidence of (a) worsening memory and learning, combined with deficits in either attention, executive functioning, expressive or receptive language skills, perceptual motor skills, or socioemotional skills, (b) slowed symptom onset, and (c) symptoms that cannot be attributed to a mix of other mental or medical syndromes and disorders

STAGES OF ALZHEIMER'S DISEASE

Alzheimer's disease begins slowly and may take a long time to become noticeable. Mild neurocognitive disorder is associated with earlier stages of Alzheimer's disease, whereas later stages are associated with major neurocognitive disorder. The stages of Alzheimer's disease are as follows:

- **Stage 1** usually comprises the first 1–3 years of the condition. Mild anterograde amnesia is experienced, especially for declarative memories. Other symptoms include diminished visuospatial skills, indifference, irritability, sadness, and anomia.
- **Stage 2** occurs between 2 and 10 years post onset, with symptoms including retrograde amnesia, restlessness, delusions, aphasia, acalculia, ideomotor apraxia (the inability to translate an idea into movement), and a generally flat mood.
- **Stage 3** usually happens between 8 and 12 years post onset and is characterized by severely impaired intellectual functioning, apathy, limb rigidity, and urinary and fecal incontinence.

TREATMENT

Individuals with Alzheimer's disease have been shown to have significant **aluminum deposits** in brain tissues, a malfunctioning **immune system,** and a low level of **acetylcholine.** Drugs that increase cholinergic activity in the brain are useful for short periods of time, including **donepezil,** which is effective for individuals in all stages of the disease, and **rivastigmine** and **galantamine,** which are approved treatments for symptoms present in the earlier stages.

Nearly all individuals in the later stages of Alzheimer's disease will exhibit **neuropsychiatric symptoms,** including but not limited to depression, anhedonia, agitation, dysphagia, incontinence, and seizures. These symptoms can be treated with medication, family and caregiver support groups, psychoeducation, family therapy, and case management. In mild cases, recommendations may include diet and nutritional services, cardiovascular exercise, psychological counseling, and socialization.

NEUROCOGNITIVE DISORDERS DUE TO TRAUMATIC BRAIN INJURY (TBI)

The diagnosis of neurocognitive disorders due to TBI includes substantiated medical evidence of an impact to the head causing brain displacement. This trauma is coupled with symptoms that may include the following:

- Loss of consciousness
- Seizures
- Loss of sense of smell (i.e., anosmia)
- Tinnitus
- Difficulty expressing thoughts
- Headaches.
- Balance and movement problems
- Confusion
- Vertigo

Individuals with TBI may also experience behavioral and emotional difficulties, including depression, anxiety, irritability, agitation, and mood swings. Treatment for TBI varies based on the areas of the brain sustaining injuries. The condition may worsen without immediate treatment provided to target or prevent neuroinflammation and cerebral hypoxia.

NEUROCOGNITIVE DISORDERS DUE TO HUMAN IMMUNODEFICIENCY VIRUS (HIV) INFECTION

Human immunodeficiency virus (HIV) can underlie major and mild neurocognitive disorders. Symptoms of HIV include deficits in cognitive, motor, and emotional functioning, including forgetfulness, impaired attention, and decelerated mental and motor processes. Other symptoms of neurocognitive disorders due to HIV include poor concentration, apathy, social withdrawal, loss of initiative, tremor, clumsiness, trouble with problem solving, and blurred vision. Individuals with mild neurocognitive disorder may not exhibit language difficulties, whereas those with major neurocognitive disorders experience difficulties such as aphasia and difficulty with fluency. Informational recall may still be intact in mild conditions.

NEUROCOGNITIVE DISORDER DUE TO VASCULAR DISEASE

In order to be diagnosed with neurocognitive disorder due to **vascular disease**, the individual must have **cognitive impairment** and either focal neurological signs or laboratory evidence of cerebrovascular disease. **Distinguishing features** include deficits in complex attention and executive functioning, making it difficult to quickly process information, engage in problem solving, and plan ahead. **Focal neurological signs** may include exaggerated reflexes, weakness in the extremities, and gait abnormalities. Symptoms may gradually increase in severity.

Risk factors for vascular neurocognitive disorder are hypertension, diabetes, smoking, and atrial fibrillation. In some cases, an individual may be able to recover from neurocognitive disorder due to vascular disease. Stroke victims, for instance, will notice a great deal of improvement in the first 6 months after the cerebrovascular accident. Most of this improvement will be in their physical, rather than cognitive, symptoms.

NEUROCOGNITIVE DISORDER DUE TO HUNTINGTON'S DISEASE

Individuals with **Huntington's disease** experience an insidious onset coupled with a slowed symptom progression. Huntington's disease is caused by the degeneration of the gamma-aminobutyric acid-producing cells in the substantia nigra, basal ganglia, and cortex. This inherited disease typically appears between the ages of 30 and 40. The **affective symptoms** of Huntington's disease include irritability, depression, and apathy. After a while, these individuals also display **cognitive symptoms**, including forgetfulness and dementia. **Motor symptoms** may also begin to emerge, including fidgeting, clumsiness, athetosis (slow, writhing movements), and chorea (involuntary quick jerks). Because the affective symptoms appear in advance of the cognitive and motor symptoms, many people with Huntington's are misdiagnosed with depression. Individuals in the early stages of Huntington's are at risk for suicide, being aware of their impending deterioration, and will have the loss of impulse control associated with the disease.

NEUROCOGNITIVE DISORDER DUE TO PARKINSON'S DISEASE

The following symptoms are commonly associated with neurocognitive disorder due to **Parkinson's disease**:

- Bradykinesia (general slowness of movement)
- Resting tremor
- Stoic and unmoving facial expression
- Loss of coordination or balance
- Involuntary pill-rolling movement of the thumb and forefinger
- Akathisia (violent restlessness)

Nearly 50% of people with Parkinson's disease will experience symptoms of depression, and 40% will experience symptoms of anxiety. Parkinson's disease is characterized by a deficiency of **dopamine-producing cells** and the presence of **Lewy bodies** in the substantia nigra. Medications such as levodopa are used to treat the symptoms of Parkinson's by increasing the amount of dopamine in the brain. Carbidopa is a decarboxylase inhibitor that is used along with levodopa to help ease the side effects of nausea and vomiting.

Major and minor neurocognitive disorders may also be due to frontotemporal lobar degeneration, Lewy body disease, substance or medication use, another medical condition, and multiple other etiologies.

PERSONALITY DISORDERS

Personality disorders occur when an individual has developed personality traits so maladaptive and entrenched that they cause personal distress or interfere significantly with functioning. Each pattern of behavior, thinking, and mood is pervasive, lifelong, and inflexible. The following are the **criteria** for personality disorders:

Criterion A	Long-term pattern of maladaptive personality traits and behaviors that do not align with the individual's culture. These traits and behaviors will be found in at least two of the following areas: • Impulse control • Inappropriate emotional intensity or responses • Inappropriately interpreting people, events, and self • Inappropriate social functioning
Criterion B	The traits and behaviors are inflexible and exist despite changing social situations.
Criterion C	The traits and behaviors cause distress and impair functioning.
Criterion D	Onset was in adolescence or early adulthood and has been enduring.
Criterion E	The behaviors and traits are not due to another mental disorder.
Criterion F	The behaviors and traits are not due to a substance.

Personality disorders are **clustered** into three groups:

Cluster A (eccentric or odd)	**Cluster B** (dramatic or excessively emotional)	**Cluster C** (fear- or anxiety-based)
Paranoid	Antisocial	Avoidant
Schizoid	Borderline	Dependent
Schizotypal	Histrionic	Obsessive-compulsive
	Narcissistic	

Differential diagnoses for **cluster A personality disorders** include but are not limited to mental disorders with symptoms of psychosis (e.g., schizophrenia), other medical conditions, other personality disorders, ASD, neurodevelopmental disorders, substance use disorders, and bipolar disorders.

Differential diagnoses for **cluster B personality disorders** include other mental and medical disorders, substance use disorders, separation anxiety, depressive disorders, bipolar disorders, and other personality disorders.

Differential diagnoses for **cluster C personality disorders** include social anxiety disorder, hoarding disorder, agoraphobia, other personality disorders, OCD, substance use, and other mental and medical disorders.

PARANOID PERSONALITY DISORDER

Paranoid personality disorder is a pervasive pattern of distrust and suspiciousness involving a belief in the malicious intentions of others. The diagnosis of paranoid personality disorder is evidenced by at least four of the following symptoms:

- Suspicion of harm, exploitation, or deceit
- Preoccupation and doubts of others' trustworthiness
- Reluctance to confide in others
- Unwarranted suspicion of infidelity
- Belief that certain remarks or events have hidden meanings
- Holds grudges
- Belief that one's character is being attacked without evidence

SCHIZOID PERSONALITY DISORDER

Schizoid personality disorder is characterized by a pervasive lack of interest in relationships with others and a limited range of emotional expression in contacts with others. At least four of the following **symptoms** must be present:

- Avoidance of or displeasure in close relationships
- Always chooses solitude
- Little interest in sexual relationships
- Takes pleasure in few activities
- Indifference to praise or criticism
- Emotional coldness or detachment
- Lacks close friends except first-degree relatives

SCHIZOTYPAL PERSONALITY DISORDER

Schizotypal personality disorder is characterized by pervasive social deficits and oddities of cognition, perception, or behavior. Diagnosis requires at least five of the following symptoms:

- Erroneous belief that random occurrences are directed toward themselves (i.e., ideas of reference)
- Odd beliefs or superstition
- Lack of close relationships except with immediate family members
- Unusual thinking and speaking (e.g., loose associations, circumstantial thinking)
- Bodily illusions or odd sensory experiences
- Suspicious of others
- Social anxiety unabated in familiar social settings
- Inappropriate or constricted affect
- Peculiarities in behavior or appearance

ANTISOCIAL PERSONALITY DISORDER

Individuals with antisocial personality disorder display an overall disregard for the rights and feelings of others. To receive a diagnosis, the individual must have had a history of the disorder starting before age 15, be at least 18 years old, and display at least three of the following symptoms:

- Unlawful behavior and disregard for social norms
- Deceitfulness and a lack of candor
- Impulsivity
- Physical aggression
- Irresponsible behavior (e.g., failure to keep a job)
- Blatant disregard for the safety of themselves and others
- Lack of remorse for harm done to others

BORDERLINE PERSONALITY DISORDER

Borderline personality disorder is a pervasive pattern of instability in social relationships, self-image, and affect, coupled with marked impulsivity. A diagnosis of borderline personality disorder requires at least five of the following symptoms:

- Desperate attempts to escape feelings of abandonment
- Unstable and intense personal relationship that vacillates between admiration and devaluation
- Dramatic shifts in self-image
- Impulsivity (e.g., spending, substance misuse)
- Suicidal ideation or non-suicidal self-harm
- Emotional instability
- Feelings of loneliness, isolation, and emptiness
- Angry outbursts and physical aggression
- Fleeting episodes of stress-induced depersonalization or paranoia

> **Review Video: Borderline Personality Disorder**
> Visit mometrix.com/academy and enter code: 550801

HISTRIONIC PERSONALITY DISORDER

Histrionic personality disorder is a pervasive and lifelong pattern of excessive emotionality and attention-seeking behavior. To diagnose a person with histrionic personality disorder, at least five of the following symptoms must be present:

- Annoyance or discomfort when not receiving attention
- Inappropriate sexual provocation
- Rapidly shifting and shallow or incongruent emotional expression
- Vague and impressionistic speech
- Exaggerated and dramatic emotional expressions
- Easily influenced by others
- Believes casual relationships are more intimate than they are
- Uses one's personal appearance to seek attention

NARCISSISTIC PERSONALITY DISORDER

Narcissistic personality disorder is grandiose behavior along with a lack of empathy and a need for admiration. The individual must exhibit at least five of the following symptoms for diagnosis:

- Grandiosity and superiority
- Fantasies of their own power and beauty

- Belief in one's personal uniqueness
- Idealized sense of self and need for extreme admiration
- Entitled to favorable treatment
- Exploitation of others
- Lack of empathy or emotional reciprocity
- Envious of others or believes others are envious of them
- Arrogant behaviors

AVOIDANT PERSONALITY DISORDER

Avoidant personality disorder is a pervasive pattern of social inhibition, feelings of inadequacy, and hypersensitivity to negative evaluation. A person with avoidant personality disorder exhibits at least four of the following symptoms:

- Fearing or avoiding work or school activities that involve interpersonal contact
- Unwillingness to associate with any person who may withhold approval
- Preoccupation with concerns about being criticized or rejected
- Conception of self as socially inept, inferior, or unappealing to others
- Risk-averse or reluctant to engage in novel experiences due to a fear of embarrassment
- Does not reveal self in intimate relationships because of shame or ridicule
- Keeps to self in new situations due to feelings of inadequacy

DEPENDENT PERSONALITY DISORDER

Dependent personality disorder is excessive reliance on others as evidenced by clinging, extreme fear of separation from an attached figure, and submissive behavior. A diagnosis of dependent personality disorder requires at least five of the following symptoms:

- Difficulty making decisions and overreliance on others' advice
- Need for others to assume responsibility for significant aspects of one's life
- Fear that disagreeing with others may result in a loss of support and acceptance
- Lacks confidence for completing tasks on their own
- Feelings of helplessness or discomfort when alone
- Goes to great lengths to get support from others
- Immediately seeks new relationships when an old one ends
- Preoccupied with the thought of having to care for themselves

OBSESSIVE-COMPULSIVE PERSONALITY DISORDER

Obsessive-compulsive personality disorder is a persistent preoccupation with organization and mental or interpersonal control. At least four of the following symptoms are required for diagnosis of obsessive-compulsive personality disorder:

- Preoccupation with rules and details
- Perfectionism that interferes with progress
- Excessive devotion to work
- Counterproductive rigidity about beliefs and morality
- Inability to throw away old objects
- Reluctance to delegate authority to others
- Rigid or stubborn
- Hoards money without spending

PARAPHILIC DISORDERS

Paraphilic disorders are intense, recurrent urges, fantasies, and behaviors involving nonhuman objects, nonconsenting partners, or pain and suffering. For a paraphilia to move from a preference to a disorder, the behavior must cause harm, interpersonal difficulty, impairment, or distress to the person or the target of the paraphilia. Paraphilic disorders can be grouped into two primary categories: (1) courtship disorders and (2) disorders directed toward atypical targets.

Anomalous sexual preferences characterize **courtship disorders**. These distressing, unusual, or divergent courtship preferences include voyeuristic disorder (spying on the private lives of others), exhibitionistic disorder (exposing one's genitalia to unsuspecting persons), and frotteuristic disorder (rubbing against nonconsensual individuals). Courtship disorders also include algolagnic disorders, in which sexual gratification involves pain or humiliation (i.e., sexual masochism disorder and sexual sadism disorder).

Paraphilic disorders also include **disorders directed toward atypical targets**. This includes pedophilic disorder, in which children younger than age 13 are targeted. Disorders **directed toward** other anomalous targets include fetishistic disorder and transvestic disorder. Fetishistic disorder involves inanimate objects (e.g., shoes, underwear), while transvestic disorder involves cross-dressing, with both requiring sexual gratification to qualify as a disorder.

Differential diagnoses for paraphilic disorders include but are not limited to normative sexual preferences and desires, bipolar disorders, neurocognitive disorders, symptoms of another medical condition (e.g., multiple sclerosis), conversion disorder, conduct disorder, substance use disorder, schizophrenia, and social phobia.

Evidence-Based Practice

CLASSES OF EVIDENCE-BASED PRACTICE

Evidence-based practice is treatment based on the best possible evidence, including a study of current research. Literature is searched to find evidence of the most effective treatments for specific diseases or injuries, and those treatments are then utilized to create clinical pathways that outline specific multi-departmental treatment protocols, including medications, treatments, and timelines. Evidence-based guidelines are often produced by specialty organizations that undertake the task of searching and analyzing literature to produce policies, procedures, and guidelines that become the standard of care for the disease. These guidelines are then used when a patient fits the disease criteria for that guideline.

Evidence-based nursing aims to improve the quality of nursing care by examining the reasons for all nursing practices and determining those that have the most positive outcomes. Evidence-based nursing focuses on the individual nurse utilizing evidence-based observations to influence decision-making.

EVIDENCE-BASED PRACTICE GUIDELINES

The creation of evidence-based practice guidelines includes the following components:

- **Focus on the topic/methodology:** This includes outlining possible interventions and treatments for review, choosing patient populations and settings, and determining significant outcomes. Search boundaries (such as types of journals, types of studies, dates of studies) should be determined.
- **Evidence review:** This includes review of literature, critical analysis of studies, and summarizing of results, including pooled meta-analysis.
- **Expert judgment:** Recommendations based on personal experience from a number of experts may be utilized, especially if there is inadequate evidence based on review, but this subjective evidence should be explicitly acknowledged.
- **Policy considerations:** This includes cost-effectiveness, access to care, insurance coverage, availability of qualified staff, and legal implications.
- **Policy:** A written policy must be completed with recommendations. Common practice is to utilize letter guidelines, with "A" being the most highly recommended, usually based on the quality of supporting evidence.
- **Review:** The completed policy should be submitted to peers for review and comments before instituting the policy.

CRITICAL PATHWAYS

Clinical/critical pathway development is done by those involved in direct patient care. The pathway should require no additional staffing and cover the entire scope of an illness. Steps include:

1. Selection of patient group and diagnosis, procedures, or conditions, based on analysis of data and observations of wide variance in approach to treatment and prioritizing organization and patient needs
2. Creation of interdisciplinary team of those involved in the process of care, including physicians to develop pathway
3. Analysis of data including literature review and study of best practices to identify opportunities for quality improvement
4. Identification of all categories of care, such as nutrition, medications, and nursing
5. Discussion and reaching consensus
6. Identifying the levels of care and number of days to be covered by the pathway
7. Pilot testing and redesigning steps as indicated
8. Educating staff about standards
9. Monitoring and tracking variances in order to improve pathways

LEVELS OF EVIDENCE IN EVIDENCE-BASED PRACTICE

Levels of evidence are categorized according to the scientific evidence available to support the recommendations, as well as existing state and federal laws. While recommendations are voluntary, they are often used as a basis for state and federal regulations.

- **Category IA** is well supported by evidence from experimental, clinical, or epidemiologic studies and is strongly recommended for implementation.
- **Category IB** has supporting evidence from some studies, has a good theoretical basis, and is strongly recommended for implementation.
- **Category IC** is required by state or federal regulations or is an industry standard.
- **Category II** is supported by suggestive clinical or epidemiologic studies, has a theoretical basis, and is suggested for implementation.
- **Category III** is supported by descriptive studies, such as comparisons, correlations, and case studies, and may be useful.
- **Category IV** is obtained from expert opinion or authorities only.
- **Unresolved** means there is no recommendation because of a lack of consensus or evidence.

OUTCOME EVALUATION

Outcome evaluation is an important component of evidence-based practice, which involves both internal and external research. All treatments are subjected to review to determine if they produce positive outcomes, and policies and protocols for outcome evaluation should be in place. **Outcome evaluation** includes the following:

- **Monitoring** over the course of treatment involves careful observation and record-keeping that notes progress, with supporting laboratory and radiographic evidence as indicated by condition and treatment.
- **Evaluating** results includes reviewing records as well as current research to determine if outcomes are within acceptable parameters.
- **Sustaining** involves discontinuing treatment but continuing to monitor and evaluate.
- **Improving** means to continue the treatment but with additions or modifications in order to improve outcomes.
- **Replacing** the treatment with a different treatment must be done if outcome evaluation indicates that current treatment is ineffective.

EVIDENCE-BASED NURSING INTERVENTIONS

Evidence-based nursing interventions enable nurses to provide high-quality patient care that is based upon research and knowledge, as opposed to giving care that is based upon tradition or information that is out of date. An evidence-based nursing approach is based on the integration of practical clinical experience with medical and clinical research; it utilizes proven clinical guidelines and assessment practices. Evidence-based nursing interventions allow nurses to make patient care decisions based on cutting-edge research that has been scientifically validated. Studies show that evidence-based nursing practice yields improved patient outcomes, enables nurses to practice up-to-date methods, improves nurse confidence and decision-making skills, and enhances Joint Commission standards.

RESOURCES

There are numerous information resources for evidence-based nursing interventions. These resources include evidence-based textbooks; databases such as CINAHL Plus, COCHRANE library, Mosby's Nursing Index, NursingConsult, and Nursing@Ovid; evidence-based nursing metasites such as the Academic Center for EBN, Joanna Briggs Institute, McGill University, ONS-EBN section, and EBN-University of Minnesota; online evidence-based nursing journals such as Clinical Nurse Specialist, Clinical Nursing Research, Evidence-Based Nursing, Journal of Nursing Care Quality, Journal of Advanced Nursing, Journal of Nursing Scholarship, Nurse

Researcher, Nursing Research, Western Journal of Nursing Research, and Worldviews on Evidence-Based Nursing; and various online tutorials.

OBTAINING RESULTS OF RESEARCH TO USE IN EVIDENCE-BASED PRACTICE

When searching for **current evidence** in print and online literature, the nurse should look for **systematic reviews, analyses, and reports**. PUBMED lists all literature and can be searched for all published articles on a particular subject. These articles can be analyzed to determine treatments that have the best evidence of efficacy. Subject and methodological terms and clinical filters can be used to find necessary information, including a specific medical subject heading (MH), subheading (SH), publication type (PT), and text word (TW). The nurse should also search the National Guideline Clearinghouse, Cochrane Databases, Agency for Healthcare Research and Quality, and US Preventive Services Task Force Recommendations for evidence and guidelines. When trials of a treatment provide evidence of effectiveness, the evidence is weighed for strength and confidence. Those that provide the strongest evidence of efficacy become recommendations and guidelines for use in the field. Research is also done on a smaller scale by specialists who publish in peer-reviewed journals their research results related to the use of a particular intervention.

Treatment Planning

SMART Technique for Goal Setting

Treatment planning is an ongoing endeavor that includes evaluation and goal setting in order to determine what path the individual wants to take as part of recovery. The nurse should develop both short-term and long-term goals with the patient, determining where the person wants to be at a point in the future, such as in 5 years. One way to determine goals and establish a plan is to utilize the SMART technique:

- **Specific**: Identifies concrete actions and desired results
- **Measurable**: Can be objectively determined to be met or not met
- **Achievable**: Is appropriate for person's abilities and situation
- **Relevant**: Pertains to a matter of importance to the patient
- **Time-based**: Has a clear time frame in view

> **Review Video: Plan of Care**
> Visit mometrix.com/academy and enter code: 300570
>
> **Review Video: SMART Goals**
> Visit mometrix.com/academy and enter code: 100378

Development of Patient Outcomes

Patient outcomes are a description of the patient's response to nursing interventions. The **outcome statement** describes what is expected and is stated in exact measurable terms. Nursing diagnosis and interventions are linked to the outcome statement. This association allows for the documentation and measurement of the effectiveness of the nursing intervention over time. Outcomes can be the actual patient response or the status of a diagnosis. Through evaluation of patient outcomes, measurable evidence is created on which nursing practice can be based. The overall goal of outcome measurement is to provide quality patient care.

Psychiatric and Mental Health Programs

A variety of **psychiatric and mental health programs** are available and should be evaluated when planning treatment, according to the needs of the individual patient.

- **Inpatient programs** provide a secure environment and comprehensive care, often with psychologists, psychiatrists, occupational therapists, social workers, and other allied health personnel. Programs may be tailored to one specific type of patient (e.g., criminally insane, substance abusers) or to a general population. They may offer short-term or long-term care.
- **Outpatient programs** provide assessment and treatment, such as group therapy, cognitive-behavioral therapy, and family therapy. Programs may be community-based, targeting specific groups of people, such as alcoholics or the homeless.
- **Partial/day hospitalization programs** provide daily inpatient care during prescribed hours (e.g., 8 a.m. to 3 p.m.) as well as outpatient services. The stay is usually short-term (1-2 weeks) and may serve as a transition from inpatient to outpatient care.

Therapeutic Frameworks

HISTORICAL IMPACT ON THERAPEUTIC INTERVENTIONS

Therapeutic interventions require the use of foundational models incorporating philosophy, theory, and practice methodologies. The disadvantage of applying past solutions is their tendency to hinder the application of unconventional solutions not found in old psychotherapy treatment manuals. Unconventional solutions may work for the individual who has not had success with a conventional method, though it may have previously worked for another patient. Mental health care has undergone a progressive development throughout time. Therapeutic trends have become part of the accepted model for mental health care. Institutions of the past have been replaced with community treatment centers that have had an innovative impact on mental health. Treatments have become more **psychologically based** as patients' surroundings have become a factor. Psychologically-trained and educationally-trained counselors have begun to specialize.

COUNSELING VS. PSYCHOTHERAPY

Some practitioners use the terms counseling and psychotherapy interchangeably to indicate the same service. However, those practitioners who believe these terms are not identical state the difference lies in the class of client that receives treatment. Other substantive differences in terminology include: the kind of therapy received, degree and nature of illness, clinical work setting or environment in which treatment is received, and the training received by the therapist. **Counseling** is a treatment that allows the client to express emotions while the therapist provides support, education, and feedback. However, **psychotherapy** is a remediation process that involves getting to the root cause of the problem. Neither counselor nor psychotherapist can make these divisions in treatment, as there is a distinctive overlap when talking with the patient.

COGNITIVE-BEHAVIORAL THERAPY

Cognitive-behavioral therapy (CBT) focuses on the impact that thoughts have on behavior and feelings and encourages the individual to use the power of **rational thought** to alter perceptions and behavior. This approach to counseling is usually short-term, about twelve to twenty sessions, with the first sessions used to obtain a history, the middle sessions used to focus on problems, and last sessions used to review and reinforce. Individuals are assigned "homework" during the sessions to practice new ways of thinking and to develop new coping strategies. The therapist helps the individual identify **goals** and then find ways to achieve those goals. CBT acknowledges that all problems cannot be resolved, but one can deal differently with problems. The therapist asks many questions to determine the individual's areas of concern and encourages the individual to question his or her own motivations and needs. CBT is goal-centered so each counseling session is structured toward a particular goal, such as coping techniques. CBT centers on the concept of unlearning previous behaviors and learning new ones, questioning behaviors, and doing homework. Different approaches to CBT include Aaron Beck's cognitive therapy, rational emotive behavior therapy, and dialectic behavior therapy.

COGNITIVE-BEHAVIORAL GROUP THERAPY FOR SOCIAL PHOBIAS

Cognitive-behavioral group therapy (CBGT) for social phobias is a form of **exposure therapy** done in a group environment, usually limited to about six patients with one or (preferably) two therapists to monitor and guide group exercises. Having an equal mix of men and women is preferred because social phobias often involve male-female interactions. Patients with different types of fears are appropriate for the group because they complement each other during therapy. The initial sessions involve psychoeducation about phobias and basic instruction in cognitive restructuring, including identifying automatic thoughts and discussing how they are errors in thinking. During exercises, such as speaking in front of the group, patients are asked to express their automatic thoughts and discuss them. The **subjective units of distress rating scale** (0–10 scale of distress) is used throughout exercises with patients giving their score every minute. Each patient is provided with individualized homework. Sessions are usually weekly for 2–3 hours for 12–24 weeks.

PERSONAL SCIENCE

Personal Science was developed in 1977 by Michael Mahoney, based on the cognitive-behavioral (CB) approach. The acronym SCIENCE is used to explain the sequential steps through which the therapist guides the patient to solve a problem:

- **S** for *specification* of the problem
- **C** for *collection* of data or facts
- **I** for *identification* of patterns or reasons for existing behaviors
- **E** for *examination* of choices that can be used to modify behavior
- **N** for *narrowing* the options and experimenting with possible modifications
- **C** for *comparing* data or facts
- **E** for *expanding*, modifying, or substituting unwanted behaviors

PSYCHOBEHAVIORAL THERAPY AND COGNITIVE-CLIENT THERAPY

Psychobehavioral therapy was developed in 1971 by George E. Woody. This is simply a combination of two psychoanalytic and behavioral techniques with a variety of eclectic approaches. Psychobehavioral therapy is based on the cognitive-behavioral (CB) approach.

Cognitive-client therapy was a cognitive-affective (CA) model designed by David Wexler in 1974. He used **information processing theory** as the foundation for his beliefs concerning cognitive roles. Wexler postulated that client-centered therapy was better established by combining affective experience with cognitive thoughts. Wexler's belief was similar to those of the cognitive-behaviorists. He believed that the client could gain control over his or her behavior through cognitive deliberations. Wexler also believed that emotional experiencing could not be accomplished without a forerunner of cognitive thought processes.

ACCEPTANCE AND COMMITMENT THERAPY

Acceptance and commitment therapy (ACT) is a "third wave" of CBT that emphasizes contextual and experiential learning through psychological flexibility. Rather than avoiding or changing dysfunctional thoughts, clients are taught to observe them without judgment or resistance. ACT uses six core processes to help clients develop psychological flexibility:

- **Cognitive defusion:** This involves detaching from thoughts their personally ascribed meanings and undesirable functions.
- **Acceptance:** This process allows thoughts, emotions, and sensations to exist without attempting to change their content or frequency.
- **Self as context:** This involves fostering an understanding that the client's thoughts do not define them.
- **Contact with the present moment:** This involves fully experiencing sensations, thoughts, and feelings while adopting an objective, nonjudgemental perspective of the here and now.
- **Values:** Therapists help clients understand that values are ongoing, dynamic, and constantly evolving principles that guide them toward living a purposeful and meaningful life.
- **Committed action:** This process involves taking proactive steps toward leading a value-driven life by integrating all five core processes into sustained behavioral change.

AARON BECK'S COGNITIVE THERAPY

Aaron Beck discovered that during psychotherapy patients often had a second set of thoughts while undergoing "free association." Beck called these **automatic thoughts**, which were labeled and interpreted, according to a personal set of rules. Beck called dysfunctional automatic thoughts **cognitive disorders**. Beck identified a triad of negative thoughts regarding the self, the environment, and the world. The key concepts in **Aaron Beck's cognitive therapy** include the following:

- **Therapist/patient relationship**: Therapy is a collaborative partnership. The goal of therapy is determined together. The therapist encourages the patient to disagree when appropriate.

- **Process of therapy:** The therapist explains the following: the perception of reality is not reality. The interpretation of sensory input depends on cognitive processes. The patient is taught to recognize maladaptive ideation, identifying observable behavior, underlying motivation, and his or her thoughts and beliefs. The patient practices distancing the maladaptive thoughts, explores his or her conclusions, and tests them against reality.
- **Conclusions:** The patient makes the rules less extreme and absolute, drops false rules, and substitutes adaptive rules.

ERIC BERNE'S TRANSACTIONAL ANALYSIS

The major concepts of **transactional analysis** according to Eric Berne are:

- **Ego State:** One's personal frame of mind
- **Parent:** Parents who exhibit feelings/behaviors learned from their parents, which may be nurturing or critical
- **Adult:** An individual who exhibits feelings/behaviors of a mature adult
- **Child:** An individual who exhibits feelings/behaviors natural to children under seven years old
- **Transaction:** Verbal and nonverbal communication between two people
- **Complementary transactions:** A message sent from the ego state of Person A which is responded to in that same ego state, or a message sent to the ego state of Person B which is responded to in that same ego state
- **Crossed transactions:** A message sent from the ego state of Person A which is responded to in another ego state, or a message sent to the ego state of Person B which is responded to from another ego state
- **Ulterior transactions:** messages that occur on two levels, the social or overt level and the hidden or psychological level

BEHAVIORISM

Behaviorists anticipate that the patient can unlearn dysfunctional behaviors. Pavlov cultivated his theories from experiments where he conditioned dogs to salivate to different stimuli. Watson and Rayner experimented on a young boy by conditioning his response to white, furry animals, causing the boy to develop a phobia. This can be related to a person's development of a phobia after a negative experience. Some people become afraid of the water after a near drowning experience. Addictive cravings, anxieties, insomnia, and pain management may be improved with relaxation training and methodical desensitization techniques. B. F. Skinner's experiments involved operant conditioning, where he proposed that feelings and actions are reinforced and rewarded. Therefore, the way to stop a behavior is to take away the reinforcement. For example, a child who exhibits misbehaviors in school may be doing so to gain the teacher's attention.

OPERANT CONDITIONING

Operant conditioning is based on feelings and actions that are reinforced and rewarded. The way to stop the behavior is to take away the reinforcement. An explanation for a client's pathological behavior is that it was reinforced. Behaviorists look for rewards that may cause their client to act out inappropriately. For example, a person who feels isolated may experience health problems out of a need to gain attention from hospital staff and or family. Token economy and contingency contractual agreements are the result of operant conditioning. Albert Bandura created **social learning theory** in 1969, based on people learning from watching others. Violence on television has been linked to real life violent acts by social learning theory. Proponents say a more functional TV model should be presented to replace the pathological behavior. Behaviorists use relaxation techniques, imagery, systematic desensitization, reinforcement contingencies, positive role modeling, and token economies.

ALBERT ELLIS'S RATIONAL EMOTIVE THERAPY

Key concepts of **Albert Ellis's rational emotive therapy** include the idea that people control their own destinies and interpret events, according to their own values and beliefs.

Forms of irrational beliefs include:

- Something is awful or terrible
- One cannot tolerate something
- Something or someone is damned or cursed

"Musturbatory" ideologies have three forms:

- I must do well and win approval or I am a rotten person.
- You must act kindly toward me or you are a rotten person.
- My life must remain comfortable or life hardly seems worth living.

Therapy consists of detecting and eradicating irrational beliefs, as follows:

- **Disputing**: Detecting irrationalities, debating them, discriminating between logical and illogical thinking, and defining what helps create new beliefs
- **Debating**: Questioning and disputing the irrational beliefs
- **Discriminating**: Distinguishing between wants and needs, desires and demands, and rational and irrational ideas
- **Defining**: Defining words and redefining beliefs

RATIONAL BEHAVIOR THERAPY

Rational behavior therapy was developed in 1977 by Maxie C. Maultsby, Jr. It is a more direct method of dealing with a patient's emotional state than Ellis' rational emotive therapy from the mid-1950's. Maultsby was Albert Ellis' student. Rational behavior is based on the cognitive-behavioral (CB) approach and has five steps, known as **emotional re-education**:

1. **Self-analysis** using rational thought helps the patient to gain intellectual insights.
2. **Changing actions** or behaviors to reflect newly gained intellectual insights.
3. **Cognitive emotive dissonance** is a refocus of attention that helps the patient bring feelings and thought patterns into alignment with each other.
4. **Rationalized feelings** promote cohesive thought patterns through consistent emotional insights.
5. **Habitual practice** of newly gained insights develops new personality traits in the patient.

MULTIMODAL BEHAVIOR THERAPY

Multimodal Behavior Therapy was invented in 1971 by Arnold Lazarus. This is a complex system that mingles client-conceptualization theories into all the human modalities of cognition, affect, and behavior that cannot be excluded from a patient's everyday life. Lazarus believed that there were exactly seven modalities. He used the acronym **BASIC ID** to explain each one:

- **B** for *behavior*
- **A** for *affect*
- **S** for *sensory*
- **I** for *imagery*
- **C** for *cognition*
- **I** for *intrapersonal*
- **D** for *drugs*

Multimodal Behavior Therapy has no guide for which technique to choose for treatment, no set therapy process, or sequential steps to take. Multimodal Behavior Therapy identifies a theme, and then the therapist utilizes the BASIC ID techniques for treating the patient.

> **Review Video: <u>Multimodal Behavior Therapy</u>**
> Visit mometrix.com/academy and enter code: 813824

RECOVERY MODEL

The **Recovery Model** approach to mental health shifts control of treatment options to the **patient** rather than the physician deciding the plan of care. This has been effective in those patients who have the capacity to make decisions to allow them to be more independent and take a more active role in the decision-making regarding their treatment plan. The goal of this model is to allow the patient to be more **autonomous** so that they may achieve the ultimate goals of finding employment and housing and living independently. The more independent the patient can become, the more they progress to making independent decisions about the treatment of their mental health issues. This model is not appropriate for those patients who are so incapacitated by their illness that they do not understand they are ill. The amount of independence and decision-making that is turned over to the patient should increase as they become more stable.

PHYSIOLOGICAL FOUNDATION FOR PSYCHOTHERAPY

The **physiological foundation for psychotherapy** is gaining momentum as research in this area advances. Biopsychological research is based on the notion that biological systems in the body are linked to human behaviors. Prescription drugs are used to alter brain chemistry to help the patient cope with imbalances in their biological systems. An alternative or supplement to drug therapy is exercise that releases endorphins and helps the patient to decrease feelings of depression. In the past, the person receiving psychological treatment was treated more like a casualty who was responsible for his or her own injured state. The mental health provider held to the belief that the patient's mental state, shortfalls involving relationships, and maladaptive behaviors were at the root of the patient's mental disorder.

ORGANIZATIONAL MODELS FOR PSYCHOECOLOGICAL DELIVERY

The **organizational models for psychoecological delivery** were identified by Seay in 1983. Care can be delivered through direct preventive interventions, remedial, or aftercare systems.

- **Direct preventive interventions** are the primary delivery target.
- **Remedial care** is the secondary delivery target.
- **Aftercare** is tertiary prevention.

These five areas are addressed:

- Residential
- Community
- Educational
- Business and political arenas
- The private sector

Services offered include:

- Individual psychotherapy
- Group psychotherapy
- Family psychotherapy
- Educational courses
- Synchronization of services
- Restructuring the patient's surroundings
- Making contacts within the community
- Advocacy
- Referral
- Ongoing professional instruction and training
- Psychodiagnostics
- Research and assessment
- Financial support

The model contains:

- Counseling/psychotherapy
- Marriage counseling services
- Family counseling services
- Drug and alcohol therapy
- Environmental restructuring
- Funding
- Community health centers
- Other approaches

This model should correct some of the organization deficiencies that are currently part of the mental health provider system.

TRAUMA-INFORMED CARE

Trauma-informed care acts on the premise that many individuals have experienced some sort of trauma, and therefore every patient should be approached with sensitivity and care. Traumatic events are deeply individualized, and what may have been traumatic to one individual, may not be to the next. Withholding judgment of what qualifies as trauma is imperative for the psychiatric-mental health nurse.

The five elements of trauma-informed care include the following:

- **Safety**: Ensuring that the patient feels emotionally and physically safe must be the first priority in order to create a conducive environment for treatment.
- **Choice**: Treatment cannot be forced and must honor the individual's right to choose.
- **Collaboration**: The patient and the nurse must work collaboratively through shared decision-making.
- **Trustworthiness**: The patient must trust the nurse in order for treatment to be effective. Trustworthiness can be established by communicating what is happening and what will happen next to the patient.
- **Empowerment**: Empower the patient with tools to cope on their own so that their recovery extends outside the walls of treatment.

PARENT-CHILD INTERACTION THERAPY

Parent-child interaction therapy (PCIT) is designed for preschool children with conduct disorder or oppositional defiant disorder. Sessions are usually 1 hour a week for 10–16 weeks. The therapist observes the parent-child interaction from outside the room (usually with a two-way mirror) and provides feedback. PCIT has two phases:

- **Child-directed interaction:** Parents learn specific skills to use when engaging children in free play, including reflecting a child's statements and describing and praising appropriate behavior while ignoring undesirable behavior. The goal is to strengthen the parent–child bond and eliminate undesirable behavior.
- **Parent-directed interaction:** During this phase, positive behaviors are increased and undesirable behaviors are decreased. Parents learn to give clear commands, provide consistent reinforcement, and use time out for noncompliance.

INCREDIBLE YEARS PROGRAM

The **Incredible Years program** for conduct disorder and oppositional defiant disorder has both a child (ages 4–7) and a parent component:

- **Child:** "Dinosaur school" is a group of children (about six children) who attend 2-hour weekly sessions for about 17 weeks. Videos and life-sized puppets are used to demonstrate ways of dealing with interpersonal problems, such as making friends, empathizing, coping with teasing, and resolving conflicts. Children practice social skills and are rewarded for positive social skills. Parents receive weekly updates and are asked to reward children for positive social skills.
- **Parent:** Parents meet in groups (about ten parents) for 2-hour sessions for 22 weeks. Parents view seventeen videos modeling appropriate methods for dealing with problem behavior and discuss them in the group. Parents learn to initiate nonthreatening play sessions, use positive reinforcement and consistent limit-setting, and learn strategies for dealing with problem behavior, such as time-outs.

PSST AND PMT

Problem-solving skills training (PSST) is designed for children 7-13 years old to address antisocial behavior, conduct disorder, and oppositional defiant disorder. Parents of these children can take a **parent management training (PMT)** course simultaneously.

- **PSST:** Children attend 50-minute individual weekly sessions for 25 weeks. The therapist presents problem situations similar to those faced by the child and then helps the child to evaluate the situation, develop goals, and alternate goals for dealing with these situations. As homework, children are assigned "super solver" tasks in which they use skills learned in therapy in real-life situations. Parents learn to assist the child in using new strategies.
- **PMT:** Parents attend a total of 16 sessions of 2 hours each over a period of 6-8 months. Parents learn techniques for managing their child's behavior, such as reinforcement, shaping, and time-outs. The therapist uses a variety of teaching methods, including instruction, modeling, and role-playing.

CONDITION-SPECIFIC THERAPEUTIC APPROACHES
HABIT REVERSAL THERAPY FOR IMPULSE CONTROL DISORDERS

Habit reversal therapy (HRT), a form of cognitive-behavioral therapy, is used to help people with tic disorders and for those with impulse control disorders, such as trichotillomania. A number of steps are involved, which are listed below.

- **Awareness:** The patient must pay attention, as behaviors are often unconscious. This often involves keeping a detailed log of the behavior, including time, duration, activity during the episode, and emotional state before, during, and after these behaviors.
- **Identification of Triggers:** The log and patient interviews help to identify triggers to help patients understand when they are at risk of the behavior and how to use stimulus control to prevent the behavior or to avoid triggers.

- **Assessment**: The patient begins to identify feelings (negative or positive) associated with the behavior and the reason for it.
- **Competitive response**: The patient carries out another action to compete with the urge to carry out the behavior, thereby preventing it.
- **Assessment of Rationalizations**: The patient must confront the rationalizations used to allow the behavior to continue.
- **Mindfulness**: The patient learns that it is not necessary to give in to the urge to carry out the behavior as urges often are of short duration.

THERAPY OPTIONS FOR OBSESSIVE-COMPULSIVE DISORDER

Therapy for obsessive-compulsive disorder aims to develop expression of thoughts and impulses in a manner that is appropriate:

Behavioral therapy (most successful):

- Combined exposure with training to delay obsessive responses; best used in conjunction with pharmacotherapy
- Steady decrease of rituals by exposure to anxiety-producing situations until patient has learned to control the related obsessive compulsion
- Reduction of obsessive thoughts by the use of reminders or noxious stimuli to stop chain-of-thought patterns, such as snapping a rubber band on the wrist when obsessive thoughts occur

Family therapy (primary issues):

- Helping the family to avoid situations that trigger OCD response
- Pointing out the tendency of family members to reassure the patient, which is apt to support the obsession
- Introducing family strategies, which involve the following:
  - Remaining neutral and not reinforcing through encouragement
  - Avoiding trying to reason logically with the patient

Pharmacologic therapy (FDA-approved medications for OCD):

- Clomipramine (Anafranil)
- Sertraline (Zoloft)
- Paroxetine (Paxil)
- Fluoxetine (Prozac)
- Fluvoxamine (Luvox)

EXPOSURE AND RESPONSE/RITUAL PREVENTION

Exposure and response/ritual prevention (ERP) is a type of therapy used to treat obsessive-compulsive disorder (OCD). ERP helps the patient learn to reduce anxiety by not performing ritualistic behavior. The goal is to habituate the person to the anxiety associated with an act so that it lessens and the ritual stops. Steps include the following:

1. **Psychoeducation**: ERP begins with education about the nature of OCD and ritualistic behavior.
2. **Ritual/fear analysis**: Fact-finding may be carried out in one or two sessions, during which a fear hierarchy is outlined regarding obsessional material starting with those that cause low anxiety and building to those that cause extremely high anxiety.

3. **Exposure and response/ritual prevention**: Exposure begins with small steps. For example, if a person is obsessed with germs, a first step might be to touch a tissue that touched a toothpick that touched a dirty tissue. The response/ritual prevention part is to avoid washing hands after touching the tissue. This may be done repeatedly to desensitize the person before moving to a high-anxiety item on the fear hierarchy.

THERAPY FOR PTSD

Individuals with **post-traumatic stress disorder (PTSD)** are usually treated with antidepressants, mood stabilizers, or antipsychotic drugs, depending on their symptoms, but one of the following therapies is essential:

- **Cognitive-behavioral therapy (CBT)**: Individuals learn to confront trauma through psychoeducation, breathing, imaginary reliving, and writing; they are taught to recognize thoughts related to their trauma and attempt a method of coping, such as distraction and self-soothing.
- **Eye-movement desensitization and reprocessing**: This form of CBT requires the individual to talk about the experience of trauma while keeping the eyes and attention focused on the therapist's rapidly moving finger. (There is no clear evidence this is more effective than standard CBT.)
- **Family therapy**: PTSD impacts the entire family, so counseling and classes in anger management, parenting, and conflict resolution may help reduce family conflict related to the PTSD.
- **Sleep therapy**: Individuals may fear sleeping because of severe nightmares. Sleep therapy teaches methods to cope with nightmares through imagery rehearsal therapy and relaxation techniques.

PSYCHOEDUCATION FOR BIPOLAR DISORDER AND SCHIZOPHRENIA

Psychoeducation, often part of cognitive-behavioral therapy, involves teaching individuals about their disease to help them manage symptoms and behavior.

- **Bipolar disorder**: Individuals are taught to understand the patterns of their disease and the triggers of mood changes so they can seek appropriate medical help. Additionally, they are taught to use self-monitoring tools, such as a daily record, to determine patterns of activity, such as sleeping, so they can maintain as consistent a schedule of eating, sleeping, and engaging in physical activities as possible; consistency tends to reduce unstable mood swings.
- **Schizophrenia**: Individuals must be taught about their disease and the effects of medications. Because medication may not eliminate all symptoms, such as hearing voices, individuals are taught methods to test reality to determine if their perceptions are correct.

DIALECTICAL BEHAVIORAL THERAPY FOR BORDERLINE PERSONALITY DISORDER

Dialectical behavioral therapy was developed for the treatment of patients with **borderline personality disorder (BPD)**. In therapy, the nurse/therapist helps patients to change behavior by replacing **dichotomous thinking** that paints the world as black or white with rational (dialectical) thinking. This therapy is based on the premise that patients with BPD lack the ability to self-regulate, have a low tolerance for stress, and encounter social and environmental factors that impact their behavioral skills. Therapy includes the following:

- **Cognitive-behavioral therapy** (once a week) focuses on adaptive behaviors that help the patient to deal with stress or trauma. Therapy focuses on a prioritized list of problems: suicidal behavior, behavior that interferes with therapy, quality of life issues, post-traumatic stress response, respect for self, acquisition of behavioral skills, and patient goals.
- **Group therapy** (2.5 hours a week) helps the patient learn behavioral skills, such as self-distracting and soothing.

MOTIVATIONAL ENHANCEMENT THERAPY FOR SUBSTANCE ABUSE

Motivational enhancement therapy (MET) is a nonconfrontational, structured approach to treatment for substance abuse that is usually done in four sessions. MET helps motivate the patient to change, accept responsibility for change, and remain committed to change. The MET therapist guides the patient through different stages of change:

1. **Pre-contemplation**: Patient does not wish to change behavior.
2. **Contemplation**: Patient considers positive and negative aspects of drug or alcohol use.
3. **Determination**: Patient makes a decision to change.
4. **Action**: Patient begins to modify behavior over time (2–6 months).
5. **Maintenance**: Patient remains abstinent.
6. **Relapse**: Patient begins the cycle again. Relapses are common.

The therapist questions, compliments, and supports the patient but avoids criticizing, labeling, or directly advising the patient. Patients, especially those who have failed previous attempts to stop using, require much encouragement. A pretreatment assessment is completed, and the patient is provided with a written report at the first meeting. The therapist uses eight strategies during sessions:

- Eliciting statements of self-motivation
- Listening empathetically
- Questioning
- Providing feedback
- Providing affirmation
- Handling or preventing resistance by reflecting, amplifying, or changing focus
- Reframing
- Summarizing

VISUALIZATION TO TREAT ANXIETY DISORDERS

Visualization (therapeutic imagery) is used to treat **anxiety disorders** primarily for relaxation, stress reduction, and performance improvement. Visualization may be used in conjunction with many other types of therapy, such as exposure therapy, which can be very stressful for some people. Visualization strives to create a visual image of a desired outcome in the mind of the patient when he or she imagines himself or herself in that place or situation. Intense concentration helps to block feelings of anxiety. For example, if the focus is on reducing anxiety, the mind focuses on that goal of therapy. All of the senses (e.g., looks, smells, feelings, sounds) may be used to imagine the feeling of relaxation in a certain place.

SINGLE-SESSION THERAPY

Single-session therapy is the **most frequent form of counseling** because individuals often attend only one session for various reasons even if more are advised. Individuals may not have insurance or believe that one session is sufficient. Sessions typically last 1 hour. The goal is to identify a problem and reach a solution in one session. The therapist serves as a facilitator to motivate the individual to view the problem as part of a pattern that can be changed and to identify a solution. The therapist may use a wide range of techniques that culminates in a **plan for the individual** (e.g., homework exercises) so the individual can begin to make changes.

SOLUTION-FOCUSED THERAPY

Solution-focused therapy aims to differentiate methods that are effective from those that are not, and to identify areas of strengths so they can be used in problem solving. The premise of solution-focused therapy is that change is possible but that the individual must identify problems and deal with them in the real world. This therapy is based on questioning to help the individual establish goals and find solutions to problems:

- **Pre-session**: The patient is asked about any differences he or she noted after making the appointment and coming to the first session.
- **Miracle**: The patient is asked if any "miracles" occurred or if any problems were solved, including what, if anything, was different and how this difference affected relationships.
- **Exception**: The patient is asked if any small changes were noted and if there were any problems that no longer seemed problematic and how that manifested.
- **Scaling**: The patient is asked to evaluate the problem on a 1-10 scale and then to determine how to increase the rating.
- **Coping**: The patient is asked about how he or she is managing.

Group Therapy

GROUP CLASSIFICATIONS

Therapy groups may be classified according to form or purpose. The following are classifications according to **form**:

- **Homogeneous**: Members chosen on a selected basis, such as abused women
- **Heterogeneous**: An assortment of individuals with different diagnoses, ages, and genders
- **Mixed**: A group that shares some key features, such as the same diagnosis, but differs in age or gender
- **Closed**: A group in which new members are excluded
- **Open**: A group in which the members and leaders change

The following are classifications according to **purpose**:

- **Task**: Emphasis on achieving a particular assignment
- **Teaching**: Developed to inform, such as teaching the rules of the unit
- **Supportive/Therapeutic**: Assisting those who share the same experience to learn mechanisms to cope with trauma and to overcome the problem, such a group for battered women
- **Psychotherapy**: Helping the patient reduce psychological stress by modifying behavior or ideas

> **Review Video: Group Work and Its Benefits**
> Visit mometrix.com/academy and enter code: 375134

GROUP DEVELOPMENTAL STAGES ACCORDING TO TUCKMAN

Tuckman's (1965) group developmental stages include:

- **Forming**: Group director takes more of an active role while members take their cues from the leader for structure and approval. The leader lists the goals and rules and encourages communication among the members.
- **Storming**: This stage involves a divergence of opinions regarding management, power, and authority. This stage may involve increased stress, and resistance may occur as shown by the absence of members, shared silence, and subgroup formation. At this point, the leader should promote and allow healthy expression of anger.
- **Norming**: It is at this stage where members express positive feelings toward each other and feel deeply attached to the group.
- **Performing**: The leader's input and direction decreases and mainly consists of keeping the group on course.
- **Mourning**: This is most deeply felt in closed groups when discontinuation of the group nears and in open groups when the leader or other members leave.

GROUP DYNAMIC ISSUES ACCORDING TO LONG AND MCMAHON

Group dynamic issues include:

- **Rank**: The position a member holds relative to other group members (Members who contribute often and enthusiastically usually rank higher in the group.)
- **Status**: Ranking given to certain positions or individuals in a group
- **Group content**: Information discussed in a group
- **Group process**: Relations within a group, such as timing of interactions, seating arrangements, and members tone of voice and body language
- **Sociogram**: The system of recording group process

Group process issues include **leadership styles**, such as:

- **Autocratic**: The leader is in charge and controls the meeting.
- **Democratic**: The leader shares responsibility with group members.
- **Laissez Faire**: The leader does not direct the course of the meeting.

Family Therapy

GOALS OF FAMILY THERAPY

Family therapy is a therapeutic modality theorizing that a client's psychiatric symptoms are a result of **pathology within the client's family unit**. This dysfunction is due to problems within the system, usually arising from conflict between marital partners. Psychiatric problems result from these behaviors. This conflict is expressed by:

- **Triangulation**, which manifests itself by the attempt of using another family member to stabilize the emotional process
- **Scapegoating**, which occurs when blaming is used to shift focus to another family member

The **goals** of family therapy are:

- To allow family members to recognize and **communicate their feelings**
- To determine the **reasons for problems** between marital partners and to **resolve** them
- To assist parents in **working together** and to strengthen their **parental authority**
- To help define and clarify **family expectations and roles**
- To learn more and different **positive techniques for interacting**
- To achieve **positive homeostasis** within the family
  - Homeostasis means remaining the same, or maintaining a functional balance. Homeostasis can occur to maintain a dysfunctional status as well.
- To enhance the family's **adaptability**
  - Adaptability is maintaining a balanced, positive stability in the family. A prerequisite for balanced stability, and a basic goal of family therapy, is to help the client family develop strategies for dealing with life's inevitable changes. Morphogenesis is the medical term often applied to a family's ability to react functionally and appropriately to changes.

THEORETICAL APPROACHES TO FAMILY THERAPY

Four theoretical approaches to family therapy are **strategic**, **behavioral**, **psychodynamic**, and **object relations** theories:

- A **strategic approach** to family therapy was proposed by Jay Haley. Haley tried to map out a different strategic plan for each type of psychological issue addressed. With this approach, there is a special treatment strategy for each malady.
- A **behavioral approach** uses traditional behavior-modification techniques to address issues. This approach relies heavily on reinforcement strategies. B.F. Skinner is perhaps the most famous behaviorist. This approach relies on conditioning and often desensitizing as well.
- The **psychodynamic approach** attempts to create understanding and insight on the part of the client. Strategies may be diverse, but in all of them the therapist acts as an emotional guide, leading the client to a better understanding of mental and emotional mechanisms. One common example is Gestalt therapy.
- **Object relations theory** asserts that the ego develops attachment relationships with external and internal objects. A person's early relationships to objects (which can include people) may result in frustration or rejection, which forms the basis of personality.

GENOGRAMS

A genogram is a visual representation of an individual's family that includes information not only regarding the members of the family, but also the status of those members and their relationships to one another. Genograms are useful in a variety of fields, including therapy, counseling, and social work. The process of creating a genogram provides value to the client by allowing them to visualize family dynamics from a macro level and step outside of those dynamics to see how their family unit functions as whole. It is also useful to the person working with the client as it allows them to better understand the client as a product of their family's structure and dynamics. Genograms can identify points of tension within the client's current family structure, or within the client's past and can be a starting point for conversation and investigation regarding any of the client's current struggles, barriers, and strengths.

GENOGRAM STRUCTURE AND SYMBOLS

Genograms rely on standardized symbols and structure to represent members of the family, their role and placement in the client's life, and their dynamics with other family members. The basic symbols and notations of genograms are outlined below. There is additional notation beyond what is included here that is sometimes used, but the particular symbols and linking methods that are used vary by convention.

Gender

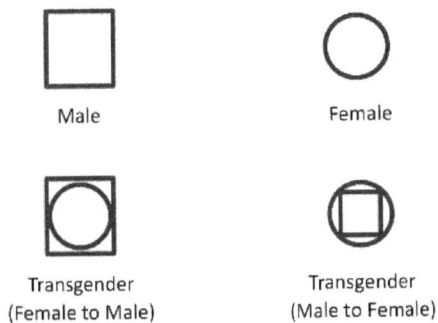

Emotional Relationships

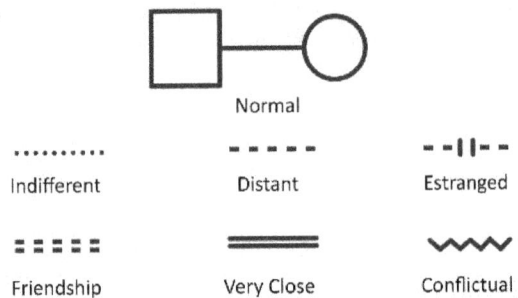

Relationships Status

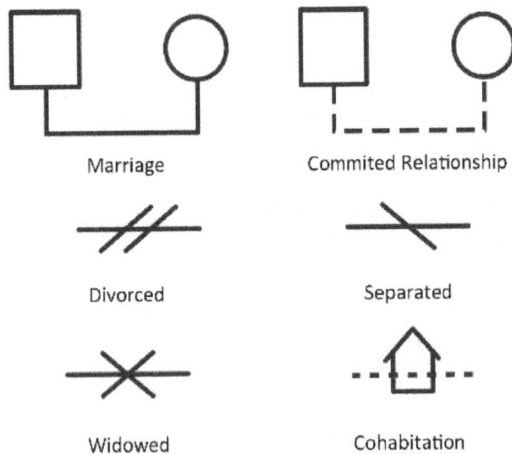

Children

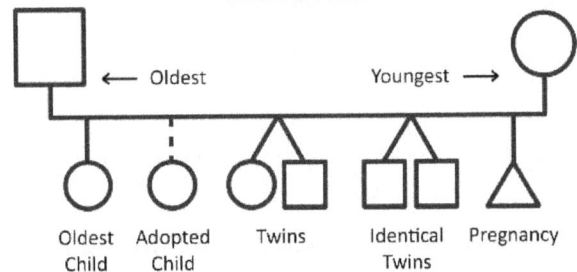

Lifespan

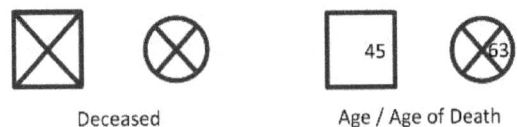

STRATEGIC FAMILY THERAPY

Strategic family therapy (Haley, 1976) is based on the following concepts:

- This therapy seeks to learn what **function** the symptom serves in the family (i.e., what payoff is there for the system in allowing the symptom to continue?).
- **Focuses**: Problem-focused behavioral change, emphasis of parental power and hierarchical family relationships, and the role of symptoms as an attribute of the family's organization.
- Helplessness, incompetence, and illness all provide **power positions** within the family. The child uses symptoms to change the behavior of parents.

Jay Haley tried to develop a strategy for each issue faced by a client. Problems are isolated and treated in different ways. A family plagued by alcoholism might require a different treatment strategy than a family undermined by sexual infidelity. Haley was unusual in that he held degrees in the arts and communication rather than in psychology. Haley's strategies involved the use of directives (direct instructions). After outlining a problem, Haley would tell the family members exactly what to do. If John would bang his head against the wall when he was made to do his homework, Haley might tell a parent to work with him and to be there while he did his homework.

VIRGINIA SATIR AND THE ESALEN INSTITUTE'S EXPERIENTIAL FAMILY THERAPY

Virginia Satir and the Esalen Institute's experiential family therapy draws on sociology, ego concepts, and communication theory to form **role theory concepts**. Satir examined the roles that constrain relationships and interactions in families. This perspective seeks to increase intimacy in the family and improve the self-esteem of family members by using awareness and the communication of feelings. Emphasis is on individual growth in order to change family members and deal with developmental delays. Particular importance is given to marital partners and on changing verbal and nonverbal communication patterns that lower self-esteem.

SATIR'S COMMUNICATION IMPEDIMENTS

Satir described four issues that impede communication between family members under stress. Placating, blaming, being overly reasonable, and being irrelevant are the **four issues which blocked family communication**, according to Virginia Satir:

- **Placating** is the role played by some people in reaction to threat or stress in the family. The placating person reacts to internal stresses by trying to please others, often in irrational ways. A mother might try to placate her disobedient and rude child by offering food, candy, or other presents on the condition that he stop a certain behavior.
- **Blaming** is the act of pointing outwards when an issue creates stress. The blamer thinks, "I'm very angry, but it's your fault. If I've wrecked the car, it's because you made me upset when I left home this morning."
- **Irrelevance** is a behavior wherein a person displaces the potential problem and substitutes another unrelated activity. A mother who engages in too much social drinking frequently discusses her split ends whenever the topic of alcoholism is brought up by her spouse.
- Being overly reasonable, also known as being a **responsible analyzer** is when a person keeps his or her emotions in check and functions with the precision and monotony of a machine.

MURRAY BOWEN'S FAMILY SYSTEMS THEORY

Bowen's family systems theory focuses on the following concepts:

- The role of **thinking versus feeling/reactivity** in relationship/family systems.
- Role of **emotional triangles**: The three-person system or triangle is viewed as the smallest stable relationship system and forms when a two-person system experiences tension.
- **Generationally repeating family issues**: Parents transmit emotional problems to a child. (Example: The parents fear something is wrong with a child and treat the child as if something is wrong, interpreting the child's behavior as confirmation.)
- **Undifferentiated family ego mass**: This refers to a family's lack of separateness. There is a fixed cluster of egos of individual family members as if all have a common ego boundary.
- **Emotional cutoff**: A way of managing emotional issues with family members (cutting off emotional contact).
- Consideration of thoughts and feelings of **each individual family member** as well as seeking to understand the family network.

Review Video: Bowen Family Systems
Visit mometrix.com/academy and enter code: 591496

FAMILY SYSTEM THEORY ASSUMPTIONS ABOUT HUMAN BEHAVIOR

Family systems theory makes several basic assumptions:

- Change in one part of the family system brings about change in other parts of the system.
- The family provides the following to its members: unity, individuation, security, comfort, nurturance, warmth, affection, and reciprocal need satisfaction.
- Where family pathology is present, the individual is socially and individually disadvantaged.
- Behavioral problems are a reflection of communication problems in the family system.
- Treatment focuses on the family unity; changing family interactions is the key to behavioral change.

MOTIVATIONS FOR CHANGE AND MEANS THROUGH WHICH CHANGE OCCURS

The **motivations for change** according to Bowen's family systems theory are as follows:

- **Disequilibrium** of the normal family homeostasis is the primary motivation for change according to this perspective.
- The family system is made up of three subsystems: the marital relationship, the parent-child relationship, and the sibling relationship. **Dysfunction** that occurs in any of these subsystems will likely cause dysfunction in the others.

The **means for change** in the family systems theory approach is the family as an interactional system.

CONTRIBUTIONS TO FAMILY SYSTEMS THEORY

The **psychodynamic theory** emphasizes multi-generational family history. Earlier family relations and patterns determine current ones. Distorted relations in childhood lead to patterns of miscommunication and behavioral problems. Interpersonal and intrapersonal conflict beneath apparent family unity results in psychopathology. Social role functioning is influenced by heredity and environment.

Don Jackson, a major contributor to family therapy, focuses on **power relationships**. He developed a theory of double-bind communication in families. Double-bind communication occurs when two conflicting messages communicated simultaneously create or maintain a no-win pathological symptom.

ASSESSMENT AND TREATMENT PLANNING IN THE FAMILY SYSTEMS THEORY

Assessment in family systems theory includes the following:

- Acknowledgement of **dysfunction** in the family system
- **Family hierarchy**: Who is in charge? Who has responsibility? Who has authority? Who has power?
- Evaluation of **boundaries** (around subsystems, between family and larger environment): Are they permeable or impermeable? Flexible or rigid?
- How does the **symptom** function in the family system?

Treatment planning is as follows:

- The therapist creates a mutually satisfactory contract with the family to establish service boundaries.
- Bowenian family therapy's goal is the differentiation of the individual from the strong influence of the family.

SAL MINUCHIN'S STRUCTURAL FAMILY THERAPY

Sal Minuchin's structural family therapy seeks to strengthen boundaries when family subsystems are enmeshed, or seeks to increase flexibility when these systems are overly rigid. Minuchin emphasizes that the family structure should be hierarchical and that the parents should be at the top of the hierarchy.

Joining, enactment, boundary making, and mimesis are four techniques used by Salvador Minuchin in structural family therapy:

- **Joining** is the therapist's attempt at greeting and bonding with members of the family. Bonding is important when obtaining cooperation and input.
- Minuchin often had his clients enact the various scenarios which led to disagreements and conflicts within families. The **enactment** of an unhealthy family dynamic would allow the therapist to better understand the behavior and allow the family members to gain insight.
- **Boundary making** is important to structural family therapies administered by Salvador Minuchin, because many family conflicts arise from confusion about each person's role. Minuchin believed that family harmony was best achieved when people were free to be themselves yet knew that they must not invade the areas of other family members.
- **Mimesis** is a process in which the therapist mimics the positive and negative behavior patterns of different family members.

THERAPEUTIC METHODS EMPLOYED BY CARL WHITAKER

Carl Whitaker, known as the dean of family therapy, developed **experiential symbolic family therapy**. Whitaker would freely interact with other family members and often played the part of family members who were important to the dynamic. He felt that experience, not information and education, had the power to change family dynamics.

Whitaker believed that in family therapy, theory was also less important than experience and that co-therapists were a great aid to successful counseling. Co-therapists freed one of the counselors to participate more fully in the counseling sessions. One counselor might direct the flow of activity while the other participated in role playing. The "psychotherapy of the absurd" is a Whitaker innovation which was influenced by the "theatre of the absurd," a popular existential art form at the time. In this context, the absurd is the unreasonable exaggeration of an idea, to the point of underscoring the underlying meaninglessness of much of human interaction. A person who repeated a neurotic or destructive behavior, for example, was being absurd. The **psychotherapy of the absurd**, as Whitaker saw it, was a method for bringing out repeated and meaningless absurdities. A person pushing against an immovable brick wall, for example, might eventually understand the psychological analogy to some problem behavior.

THEORIES OF CAUSALITY

Multiple theories of causality exist in the interpretation of family dynamics, which are then applied to the selection of therapeutic interventions. While linear causality (the concept that one cause equals one effect) uses a direct line of reasoning and is commonly used in individual counseling, **circular/reciprocal causality** is often used in family therapy and refers to the dynamic interactions between family members in which actions and reactions are self-reinforcing. Consider a dynamic in which parents are struggling with a rebellious and defiant adolescent child. In reaction to this, the parent's express anger and frustration through lectures that often escalate to shouting. The adolescent's response to shouting is to retreat and to continue to act defiantly. Due to this, the parents are quicker to escalate frustration, and the adolescent become more defiant. Interventions are targeted to disrupt this unhealth cycle by targeting assumptions and behaviors that feed the behaviors and replace them with those that foster trust and safety.

PARADOXICAL INTERVENTION STRATEGIES

Paradoxical intervention strategies involve the use of the client's disruptive behavior as a treatment itself, requiring the client to put the behavior in the spotlight to then motivate change. This technique tries to accomplish the opposite of what it suggests on the surface. Interventions include the following:

- **Restraining** is advising that a negative behavior not be changed or be changed only slightly or slowly. This can be effectively used in the context of couples therapy when a couple is struggling with intimacy issues. The therapist may challenge the couple to refrain from sexual intimacy for a period of time, thus removing certain stressors from that dynamic, possibly resulting in a positive intimate experience that occurs naturally and spontaneously.
- **Positioning** is characterizing a negative behavior in an even more negative light through the use of exaggeration. "David, do you feel you are not terrifying your family enough with your reckless driving or that you ought to drive faster in order to make them worry more about your wellbeing? Perhaps that way you will know that they care about you," says the therapist using positioning as a technique. It is important that this technique be used only with great care, as it can be harmful to clients with a negative self-image. It is generally used in situations where the client is behaving in a certain negative way in order to seek affirmation or attention.
- **Prescribing the symptom** is another paradoxical technique used by therapists to obtain an enlightened reaction from a client. A therapist using this technique directs the client to activate the negative behavior in terms that are absurd and clearly objectionable. 'John, I want you to go out to that sidewalk overpass above the freeway and yell as loud as you can at the cars passing below you. Do it for at least four hours." The therapist prescribes this activity to cure his client's dangerous tendency toward road rage.
- **Relabeling** is recasting a negative behavior in a positive light in order to get an emotional response from the client. "Perhaps your wife yells at you when you drink because she finds this behavior attractive and wants your attention," the therapist might say. The therapist might even support that obviously illogical and paradoxical argument by pointing out invented statistics, which support the ridiculous assertion.

EXTINCTION, TIME OUT, AND THOUGHT STOPPING

Behavior modification is a term used in facilities like schools and jails to bring behavior into line with societal or family rules:

- **Extinction** is the process of causing a behavior to disappear by providing little or no reinforcement. It is different from punishment, which is negative reinforcement rather than no reinforcement at all. Very often, a student will be removed from the general population and made to sit alone in a quiet room. In schools, this goes by various names, but is often called in-school suspension (ISS). It is hoped that, through lack of reinforcement and response from outside, the offensive behavior will become extinct.
- **Time out** is another extinction technique, generally applied to very young children. A disobedient child will be isolated for a specified, usually short time whenever he or she misbehaves. The method's operant mechanism assumes that we are all social animals and require the reinforcement of the outside world. Deprived of this, we adapt by altering our behavior.
- **Thought stopping** is a learned response which requires the participation and cooperation of the client to change a negative behavior. When it is successful, the client actively forbids negative thoughts from entering his or her mind.

SPECIFIC FAMILY THERAPY INTERVENTIONS
FAMILY THERAPY INTERVENTIONS USED WITH OCD

Family therapy interventions used to treat individuals with **obsessive-compulsive disorder (OCD)** include therapy oriented to develop expression of thoughts and impulses in a manner that is appropriate. This approach assumes that family members often:

- Attempt to avoid situations that trigger OCD responses
- Constantly reassure the individual (which often enables the obsession)

Family therapy to address these issues involves:

- Remaining neutral and not reinforcing through encouragement
- Avoiding attempts to reason logically with individual

FAMILY THERAPY INTERVENTIONS FOR PANIC DISORDERS

Family dynamics and therapy interventions for **panic disorders** include:

- Individuals with agoraphobia may require the presence of family members to be constantly in close proximity, resulting in marital stress and over-reliance on the children.
- Altered role performance of the afflicted member results in family and social situations that increase the responsibility of other family members.
- The family must be educated about the source and treatment of the disorder.
- The goal of family therapy is to reorganize responsibilities to support family change.

FUNCTIONAL FAMILY THERAPY FOR ADOLESCENTS WITH ANTISOCIAL BEHAVIOR

Functional family therapy (FFT) is designed for adolescents (11–17 years of age) with **antisocial behavior**. FFT uses the principles of family systems theory and cognitive-behavioral therapy and provides intervention and prevention services. While the therapy has changed somewhat over the past 30 years, current FTT usually includes three phases:

1. **Engagement/motivation:** The therapist works with the family to identify maladaptive beliefs to increase expectations for change, reduce negativity and blaming, and increase respect for differences. Goals are to reduce dropout rates and establish alliances.
2. **Behavior change:** The therapist guides the parents in using behavioral interventions to improve family functioning, parenting, and conflict management. Goals are to prevent delinquent behavior and build better communication and interpersonal skills.
3. **Generalization:** The family learns to use new skills to influence the systems in which they are involved, such as school, church, or the juvenile justice system. Community resources are mobilized to prevent relapses.

MULTISYSTEMIC THERAPY FOR ADOLESCENTS WITH ANTISOCIAL BEHAVIOR

Multisystemic therapy (MST) is a **family-focused program** designed for adolescents (11–17 years of age) with antisocial and delinquent behaviors. The primary goal is **collaboration** with the family to develop strategies for dealing with the child's behavioral problems. Services are delivered in the family's natural environment rather than at a clinic or office with frequent home visits, usually totaling 40–60 hours over the course of treatment. Sessions are daily initially and then decrease in frequency. A variety of different therapies may be used, including family therapy, parent training, and individual therapy. Therapists use different approaches but adhere to basic principles, including focusing on the strength of the systems, delivering appropriate treatment for developmental level, and improving family functioning. The goals of therapy are to improve family relations and parenting skills, to engage the child in activities with nondelinquent peers, and to improve the child's grades and participation in activities, such as sports.

THERAPEUTIC METHODS FOR COUNSELING AN ADOLESCENT WITH BEHAVIORAL PROBLEMS

When an **adolescent's behavior** is a problem, some parents have him or her sign an agreement to perform in a specified manner. The agreement may state that a reward will be provided to the adolescent so long as the contract is upheld. The therapist can help parents and children write an effective contract. Another time-honored method of behavior conditioning is the withholding of leisure activity until chores are done. In a family therapy session, the therapist might advise stating the case like this: "Your television has a parental guide lock which will not be turned on unless you can demonstrate that all your homework is complete."

ROLE OF THE THERAPIST

The role of the therapist in family therapy is to interact in the here and now with the family in relation to current problems. The therapist is a consultant to the family. Some aspects of the therapist's role differ according to school of thought:

- **Structural**: The therapist actively challenges dysfunctional interaction.
- **Strategic and Systemic**: The therapist is very active.
- **Milan School**: Male/female clinicians are co-therapists; a team observes from behind a one-way mirror and consults and directs the co-therapists with the clients.
- **Psychodynamic**: The therapist facilitates self-reflection and understanding of multi-generational dynamics and conflicts.
- **Satir**: The therapist models caring, acceptance, love, compassion, nurturance in order to help clients face fears and increase openness.

KEY CONCEPTS OF FAMILY THERAPY

Key **concepts of family therapy** include the following:

Behavior modeling	The manner in which a child bases his or her own behavior on the behavior of his or her parents and other people. In other words, a child will usually learn to identify acceptable behaviors by mimicking the behavior of others. Some children may have more difficulty with behavior modeling than others.
Boundaries	The means of organization through which system parts can be differentiated both from their environment and from each other. They protect and improve the differentiation and integrity of the family, subsystems, and individual family members.
Collaborative therapy	Therapy in which a different therapist sees each spouse or member of the family.
Complementary family interaction	A type of family relationship in which members present opposite behaviors that supply needs or lacks in the other family member.
Complementarity of needs	Circular support system of a family, in which reciprocity is found in meeting needs; can be adaptive or maladaptive.
Double-bind communication	Communication in which two contradictory messages are conveyed concurrently, leading to a no-win situation.
Family of origin	The family into which one is born.
Family of procreation	The family which one forms with a mate and one's own children.
Enmeshment	Obscuring of boundaries in which differentiation of family subsystems and individual autonomy are lost. Similar to Bowen's "undifferentiated family ego mass." Characterized by "mind reading" (partners speak for each other, complete each other's sentences).
Heritage	The set of customs, traditions, physical characteristics, and other cultural artifacts that a person inherits from his or her ancestors.
Homeostasis	A state of systemic balance (of relationships, alliances, power, authority).
Identified patient	The "symptom bearer" in the family.
Multiple family therapy	Therapy in which three or more families form a group with one or more clinicians to discuss common problems. Group support is given and problems are universalized.
Scapegoating	Unconscious, irrational election of one family member for a negative, demeaned, or outsider role.

Psychopharmacotherapeutic Management

LITHIUM

WORK-UP REQUIRED BEFORE STARTING PATIENTS ON LITHIUM

Lithium has a very narrow **therapeutic window**, and **lithium toxicity** is a medical emergency and can lead to death. Lithium is cleared from the body by the kidneys and can negatively affect thyroid function. An initial assessment should include an evaluation of kidney function. This would be determined through a urinalysis (UA), BUN and creatinine levels, an electrolyte panel, 24-hour urine for creatinine clearance, screening for diabetes, hypertension, and any history of diuretic medications or overuse of analgesics. Thyroid function must also be evaluated. A TSH, T3, T4, and free thyroxine index should be drawn. A complete physical along with a complete family and patient history should be obtained. Other tests should include a 12 lead ECK, fasting blood sugar, and CBC.

SIDE EFFECTS AND ADVERSE REACTIONS

There can be many side effects and adverse reactions associated with the use of lithium. As **serum levels** of lithium increase, so do associated side effects. If **plasma levels** are kept at the lower therapeutic end, many of the associated symptoms are mild and may resolve after a few weeks of treatment. Some of the side effects include the following: weight gain, fine motor tremors, fatigue, headaches, inability to concentrate, outbreaks of acne, a maculopapular rash, GI upset, diarrhea, decrease in appetite, polyuria, polydipsia, or swelling. GI symptoms can be decreased if the dosage is taken with food or milk. Lithium is contraindicated in pregnancy, especially during the first trimester.

TOXICITY

Because lithium has a very narrow therapeutic window, **plasma levels** must be frequently monitored. The normal therapeutic range is 0.6-1.2 mEq/L for adults. Lithium toxicity is an emergency and can lead to patient death. Plasma levels will usually decrease to an acceptable level within 48 hours after discontinuation of the medication; however, in severe cases involving acute renal failure, dialysis may be necessary. A complete initial assessment, ongoing assessments, frequent evaluations of lithium levels, and patient education are all an essential part of the treatment plan and prevention of toxicity. A patient must be able to tell the difference between side effects and symptoms of toxicity.

CAUSES

Lithium replaces sodium in the **sodium-potassium pump** within the body and is retained more readily than sodium within the cell. Therefore, any physical change that would affect **sodium levels** would affect lithium levels. Decrease in dietary sodium intake, vomiting, diarrhea, diaphoresis, fever, or greatly decreased fluid intake can lead to an increase in plasma lithium levels. The use of certain medications, such as loop or thiazide diuretics, ACE inhibitors, alcohol, carbamazepine, haloperidol, or NSAIDs, can also cause an increase in lithium levels. Lithium levels can also be decreased by increased dietary intake of sodium, caffeine, osmotic diuretics, or use of acetazolamide.

SYMPTOMS

The symptoms associated with lithium toxicity can be similar to many of the side effects. It is vital that the patient and provider be well educated on the differences between the two. **Early detection** of toxicity can prevent devastating patient outcomes. Symptoms of mild toxicity associated with blood levels of 1.5-2.0 mEq/L can include severe vomiting and diarrhea, increased muscle tremors and twitching, lethargy, body aches, ataxia, ringing in the ears, blurry vision, vertigo, or hyperactive deep tendon reflexes. More severe symptoms associated with blood levels greater than 2.0 mEq/L can include elevated temperature, low urine output, hypotension, ECG abnormalities, and decreased level of consciousness, seizures, coma, or death.

NURSING INTERVENTIONS FOR SIDE EFFECTS

Nursing interventions and patient education about these interventions can help ease some of the side effects associated with the use of lithium. For **edema**, elevate the hands or feet, monitor for weight gain, monitor I&O for decreased urine output, and monitor salt intake. For **tremors**, provide reassurance as stress can increase the tremors. If the tremors interfere with daily functioning, notify the ordering provider. **Mild diarrhea or GI upset** can be decreased with smaller, more frequent dosing of lithium taken with food. If diarrhea worsens, notify the healthcare provider and monitor for signs of toxicity. The patients experiencing the side effects of **weakness, fatigue, and inability to concentrate** will need reassurance that these symptoms usually resolve in a few weeks. Sugarless hard candy can help reduce symptoms of dry mouth or a metallic aftertaste. Encourage regular oral care to protect mucous membranes.

ANTIPSYCHOTIC CLASS OF MEDICATIONS

TYPICAL AND ATYPICAL ANTIPSYCHOTIC MEDICATIONS

With recent research and development of new antipsychotic medications, there has developed a need to differentiate between the older and newer drugs.

- The drugs originally utilized to treat psychosis are often referred to as the **typical antipsychotic medications**. These medications are also known as neuroleptics or major tranquilizers. Drugs of this class include medications such as Thorazine and Haldol.
- The newer medications created within the last 20 years are referred to as **atypical antipsychotic medications**. The newer drugs have fewer side effects and unwanted associated neurologic symptoms, such as tardive dyskinesia. Drugs of this class include medications such as Risperdal and Zyprexa. The atypical class of medications is now considered the first-line drug therapy choice.

> **Review Video: Antipsychotic Drugs**
> Visit mometrix.com/academy and enter code: 369601

TARGETED SYMPTOMS

The typical antipsychotic medications will only affect the positive targeted symptoms, while the newer atypical antipsychotic medications will affect both the positive and negative targeted symptoms.

- The **positive targeted symptoms** are associated with an excess of normal function and mainly affect the psychotic thinking processes and disorganization of speech, motor movements, and social behaviors. Examples of these can include delusions, hallucinations, incoherence, catatonic motor movements, or unacceptable social behaviors.
- The **negative targeted symptoms** are associated with a reduction of normal function and mainly affect mood, cognition, and socialization. Examples of these can include a flat affect, a reduction in thought and speech, inability to focus or experience pleasure, or apathy.

INDICATION AND MECHANISM OF ACTION

The most common indicator for the use of antipsychotic drugs is the **treatment of psychosis**. This class of medication is also used in the treatment of schizophrenia, organic brain syndrome, delusional disorders, agitation associated with the progression of Alzheimer's disease, substance-induced psychosis, severe depression with associated psychosis, and disruptive behaviors associated with dementia or delirium. The typical antipsychotic medications are **postsynaptic dopamine antagonists** with the new atypical class blocking serotonin and dopamine receptors. The difference in their mechanism of action results in a different patient response and targeted symptom treatment.

SIDE EFFECTS

CARDIOVASCULAR SIDE EFFECTS

There are many different side effects that may occur with the use of antipsychotic medications. One of the most dangerous side effects includes those involving the **cardiovascular system**. Symptoms can include orthostatic hypotension and ECG changes. **Orthostatic hypotension** is produced because certain antipsychotic medications bind with alpha adrenergic receptors. Medications such as chlorpromazine, thioridazine, and clozapine have been associated with causing orthostatic hypotension. The **ECG changes** that can occur include a prolonged Q-T interval within the QRS complex. Medications such as thioridazine and ziprasidone have been associated with this ECG abnormality.

UNWANTED WEIGHT GAIN

Certain antipsychotic medications can cause an increase in hunger and therefore lead to unwanted weight gain. The lower potency antipsychotics are more commonly associated with this side effect, with clozapine and olanzapine as common culprits. Patients should be educated that increased weight leads to increased risks for cardiovascular disease and diabetes. They should be encouraged to start a diet and exercise program as soon as this side effect becomes evident. Alternative medications such as ziprasidone and quetiapine should be considered because they have shown no indication of causing unwanted weight gain.

ANTICHOLINERGIC SIDE EFFECTS

Anticholinergic side effects are due to the **blocking of acetylcholine**. These side effects can be seen with both typical and atypical antipsychotic medications. Symptoms can include dry mouth and mucous membranes, decreased gastric motility and constipation, urinary retention and/or hesitancy, blurry vision, confusion, or memory loss. These types of side effects can be seen with many psychiatric medications. The patients should be reassured that many of these side effects are only temporary. They should be encouraged to perform good oral hygiene, use lip balm, eat a high fiber diet, and to postpone any eye exams for approximately 3 weeks after a consistent medication dosage has been determined.

POTENTIAL FOR DEVELOPING A BLOOD DISORDER

Blood disorders associated with the use of antipsychotic medications do not occur often but can be very dangerous. The use of **clozapine** has been associated with increased risk of developing what is called **agranulocytosis**. This is an acute reduction in the normal level of WBC's and neutrophils. Their reduction increases the risk for life threatening infections. A patient who develops agranulocytosis may need to be hospitalized so they can be closely monitored and placed in reverse isolation. Common symptoms include fever of unknown origin, malaise, sore throat, and mouth sores. The patient will need to have blood drawn to check these levels once a week for approximately the first 6 months and then every 2 weeks for the duration of the medication therapy. Prescriptions should only be given for one week at a time. Once clozapine has been stopped, blood samples should be checked for an additional 4 weeks. The patient should be educated to report any fever, sore throat, or mouth sores immediately and discontinue the medication until a CBC can be drawn.

INCREASED RISK FOR SEIZURES AND WATER TOXICITY

In patients with undiagnosed underlying seizure disorder, the use of antipsychotic medications can lower their **seizure threshold**. This can lead to the onset of **seizure disorder**. Patients with already diagnosed seizure disorder should be very closely monitored for increased seizure activity. One of the more serious side effects associated with use of antipsychotic medications is water toxicity. This can develop over time and leads to ingestion of large quantities of water. The patient will develop polydipsia and polyuria and may appear puffy in the face or around the eyes. Hyponatremia will develop, which can cause confusion, agitation, abdominal distention, or if untreated, death. These patients should be weighed daily and serum sodium levels monitored closely.

PHOTOSENSITIVITY AND PIGMENT CHANGES

Photosensitivity can occur while taking certain antipsychotic medications. Patients using low-potency antipsychotics should be aware that they are at increased risk of developing severe **sunburns or rashes**

related to sun exposure. They should be educated to wear sun block lotion or cover all exposed skin and to wear dark sun glasses when outdoors.

Pigment changes can also occur with sun exposure. These areas of skin can become discolored due to pigment deposits and may range in color from orange to bluish grey. The face and neck areas are at the greatest risk for this discoloring. Patient's taking high doses of the drug **thioridazine** may experience pigment changes in the eyes called retinitis pigmentosa. This condition can lead to a severe decrease in vision. Recommended doses of thioridazine are 800 mg/day or less.

Neuroleptic Malignant Syndrome

Neuroleptic malignant syndrome (NMS) is one of the most serious complicating side effects associated with the use of antipsychotic medications. This potentially fatal and rare condition can result with one single dosage of medication. The highest risk medications fall into the **high-potency** category. Symptoms occur acutely and can include high fever, tachycardia, diaphoresis, rigid muscles, shaking, incontinence, confusion and decreased level of consciousness, renal failure, and elevated CPK levels. It is very important to always monitor a patient's **temperature** with the use of antipsychotics. The patient may require supportive care in the form of resuscitation, mechanical ventilation, hydration, and fever reducing actions. All antipsychotic drugs must be discontinued and the patient may be treated with dantrolene or bromocriptine. Development of this side effect does not exclude the patient from future treatment with antipsychotic medications.

Tardive Dyskinesia

Tardive dyskinesia (TD) is a chronic syndrome that can develop as a result of the long-term use of antipsychotic medications. The **elderly population** is at the highest risk for development of this syndrome. There is currently no effective treatment and the best defense is early detection and prevention of symptoms. Use of the lowest effective dosage of an atypical antipsychotic is often recommended for prevention. Frequent assessments for development of these symptoms are vital due to the fact that many of the patients are unaware that the symptoms may be occurring in the early phases. Symptoms can include involuntary movements of the face, such as tongue protrusion, lip smacking, blinking, grimacing, or chewing. Patients can also experience choreiform movements of the extremities and trunk of the body such as repetitive finger movements or irregular breathing patterns and swallowing air, which causes frequent belching and grunting to occur.

Extrapyramidal Symptoms (EPS)

Extrapyramidal symptoms (EPS) occur commonly with the use of antipsychotic medications. There are **three main syndromes** that fall into this category. They include dystonia, pseudoparkinsonism, and akathisia. These symptoms usually develop early in treatment and resolve by approximately 3 months. Many times, these symptoms are frightening to patients, causing them to stop their medications. They can also be confused with anxiety related symptoms. Assessment and symptom recognition are vital to the successful treatment of the patient. Some treatment options may include a reduction in the dosage of medication, a change to a different medication, or adding a new drug to specifically treat the symptoms. Patient reassurance, support, and education about these syndromes can help to decrease stress and anxiety.

Dystonia

Dystonia is a syndrome associated with EPS that can occur with the use of antipsychotic medications. This is often the first of the associated syndromes to occur and usually appears within the first few dosages of medication. Symptoms include **spasms** of the large muscle groups of the head, neck, and back. Patient complaints may also include a **thick tongue** or **stiff neck**. These symptoms can have an abrupt and painful onset. If untreated, this syndrome can lead to more severe symptoms, such as a protruding tongue, oculogyric crisis, torticollis, laryngopharyngeal constriction, or extreme abnormal posturing of the upper body. If the muscle spasms become sustained, this can lead to impaired respiratory status and a medical emergency. These symptoms are more often seen in children and young men.

PSEUDOPARKINSONISM

With pseudoparkinsonism, many of the symptoms are the same as Parkinson's disease, but the cause is different. Parkinson's disease occurs due to the loss of **dopaminergic cells**, while pseudoparkinsonism is a **medication-induced state**. Symptoms may include rigidity, slowing movements associated with akinesia, and tremors. Many times, muscle rigidity is first noticed in the upper extremities. Increased salivation, mask-like facial expressions, and a decrease in reflexes or initiation of movements may also occur. Pseudoparkinsonism occurs more commonly in men and the elderly population. Symptoms usually appear within the first month of treatment and unfortunately there is usually no development of tolerance or resolution of symptoms. Treatment of symptoms with amantadine may help; however, the patient must have good renal function to take this medication.

AKATHISIA

The primary **symptom** of akathisia associated with the use of antipsychotic medications is an inability of the patient to remain still. They will often exhibit **repetitive motions**, such as pacing or rocking back and forth. They will often feel restless and the only way to relieve this restlessness is by moving. It is also possible for the individual to feel inner restlessness and not exhibit outward symptoms. They may be **unable to relax** and experience **high levels of anxiety**. Many times, the patient will be unable to explain their need to move about. Akathisia symptoms can be difficult to treat. Limited success has been seen with use of beta-adrenergic blockers, anticholinergics, antihistamines, and low-dose anti-anxiety medications. The patient should be switched to an atypical antipsychotic. If unable to change medications, the lowest effective dose of a typical antipsychotic can be used.

A complete **baseline assessment** is vital information to help differentiate between akathisia and an increase in psychotic symptoms. Akathisia can often be confused with agitation or an exacerbation of the patient's psychotic symptoms. Often the patient will have their medication dosages increased, only to find that there has been an increase in symptoms. Agitation associated with psychotic behavior does not usually just acutely appear after the initiation of antipsychotic medication. If possible, the provider should try to distinguish between muscle restlessness associated with akathisia and mental restlessness associated with agitation. The patient needs **reassurance** and validation that the symptoms are a treatable side effect of their medication.

ANTIDEPRESSANTS

The main indicator for use of an antidepressant is simply **depression**. This can be further expanded to include major depression, atypical depression, and anxiety disorders. Depression type symptoms commonly include loss of interest in usual or pleasurable activities, decreased levels of energy, having a depressed mood, decreased ability to concentrate, loss of appetite, or suicidal thoughts. Antidepressants are also commonly used to treat **anxiety disorders** that include panic attacks, obsessive-compulsive disorder (OCD), social phobias, anxiety attacks, or post-traumatic stress disorder. They may also be beneficial in treating chronic pain syndromes, premenstrual syndrome, insomnia, attention deficit hyperactivity disorder, or bed wetting.

SSRIs

Selective serotonin reuptake inhibitors (SSRIs) prevent the reuptake of serotonin at the presynaptic membrane. This increases the amount of serotonin in the synapse for neurotransmission. This class of antidepressants has been shown to reduce depression and anxiety symptoms, and is currently the first line treatment for generalized anxiety disorder. Common side effects are usually short in duration and include headache, GI upset, and sexual dysfunction. They do not cause significant anticholinergic, cardiovascular, or significant patient sedation side effects. Examples of SSRIs include citalopram (Celexa), escitalopram (Lexapro), fluoxetine (Prozac), Fluvoxamine (Luvox), paroxetine (Paxil), and sertraline (Zoloft). These drugs are not highly lethal in overdose.

> **Review Video: So Sad**
> Visit mometrix.com/academy and enter code: 620613

TRICYCLIC ANTIDEPRESSANTS
SIDE EFFECTS

Tricyclic antidepressants not only block the reuptake of serotonin and norepinephrine, they also act to block muscarinic cholinergic receptors, histamine H1 receptors, and alpha1 noradrenergic receptors. These receptors do not affect depression symptoms, but their blockade is implicated in some of the side effects associated with tricyclics. The blockade of the muscarinic receptors produces anticholinergic side effects such as dry mouth, blurred vision, constipation, urinary retention, and tachycardia. The blockade of the histamine receptors is associated with drowsiness, low blood pressure, and weight gain. The alpha-1 noradrenergic receptor blocking action produces the side effects associated with orthostatic hypotension, vertigo, and some memory disturbances.

MECHANISM OF ACTION AND NECESSARY EVALUATIONS

Most of the tricyclic antidepressants have very similar mechanisms of action and side effects. Although their exact mechanism of action is unknown, they are believed to act to inhibit the reuptake of both serotonin and norepinephrine. These drugs have a high **first-pass rate of metabolism** and are excreted by the kidneys. A complete **physical and history** should be obtained before starting a patient on tricyclic drugs. Because this class of antidepressants can cause death with an overdose, an initial **suicide risk assessment** must be obtained, and continued assessments for this risk are a necessity. This class of drug can cause a prolongation in the electrical conduction of the heart. Therefore, a **baseline ECG** should be performed in children, young teenagers, anyone with cardiac electrical conduction problems, and adults over age 40.

MAOIs

The mechanism of action for monoamine oxidase inhibitors (MAOIs) is exactly what their name indicates. These drugs act to inhibit the enzyme **monoamine oxidase (MAO)**. There are actually two of these enzymes, **MAO A** and **MAO B**, and this class of medication inhibits both. These enzymes act to metabolize serotonin and norepinephrine. By inhibiting the production of these enzymes, there are increased levels of **serotonin** and **norepinephrine** available for neurotransmission. Medications that selectively inhibit MAO B have no antidepressant effects and can be used to treat disease processes such as Parkinson's.

SIDE EFFECTS

Side effects associated with the use of monoamine oxidase inhibitors (MAOIs) are extensive due to their action on multiple neurotransmitters. For this reason, they are not the preferred option in the treatment of depression. They can include symptoms such as GI upset, vertigo, headaches, sleep disturbances, sexual dysfunction, dry mouth, visual disturbances, constipation, peripheral edema, urinary hesitancy, weakness, increased weight, or orthostatic hypotension. The elderly population is at greatest risk for problems with **orthostatic hypotension** and should have lying, sitting, and standing blood pressure checks to monitor for this side effect. Orthostatic hypotension can lead to injuries related to falls such as fractures. The most dangerous side effect can be an extreme elevation in blood pressure.

SIDE EFFECT OF HYPERTENSION

Monoamine oxidase inhibitors (MAOIs) are associated with many different side effects; however, the most dangerous side effect is the development of a **severe increase in blood pressure** or a **hypertensive crisis**. Hypertension can develop due to the presence of increased levels of **tyramine**. These levels increase because **monoamine oxidase**, which normally metabolizes tyramine, is inhibited. Increased levels of tyramine produce a vasoconstrictive response by the body that leads to increased blood pressure. Symptoms associated with hypertensive crisis can include severe occipital headache, palpitations, chest pain, diaphoresis, nausea and vomiting, flushed face, or dilated pupils. Complications associated with hypertensive crisis include hemorrhagic stroke, severe headache, or death. In depth patient education is vital and should include symptoms of hypertension, close monitoring of blood pressure, and low-tyramine diet.

DIET RESTRICTIONS

Monoamine oxidase inhibitors can lead to increased levels of **tyramine** in the nerve cell. These increased levels can lead to a dangerous and possibly fatal increase in **blood pressure**. Certain **foods that contain tyramine** should be avoided to help prevent hypertensive episodes. These foods include any cheeses except for fresh cottage, ricotta, processed cheese slices, or cream cheese, and any meat, fish, or poultry that has been improperly stored, fermented, or dried, including pepperoni, salami, summer sausage, pickled, or smoked fish. Other foods include fava or broad bean pods, sauerkraut, overripe fruit, banana peels, all tap beers, beef and chicken liver, any fermented product, products containing monosodium glutamate, or soybean condiments such as soy sauce. Red wine can produce the side effect of headache unrelated to hypertension and should also be avoided.

MONITORING ANTIDEPRESSANTS

TRICYCLICS AND HETEROCYCLICS

The monitoring of tricyclics and heterocyclics includes the following:

- Observe for toxicity.
- Inform patients not to take with monoamine oxidase inhibitors.
- Observe for decreased therapeutic response to hypertensives (e.g., clonidine, guanethidine).
- Monitor other medications; patient should avoid other central nervous system depressants, including alcohol. Some medications potentiate the effects of tricyclics, including bupropion, cimetidine, haloperidol, selective serotonin reuptake inhibitors, and valproic acid.
- Inform patient to avoid prolonged exposure to sunlight or sunlamps.
- Administer major dosage of drug at bedtime if patient experiences drowsiness.
- Monitor for sedation, cardiac arrhythmias, insomnia, gastrointestinal upset, and weight gain.

SELECTIVE SEROTONIN REUPTAKE INHIBITORS

The monitoring of SSRIs includes the following:

- Monitor for increased depression and suicidal ideation, especially in adolescents.
- Inform patients of the following:
  - Smoking decreases effectiveness.
  - Fatal reactions may occur with monoamine oxidase inhibitors.
  - Taking SSRIs with benzodiazepines or alcohol has an additive effect.
  - Some drugs, such as citalopram, may increase the effects of β-blockers and warfarin.
- Avoid cimetidine, which is prescribed for ulcers and gastroesophageal reflux disease, and St. John's wort.
- Inform patients of possible decreased libido and sexual functioning.
- Monitor for insomnia and gastrointestinal upset.

ANTI-ANXIETY AND SEDATIVE-HYPNOTIC MEDICATIONS

Antianxiety medications are indicated when symptoms of anxiety are out of proportion for the situation. **Physical disease processes or illness** should be ruled out first before determining that the anxiety should be treated as a **psychiatric problem**. Disease process such as hypothyroid, hypoglycemia, cardiovascular disease, or pulmonary disease can produce anxiety symptoms. Other medications or substance abuse should also be ruled out as possible causes. Many times, anxiety occurs along with other psychiatric disturbances; therefore, the patient should be screened for other **disorders** such as depression or schizophrenia. Many times, the anxiety symptoms will resolve if the main psychiatric disorder is treated appropriately.

> **Review Video: Sedatives, Hypnotics, and Insomnia Management**
> Visit mometrix.com/academy and enter code: 666132
>
> **Review Video: Chronic Insomnia**
> Visit mometrix.com/academy and enter code: 293232

BENZODIAZEPINES

INDICATIONS

Benzodiazepines prescribed for **anxiety**, though current recommendations recommend the use of SSRIs and buspirone prior to prescribing benzodiazepines for anxiety due to side effects and addiction potential. Some of the more commonly prescribed include chlordiazepoxide, lorazepam, diazepam, flurazepam, and triazolam. Benzodiazepines act to enhance the neurotransmitter **GABA**. This neurotransmitter inhibits the firing rate of neurons and therefore leads to a decline in anxiety symptoms. Indications for their use can include anxiety, insomnia disorders, alcohol withdrawal, seizure control, skeletal muscle spasticity, or agitation. They can also be utilized to reduce the anxiety symptoms pre-operatively or before any other type of medical procedure such as cardiac catheterization or colonoscopy. This class of drug is also the treatment of choice for alcohol withdrawal.

SIDE EFFECTS

There are several common side effects associated with the use of benzodiazepines. One of the most common is the effect of **drowsiness**. Patients should be advised to use caution when operating motor vehicles or machinery. Activity will help decrease this effect. Other side effects include feelings of detachment, irritability, emotional lability, GI upset, dependency, or development of tolerance. The elderly population is at high risk for development of **dizziness** or **cognitive impairment**, which places them at high risk for falls with associated injuries. When discontinuing a benzodiazepine after long-term use, the drug should be weaned off to prevent withdrawal side effects.

TREATMENT OF INSOMNIA

Benzodiazepines are used to treat insomnia because of their **sedative-hypnotic effects**. There are three different types of insomnia, which include the inability to fall asleep, inability to stay asleep, or the combination of both. Many times, insomnia can be helped by a change in habits or talking about worries or stress the patient may be experiencing. When using a sedative-hypnotic to treat sleep disturbances, the medication should have rapid onset and allow the patient to wake up feeling refreshed instead of tired and groggy. When administered at bedtime, most benzodiazepines will produce a sleep-inducing effect and should be used on a short-term basis.

USE OF BUSPIRONE FOR TREATMENT OF ANXIETY

Due to the addictive potential of benzodiazepines, the use of nonbenzodiazepines to treat anxiety has increased. Buspirone is recommended as a second-line treatment for generalized anxiety disorder, either as monotherapy or in addition to SSRIs (the first-line treatment). This medication is highly effective in treating anxiety and its associated symptoms such as insomnia, poor concentration, tension, restlessness, irritability, and fatigue. Buspirone has no addiction potential, is not useful in alcohol withdrawal and seizures, and is not known to interact with other CNS depressants. Because it may take several weeks of continual use for the effects of this drug to be realized by the patient, it cannot be used on an as needed basis. Buspirone does not increase depression symptoms and therefore is useful in treating anxiety associated with depression. Side effects associated with medication can include GI upset, dizziness, sleepiness, excitement, or headache.

STIMULANT MEDICATIONS

Stimulant medications are utilized to treat **attention deficit hyperactivity disorder**, **narcolepsy**, and **obesity** that persist despite trying other treatment options. They are also used along with other medications to treat **fatigue** common in depression or other mood disorders. These stimulants lead to an increased level of **catecholamines** in the synapses. They increase the levels released as well as block their reuptake. They mainly affect **dopamine and norepinephrine levels**. Side effects of these medications can include decreased appetite, sleep disturbances, vertigo, irritability, GI upset, headache, palpitations, tachycardia, irregular heart rate, dry mouth, or constipation.

MEDICATION MANAGEMENT OF BIPOLAR DISORDER

PHASES OF MANAGEMENT

During the **acute phase** of bipolar, the main goal is the elimination of symptoms and stabilization of mood. To achieve this, mood stabilizer may need to be used in polypharmacy therapy with antipsychotics or benzodiazepines if the patient is psychotic or experiencing agitation or insomnia.

During the **continuation phase**, the main goal is to prevent relapse of the manic or depressive episode and to prevent the patient from swinging over to the opposite pole. This phase can last approximately 2-9 months and consists of close monitoring and continuation of the mood stabilizing medication.

During the **maintenance phase**, the outcome goal is to continue remission of the disorder and enhance quality of life. This phase may consist of life-long treatment with a mood stabilizer

MEDICATION ASSESSMENTS

Medication treatment regimens for bipolar patients should be consistently **evaluated**. It is possible for the antidepressant medication used for the depressed episode to actually cause a manic episode. If this occurs the medication should be discontinued. **Patient medication compliance** is also very important. Many times, the patients will feel as if they no longer need their medications and self-discontinue leading to a manic or depressive episode. Patients should be well educated on interactions with other substances or alcohol and they may need to have regular drug testing to rule out substance abuse.

MOOD STABILIZING MEDICATIONS USED IN PATIENTS WITH BIPOLAR AFFECTIVE DISORDERS

Mood stabilizing medications are most commonly utilized to treat **bipolar disorder**. This disorder is characterized by recurrent periods of mania and if left untreated, is associated with increased rates of morbidity and mortality. The goal of treatment with mood stabilizing medications is to prevent recurrence of acute episodes while functioning at an optimal level of production in daily life. Lithium remains the treatment of choice; however, some anticonvulsants such as carbamazepine and valproate have shown some mood stabilizing properties. In addition, calcium-channel blockers have also been used in conjunction with other medication choices to control symptoms. FDA-approved medications for treatment of bipolar disorder include lithium, olanzapine, and valproic acid.

SIDE EFFECTS OF DIVALPROEX IN TREATMENT OF BIPOLAR DISORDER

Divalproex (Depakote), a derivative of valproic acid, has the **fewest side effects** and **adverse reactions** and the **lowest potential for toxicity** of all anticonvulsants used to treat bipolar disorder. This medication has become the **first-line medication choice** for treatment of bipolar disorder because of its low potential for toxicity and effective treatment in several subgroups of bipolar disorder. It is usually well tolerated by the patient with side effects including GI upset, tremors, drowsiness, headache, vertigo, and ataxia. It has also been associated with increased appetite and weight gain. The appearance of unexplained bruising, petechiae, or bleeding can indicate thrombocytopenia, and the drug must be stopped. The most dangerous adverse side effect to this medication is severe liver damage. Liver function tests are obtained before starting the drug, then every 1-4 weeks for 6 months, followed by routine evaluations every 3-6 months throughout treatment. This medication is contraindicated during pregnancy.

INDICATIONS FOR USE OF ANTICONVULSANTS TO TREAT BIPOLAR AFFECTIVE DISORDER

Anticonvulsant medications are most commonly used to treat seizure disorder. However, they have also shown effectiveness in a reduction of mania symptoms associated with **bipolar affective disorder**. There are several anticonvulsant medications that are utilized in the treatment for mania. They include the following: valproic acid, gabapentin, carbamazepine, topiramate, lamotrigine and oxcarbazepine. These medications are often second-line drugs for patients unresponsive to lithium or Depakote, with valproate being the most widely recommended second-line medication used. Patients with mixed or dysphoric mania have been found to benefit most from use of anticonvulsants to treat their symptoms of high anxiety and agitation.

DOSE CALCULATIONS
CALCULATING DOSES AND MONITORING ANTIANXIETY AGENTS

Classes include the following:

- Antihistamines (hydroxyzine)
- Benzodiazepines (alprazolam, bromazepam, chlordiazepoxide, clonazepam, clorazepate, diazepam, lorazepam, oxazepam)
- Tranquilizers (meprobamate)
- Azapirones (buspirone)

Doses are calculated, according to a daily dosage range, which varies for different drugs (e.g., alprazolam, 0.75-4.0 mg daily; diazepam 4-40 mg daily). The usual procedure is to start with a low initial dose and then slowly increase the strength every 3–4 days or longer if the response is inadequate. Buspirone has a delayed onset, so the initial response does not occur for up to 2 weeks.

- Administer with food or milk, but avoid grapefruit juice.
- Inform patient that abrupt discontinuation may cause life-threatening effects.
- Observe for reduced anxiety, exacerbation of depression, or paradoxical excitement.
- Monitor for orthostatic hypotension and blood dyscrasias (e.g., sore throat, bruising, bleeding).
- Provide ice chips, sugarless gum, and hard candy for dry mouth.
- Provide stool softeners for constipation.
- Inform patient to avoid central nervous system depressants, such as alcohol.

CALCULATING DOSES OF ANTIDEPRESSANTS
TRICYCLICS AND HETEROCYCLICS

Doses are calculated according to a **daily dosage range**, which varies for different drugs (amitriptyline, 50–300 mg daily; nortriptyline, 30–150 mg daily, bupropion, 200–450 mg daily). The initial dose is usually a fairly low one, depending on the degree of depression (somewhat higher for inpatients than outpatients), and may be given in a single dose or divided doses. Slow titration is necessary because response may take 1–4 weeks.

Classes include the following:

- **Tricyclics** (amitriptyline, amoxapine, clomipramine, desipramine, doxepin, imipramine, nortriptyline, protriptyline, trimipramine)
- **Heterocyclics** (bupropion, maprotiline, mirtazapine, trazodone)

SSRIs

Doses are calculated according to a **daily dosage range**, which varies for different drugs (citalopram, 20–40 mg; sertraline, 50–200 mg). The **initial dose** is usually low and titrated as necessary. For patients with comorbid anxiety, a low initial dose is essential. Because response often takes up to 4–6 weeks, the initial dose should not be increased for several weeks. If adverse effects occur, a lower dose should be given. If symptoms subside, the dose may be increased at a later time if necessary. If no response occurs after 4–6 weeks, then a different medication should be considered. Common SSRIs include the following:

- Citalopram (Celexa)
- Escitalopram (Lexapro)
- Fluoxetine (Prozac)
- Fluvoxamine (Luvox)
- Paroxetine (Paxil)
- Sertraline (Zoloft)

Complementary Interventions

ALTERNATIVE AND COMPLEMENTARY MEDICINE

Complementary and alternative medicine (CAM) focuses on the whole person, including not just the physical aspects but the **spiritual and psychosocial aspects** as well. This approach utilizes many different philosophies and therapies that work together to help incorporate all aspects of the person as a whole in the healing process. Alternative medicine is used alone, whereas complementary medicine is used in conjunction with conventional Western medicine. There are **five major categories** of complementary and alternative medicine. These include alternative medical systems, mind-body interventions, biologically based therapies, manipulative and body-based methods, and energy therapies.

ALTERNATIVE MEDICAL SYSTEMS

Alternative medical systems are complete systems of theory and practice. These systems have come into being and progressed apart from the more conventional biomedical approach. Many of these systems were already in existence for hundreds or thousands of years before the inventions of conventional medicine. Examples of these systems include traditional oriental medicine, Ayurveda, homeopathy, and naturopathy.

- **Ayurveda** promotes good health and disease prevention through a healthy lifestyle. This system utilizes massage, meditation, yoga, a healthy diet, and herbal medicine.
- **Homeopathy** operates under the belief that the body can heal itself. This system believes that if a certain substance causes symptoms, then giving the same substance in small diluted doses to the body can cure the symptoms by enhancing the body's natural healing processes.
- **Naturopathic medicine** also believes the body can heal itself and promotes health and healing through the use of organic food, exercise, and a well-balanced healthy lifestyle.

MIND-BODY INTERVENTIONS

The domain of mind-body interventions utilized with complementary and alternative medicine (CAM) incorporates a variety of techniques designed to improve the **mind's** ability to alter **physical symptoms** of diseases. This system believes that the mind can help keep the body healthy. Some of these interventions, such as support groups and cognitive-behavioral therapy, are now utilized in more mainstream Western style medicine. Other examples of these types of interventions are still considered to belong to the realm of CAM and can include meditation; guided imagery; relaxation techniques; aromatherapy; hypnosis; prayer; and art, humor, light, music, or dance therapy. Many of these therapies are widely utilized as alternative treatments or in complement with conventional medicine to treat chronic pain.

BIOLOGICALLY BASED THERAPIES

The domain of biologically based therapies in complementary and alternative medicine (CAM) utilizes products found in **nature**. These practices include the use of interventions and products that may be sometimes utilized by conventional medicine, such as the use of dietary supplements. Other examples of these products can include herbal treatments or special nature-based diets. Some of these therapies, such as use of shark cartilage to treat cancer, are controversial and lack any scientific evidence to support their use.

MANIPULATIVE AND BODY-BASED METHODS AND ENERGY THERAPIES

The domain of manipulative and body-based methods in complementary and alternative medicine is based upon the **manipulation and movement of parts of the body**. Some examples of this domain include massage therapy, chiropractic or osteopathic manipulation, and reflexology.

The domain of **energy therapies** focuses on energy fields. Within this domain there are two different types of energy fields.

- The first type is **biofield therapy**, which affects the energy fields that surround the body or are derived from within the body. Examples of biofield therapy include qi gong, Reiki, and therapeutic touch.
- The second type of energy field is **electromagnetic based therapies**, which use energy from sources outside the body. Examples of these types of therapies include pulsed fields, magnetic fields, alternating current, or direct current fields.

ACUPUNCTURE

One of the main uses for acupuncture is for the treatment of **pain**. This treatment originated in China in the sixteenth century and has been recognized by the World Health Organization to assist with symptom relief of over 30 disease processes or conditions. This treatment involves the insertion of stainless-steel needles into 14 acupoints found along the body's energy channels or meridians. The belief is that this treatment restores the balance of energy within the body. The insertion of the needles induces an ache within the stimulated muscle, which then sends a message to the central nervous system to release endorphins, which block pain, along with serotonin and norepinephrine.

IMPLEMENTING RELAXATION SKILLS ON THE PSYCHIATRIC UNIT

On the psychiatric unit, there are several different patients who are at different **levels of severity** in their mental illness. This can occasionally create a potentially volatile environment when there are conflicting personalities. **Decreasing the stimuli** on the unit can have a calming effect on some. This would include lowering the volume on a television or stereo. Decreasing the noise at the nurse's station or amongst staff on the floor can also help to decrease some of the stimuli which patients are exposed to. Playing soft music can be soothing. Soft, neutral colors within the interior of the unit can create a more calming environment, as well. When a patient appears to be escalating or becoming more agitated, engaging them in another activity to **redirect their energy** can be helpful. This can include removing them from a disagreement with another patient, finding an outlet for their energy to encourage their focus on something else, or speaking calmly to them to help with relaxation.

ST. JOHN'S WORT FOR TREATMENT OF DEPRESSION

The use of complementary and alternative medicine for the treatment of **depression** is very common. One of the most widely utilized and studied herbal therapies for the treatment of depression is **St. John's wort** or hypericum. This particular herb is widely utilized to treat depression symptoms in both the United States and in European countries. It has shown some effectiveness in treating moderate depression, anxiety disorder, insomnia, or seasonal affective disorder. Medical providers should be aware if the patient is taking this herb due to its contraindications with many commonly prescribed medications such as birth control pills, statins used to treat hyperlipidemia, protease inhibitors, antineoplastics, SSRIs, anticonvulsants, theophylline, and anticoagulants such as coumadin.

ECT

Electroconvulsive therapy (ECT) is a treatment in which the use of a brief electrical shock is utilized to induce a **seizure**. Although it is not certain exactly how ECT works, it is believed that the seizure acts to alter certain electrochemical processes in the brain. ECT is not for everyone. Psychiatrists only administer this procedure to selective patient populations. ECT is recommended for individuals with severe depression that is unresponsive to medications or accompanied by suicidal ideations, psychosis, insomnia, homicidal ideations, or guilt and hopelessness. It is also recommended for schizophrenia or mania that is unresponsive to medications. It may also have some limited indications for use in catatonia, schizoaffective disorder, Parkinson's disease, or the individual in which certain medications are contraindicated. Use of ECT on the elderly population should be performed with great caution due to the coexistence of many contraindicated disease processes with this population. This population often has preexisting heart disease.

PRE- AND POST-PROCEDURAL EVALUATION AND TEACHING

Before preparing for electroconvulsive therapy (ECT) the individual must first have a complete **history and physical**. This should include lab tests, EKG, and careful blood pressure evaluation for hypertension. The individual must be physically capable of tolerating the procedure. An anesthesiologist will also be consulted to evaluate for any contraindications to the use of **anesthesia**. After the procedure the individual will be taken to a recovery area where they will be monitored and the anesthetic is allowed to wear off. The patient usually begins to awaken 5-10 minutes after the procedure is completed. A short period of confusion lasting up to a few hours is not uncommon. Once completely awake, the patient may then dress, eat, and return home or to their room in the hospital.

INFORMED CONSENT

An informed written consent must be obtained prior to the use of electroconvulsive therapy (ECT). This involves using clear and understandable language to **educate** the person about ECT, including what to expect before, during, and after the procedure; any benefits, risks, or side effects; how many treatments are expected; and any optional treatments available. Any and all questions are encouraged and clearly answered. A simple and concise video may also be a very useful educational tool to assist the individual in understanding what to expect with ECT. The individual should be updated on the progress of the treatments with each procedure and may withdraw consent to continue at any point during the course of treatment. If the person is unable to make decisions for him or herself, most local laws provide for the court to appoint a legal guardian to provide consent.

PERFORMANCE OF TREATMENTS AND MONITORING

Electroconvulsive therapy (ECT) is performed in a **hospital setting**. The individual may be inpatient or outpatient. ECT is performed up to 3 times per week with the total number of treatments ranging from 6 to 12. ECT is administered in the **morning** with the patient having been NPO to reduce the risk of vomiting and subsequent aspiration. The treatment is performed by a **psychiatrist** with an **anesthesiologist** present to administer short-acting anesthesia and muscle relaxant intravenously. The procedure itself takes approximately 10-15 minutes. Electrode pads are placed on the side of the head and the shock, lasting 1-2 seconds, can be administered unilaterally or bilaterally causing a brief seizure. The seizure usually lasts 30-60 seconds and is monitored by use of an EEG. A few minutes after the procedure is completed the patient begins to awaken.

POTENTIAL RISKS

The **risks** associated with ECT are the same as many other medical procedures involving **anesthesia**. There are also risks involved with the introduction of an **electrical shock** into the body. The pre-procedural history and physical are very important in determining any preexisting contraindicated medical conditions such as heart disease, cardiac arrhythmias, pulmonary disease, central nervous system problems, hypertension, or previous reaction to anesthesia. ECT may cause an increase in heart rate and blood pressure and could in rare cases, as in any medical procedure, lead to death.

SIDE EFFECTS

The side effects associated with electroconvulsive therapy (ECT) can originate from the administration of the **electrical shock**, the **anesthesia**, or more likely from a combination of both. Immediately after the treatment side effects may include headaches, transient confusion, muscle soreness, nausea, vomiting, or jaw pain. ECT can also cause some **memory loss**. This side effect may worsen over the course of treatment and may include **retrograde amnesia**, causing partial or complete memory loss of events occurring days, weeks, months, or occasionally years before the procedure. Memory loss during the actual time of the treatments may also occur. For most people, this amnesia will resolve within a few months after treatment has ended.

191

Evaluating Intervention Effectiveness

PURPOSE OF EVALUATING PATIENT OUTCOMES

The main purpose of evaluating patient outcomes is to assure the delivery of **quality care**. Patient outcome measures drive the process of quality improvement. These outcomes provide a framework for an expected patient response based on current medical knowledge. By monitoring and documenting patient outcomes, **negative trends or variations** can be identified and then measures put in place to decrease these trends. Through identification of negative variables, nursing interventions can be added or removed to positively affect patient outcomes. Patients can also utilize outcome measurements to achieve feelings of success when they attain a specific outcome.

DOCUMENTATION OF PATIENT OUTCOMES

Psychiatric nurses are not only responsible for creating nursing diagnoses and interventions and evaluating outcomes, but they are also responsible for their proper **documentation**. This documentation is utilized to determine the success of the treatment as well as its cost effectiveness. These outcomes are measured against multiple factors that may affect the patient during treatment, such as physical illness, coping abilities, functional status, and overall patient and family satisfaction. This data collection can be utilized to determine program development, budgets, and staffing related issues. The main outcomes to be evaluated include clinical, satisfaction, functional, and financial outcomes.

COLLABORATION IN DEVELOPING AND UPDATING A CARE PLAN

One of the most important forms of collaboration in developing and updating a care plan is between the nurse, the patient, and his or her family, but this type of collaboration is often overlooked. Nurses and others on the health care team must always remember that the point of collaborating is to improve patient care. This means that the patient and the patient's family are central to all planning. Including the family may initially be time-consuming, but asking and evaluating the wants of the patient and the family can provide valuable information that can facilitate planning and improve the allocation of resources. Families, including young children, often feel validated and more positive toward the medical system when they are included in the decision-making process.

EXPECTED DEVELOPMENTAL RESPONSE TO ILLNESS AND HOSPITALIZATION IN PATIENTS
PEDIATRIC PATIENTS

Many pediatric patients who suffer from chronic illness are much more knowledgeable about the healthcare process than other children. There can seem to be a "loss of innocence" about them as they navigate through the process of doctor's appointments, treatment appointments, various therapy obligations, and other necessary treatments. Unfortunately, pediatric patients with a chronic illness are often not able to participate in many of the **normal activities** seen performed by healthy children. There may be **anger** expressed by these patients because of their situation. **Depression** can also occur because of the sense of loss they experience with the absence of normal age-appropriate activities and friends. Because they are often not exposed to the normal activities of others in their age group, they may experience a **sense of loss** for missing out on these experiences. This can lead to feelings of hopelessness and helplessness if they do not have any control over the lives.

ADOLESCENT PATIENTS

Delayed growth and puberty are common results of most chronic illnesses. This may be transient with normal development by adulthood. For those adolescents with chronic mental health issues, they may adopt the sick role as a way of identifying themselves. This can develop into **egocentricity** that can carry into adulthood. **Sexual development** may be delayed as well, as they develop a sense that they are not attractive to others. Their sense of independence may be delayed and they may suffer from **social isolation** due to their chronic illness. If their chronic illness interferes with formal education, this can lead to failure to develop a **vocation**, which can prevent them from living independently later in life.

ELDERLY PATIENTS

Elderly patients who suffer from chronic illnesses that require frequent hospitalization are at high risk for developing **depression** and **anxiety**. They may have fears pertaining to end-of-life issues and a sense of loss due to the limitations of their body due to the chronic illness. Many of these patients may have already lost a spouse or someone else who was a vital part of their support team, which can contribute to feelings of helplessness and hopelessness. They may also be facing regrets for those things they have lost or things they wish they could do. All of these factors can combine to contribute to feelings of despair and thoughts that life is no longer worth living. Many elderly patients may feel like they are a burden with their health issues and feel like giving up because they are not as independent as they had been.

Psychotherapy and Related Theories

Psychotherapy Principles and Theoretical Frameworks

IMOGENE KING'S THEORY OF GOAL ATTAINMENT

King organizes her **theory of goal attainment** within three systems as follows:

- **Personal systems**: Each individual is a personal system.
- **Interpersonal systems**: Interpersonal systems are the interactions among people.
- **Social systems**: A social system is an organized system of roles, behaviors, and practices.

King's theory states that people come together to help and to be helped. Key concepts of the theory are as follows:

- **Interaction**: Goal-directed communication
- **Perception**: Organizing, processing, storing, and exporting information
- **Communication**: Information sharing among individuals
- **Transaction**: Observable behaviors of people interacting with their environment
- **Role**: A set of behaviors expected of a person occupying a certain position
- **Stress**: A response to a stressor
- **Growth and development**: Continuous changes which occur in life
- **Time**: The passage of events which move toward the future
- **Space**: A physical area or territory

SISTER CALLISTA ROY'S ADAPTATION MODEL

According to **Roy's adaptation model**, each person is an adaptive system with four adaptive elements.

- **Input**: Internal or external stimuli
- **Internal processes (coping mechanisms)**:
  - The regulator subsystem—chemical, neural, and endocrine transmitters
  - The cognator subsystem—perception, information processing, judgment, and emotion
- **Adaptive modes (system effectors)**:
  - Physiological function mode—identifies patterns of physiological functioning
  - Self-concept mode—identifies patterns of values, beliefs, and emotions
  - Role function mode—identifies patterns of social interaction
  - Interdependence mode—identifies patterns of human values, affection, and love
- **Individual output**: Adaptive response or ineffective response

The goal of nursing is the promotion of adaptive responses in relation to adaptive modes. Health is the process of being and becoming an integrated person. Environment includes the conditions, circumstances, and influences affecting the growth and behavior of a person.

According to Roy, the **nursing process levels** consist of the following:

- **First-level assessment**: Includes behavioral assessment and the assessment of the four adaptive models
- **Second-level assessment**: Includes identification of focal, contextual, and residual stimuli, along with identification of ineffective responses
  - The identification of the nursing diagnosis
  - Goal setting with the client
  - Implementation by manipulating focal, contextual and/or residual goals
  - The evaluation of goal behaviors and possible readjustment of goals and interventions

MARTHA ROGERS' THEORY OF UNITARY HUMAN BEINGS

Nursing theory, according to **Rogers' theory of unitary human beings**, is defined as the phenomenon central to nursing the life process of human beings. Rogers' assumptions are as follows:

- The human being is a unified whole, processing integrity and manifesting characteristics that are more than and different from the sum of his or her parts.
- The person and environment are continually exchanging matter and energy with each other.
- The life process revolves irreversibly and unidirectionally along the time-space continuum.
- Patterns and organization identify individuals and reflect their wholeness.
- Human beings are characterized by their capacity for abstraction and imagery, language, thought, sensation, and emotion.

The **foundational concepts** of Rogers' theory are as follows:

- **Energy field**: An electrical field that is in a continuous state of flux.
- **Openness**: Energy fields are open to exchange with other energy fields.
- **Pattern**: Energy fields have patterns that change as required.
- **Four-dimensionality**: Energy fields are embedded in a four-dimensional space-time matrix.

Rogers' **principles of homeodynamics** are as follows:

- **Integrality**: The continuous, mutual simultaneous interaction between humans and environmental fields
- **Resonancy**: The identification of human and environmental fields by changing wave patterns
- **Helicy**: The evolving innovative repatterning growing out of the mutual interaction of man and environment

DORTHEA OREM'S THEORY OF SELF-CARE DEFICIT

According to Dorthea Orem, self-care refers to activities that maintain life, health, and wellbeing. The three **categories of self-care fundamentals** are:

- **Universal**: Activities of daily living (ADLs)
- **Developmental**: Specialized activities related to a specific task or event
- **Health deviation**: Activities required by illness, injury, or disease

Self-care deficit refers to the inability to provide complete self-care. Someone with a self-care deficit requires nursing care. Nursing care involves the following:

- Entering into and maintaining the nurse-patient relationship
- Assessing how the patient can be helped
- Responding to patients' needs and requests

- Prescribing, providing, and regulating direct help
- Coordinating and integrating nursing care with other services

Nursing system refers to the amount of nursing care a patient requires, categorized as follows:

- **Wholly compensatory**: Nurse provides all care
- **Partly compensatory**: Nurse and patient collaborate in care
- **Supportive-educative**: Patient provides needed care, while nurse educates and promotes the patient as a self-care agent

MADELEINE LEININGER'S THEORY OF CULTURE CARE DIVERSITY AND UNIVERSALITY

Madeleine Leininger notes in the **theory of culture care diversity and universality** that "care is the essence of nursing and the central, dominant and unifying focus" (Leininger, 1991). Other definitions and concepts include:

- **Culture**: The learned, shared, and transmitted values, beliefs and norms of a group that guide their actions and decisions
- **Cultural care diversity**: Refers to differences in meanings, patterns, values and/or symbols of care, within or between collectivities, related to expressions of human care
- **Cultural care universality**: Refers to uniform meanings, patterns and/or symbols of a group that are manifest in many cultures and reflect ways to help people
- **Cultural and social structure dimensions**: Refer to patterns of structural and organizational factors of a particular culture, which include religious, social, kinship, economic, political, legal, educational, technological, and ethno-historical factors

Key terms in the theory of culture care diversity and universality include:

- **Cultural care preservation or maintenance**: Refers to the actions and decisions that help people retain relevant cultural care values and maintain wellbeing, recover from illness, and face handicaps or death
- **Cultural care accommodation or negotiation**: Refers to actions and decisions that help people of a designated culture negotiate for a beneficial outcome with health caregivers
- **Cultural care re-patterning or restructuring**: Refers to actions and decisions that help clients modify their "lifeways" for beneficial health care while respecting their cultural values and beliefs
- **Cultural congruent nursing care**: Refers to actions and decisions that are tailored to fit cultural patterns and beliefs

THEORIES OF CARL JUNG

Jung's archetypes are the images and concepts that develop the collective unconscious of humanity. The main archetypes are:

- **The Way**: The image of a journey or voyage through life
- **The Self**: The aspect of the mind that unifies and orders experience
- **Animus and Anima**: The image of gender
- **Rebirth**: The concept of being reborn, resurrected or reincarnated
- **Persona**: The role or mask one shows to others
- **Shadow**: The dark side of one's personality
- **Stock characters**: Dramatic roles that appear over and over in folktales
- **The Hero**: The character who vanquishes evil and rescues the downtrodden
- **The Trickster**: The character who plays pranks or works magic spells
- **The Sage**: The wise old person

- **Power**: A symbol such as the eagle or the sword
- **Number**: Certain numbers appear throughout history and across cultures

The two **attitudinal types** according to Jung are:

- **Introvert**: One oriented toward the inner, subjective world
- **Extrovert**: One oriented toward the outer, external world

The four **functional types** according to Jung are:

- **Thinking**: An intellectual process involving ideas
- **Feeling**: An evaluative function involving value or worth
- **Sensing**: A function involving recognition that something exists, without categorizing or evaluating it
- **Intuiting**: A function involving creative inspiration without having all the facts

THEORIES OF SIGMUND FREUD
PSYCHOANALYTIC/PSYCHODYNAMIC PERSONALITY THEORY

Sigmund Freud, commonly known as the father of psychoanalysis, based his practice on **psychoanalytic and psychodynamic personality theories**. The foundations of these theories are based on the following concepts.

Levels of awareness:

- **Conscious**: Thoughts, feelings, desires of which a person is aware and able to control
- **Preconscious**: Thoughts, feelings, desires not in immediate awareness but can be recalled to consciousness
- **Unconscious**: Thoughts, feelings, desires not available to the conscious mind

Stages of development: Each person passes through stages of psychosexual development (can become trapped in any stage):

- **Oral**: Focus on sucking and swallowing
- **Anal**: Focus on spontaneous bowel movements or control over impulses
- **Phallic**: Focus on genital region, and identification with parent of same gender
- **Latency**: Sexual impulses are dormant, focus on coping with the environment
- **Genital**: Focus on erotic and genital behavior, leading to development of mature sexual and emotional relationships

Personality structure: The personality has three main components:

- **Id**: Unconscious pleasure principle, manifest by a desire for immediate and complete satisfaction with disregard for others
- **Ego**: Rational and conscious reality principle, which weighs actions and consequences
- **Superego**: Conscious and unconscious censoring force of the personality, which evaluates and judges behavior

Common **Freudian psychiatric terms** include:

- **Oedipus Complex or Electra Conflict**: At the age of four or five, the child falls in love with the parent of the opposite sex and feels hostility toward the parent of the same sex.
- **Defense mechanisms**: Conscious or unconscious actions or thoughts designed to protect the ego from anxiety.
- **Freudian slips**: Also known as parapraxes, these are overt actions with unconscious meanings.

- **Free association**: A method designed to discover the contents of the unconscious by associating words with other words or emotions.
- **Transference**: Transference takes place when feelings, attitudes and/or wishes linked with a significant figure in one's early life are projected onto others in one's current life.
- **Counter-transference**: This happens when the feelings and attitudes of the therapist are projected onto the client inappropriately.
- **Resistance**: Resistance is anything that prohibits a person from retrieving information from the unconscious.
- **Fixation**: Someone who is bogged-down in one stage of development has a fixation.

Review Video: Sigmund Freud
Visit mometrix.com/academy and enter code: 473747

FREUD'S CONCEPT OF SUPEREGO

Freud coined the word *superego* to make sense out of the rules imposed upon us by our parents. Rules involving parents, family, religion, and culture contribute to our sense of right and wrong. The problem arises whenever a rule has been imposed that is unrelenting and harsh. Freud linked this to his interview of female clients. Victorian women had difficulty accepting their sexual urges as a natural occurrence. This conflict of right and wrong caused the females to experience hysterical paralysis and other notable anxiety disorders. However, symptoms were alleviated when the clients gained insight and emotional release from their inner turmoil. **Free association** is the client's expression concerning secretive and painful thoughts, feelings, and memories in a non-judgmental therapy session. The therapeutic bond or relationship is imperative in this technique. Free association used in this way can still be beneficial today.

Review Video: Interaction of the Id, Ego, and Superego
Visit mometrix.com/academy and enter code: 690435

FREUD'S CONCEPT OF TRANSFERENCE

Freud's concept of **transference** can be applied to the exchanges that take place between the modern client and the mental health care provider. The client's propensity is to behave toward the provider as one would a key authority figure. The provider can help the client understand this propensity and work to help the client alter this unconscious transference to other people. Awareness of transference must become a part of the client's conscious thought. The client must be aware when this has happened and seek to change the behavior on a conscious level. Cognitive rethinking techniques and behavioristic role plays enable the provider's efforts to get the client to work through a maladaptive behavior. The provider can also use a variety of techniques to help the client internalize positive feelings and thought patterns.

UNCONSCIOUS MIND IN CONJUNCTION WITH PSYCHODYNAMIC THEORIES

Sigmund Freud's theories involve getting at **unconscious thoughts** that cause behaviors. The client must come to terms with unconscious thoughts rather than bottle up those feelings, and thus deal with issues in a more functional manner. **Psychodynamic theorists** of today try to help the client make a connection between the past and existing problems. However, a cognitive-behavioral approach may need to be supplemented with in-depth counseling. Some topics that may require further investigation are the client's family and parental interactions, unresolved issues, unconscious practices, and defensive mechanisms. Freud believed pathological thinking was at odds with the id instincts of Eros and Thanatos. Eros stands for the life processes involving love and relationships. Thanatos stands for death processes involving negative emotions and the fighting response. The mind is trying to manage these forces, which causes anxiety and the client forms phobias or conversion disorders.

OBJECT-RELATIONS SCHOOL

The **Object-Relations School** looks at the primary caregiver relationship in a child's early years of growth. A positive parental relationship leads the infant to understand about safety, security, self-worth, nurturance, and caring. The infant grows into a child with a positive self-identity and is better able to form healthy relationships with others. Those infants that have a negative parental relationship feel unloved, detested, valueless, insignificant, inferior, and shamed. These images form the person's personality and behaviors. The inner belief system is referred to as the schema in the cognitive therapy model. It is known as the **incorporated object relation** in the psychodynamic model. Object-relations take into account the Freudian theories regarding instinctive urges. These urges are the driving force to form either loving or destructive relationships. The client explores the repressed feelings in front of a provider who has created a safe and trusted setting.

ALFRED ADLER'S THEORY OF INDIVIDUAL PSYCHOLOGY

Adler's **key concepts** include:

- Inferiority feelings are the source of all human striving.
- Personal growth results from one's attempts to compensate for this inferiority.

Two types of **complexes** exist:

- **Inferiority**: An inability to solve life's problems
- **Superiority**: An exaggerated opinion of one's abilities and accomplishments in an attempt to compensate for an inferiority complex

The goal of life is to strive for superiority. Lifestyle is the unique set of behaviors created to compensate for inferiority and to achieve superiority.

Adler also theorized that **birth order** affects personality:

- **First born**: Happy, secure, and the center of attention until dethroned by the second child; interested in authority and organization
- **Second born**: Born into a more relaxed atmosphere and has the first-born as a model; interested in competition
- **Youngest child**: Pet of the family and may retain a sense of dependency

FRITZ PERLS' GESTALT THERAPY

The removal of masks and facades is the goal of Gestalt therapy, according to Perls. A creative interaction needs to be developed so the client can gain an ongoing awareness of what is being felt, sensed, and thought. **Boundary disturbances** (lack of awareness of the immediate environment) may occur:

- **Projection**: Fantasy of what another person is experiencing
- **Introjection**: Accepting the beliefs and opinions of others without question
- **Retroflection**: Turning back on oneself that which is meant for someone else
- **Confluence**: Merging with the environment
- **Deflection**: Interfering with contact, used by receivers and senders of messages

Goal of therapy is integration of self and world awareness. **Techniques** of therapy include:

- **Playing the projection**: Taking on and experiencing the role of another person
- **Making the rounds**: Speaking or doing something to other group members to experiment with new behavior
- **Sentence completion**: "I take responsibility for…"
- **Exaggeration** of a feeling or action to clarify the purpose or intent

- **Empty chair dialogue**: Having an interaction with an imaginary provocateur
- **Dream world**: Explored by describing and playing parts of a dream

CARL ROGERS' CLIENT CENTERED THEORY

Key concepts in **Carl Rogers' client centered theory** include:

- The **attributes** of the therapist
- **Congruence**: inner feelings match outer actions
- **Unconditional positive regard**: therapist sees the client as a person of intrinsic worth and treats the client non-judgmentally
- **Empathic understanding**: therapist is a sensitive listener

The **goal of therapy** is helping the client become a fully functioning person, achieving this goal by:

- Relinquishing facades
- Banishing "oughts"
- Becoming a non-conformist by moving away from cultural expectations
- Becoming self-directed as opposed to pleasing others
- Dropping defenses
- Trusting one's own intuition
- Accepting others

NEUROLINGUISTIC PROGRAMMING

The major concepts of **neurolinguistic programming (NLP)** according to Bandler and Grinder include:

- **Representational Systems**: Sensory models through which people access information, such as audio, visual and kinesthetic models. Cues to representational systems are patterns which can be heard or observed.
  - Preferred predicates: a "view" that suggests a visual system
  - Eye-Accessing cues: looking upward suggests a visual system
  - Hand movements: pointing toward the ear suggests an auditory system
  - Breathing patterns: suggest a kinesthetic system
  - Speech pattern/tone: suggests an auditory system
- **Language structure**:
  - Surface structure: sentences that native speakers of a language speak and write
  - Deep structure: the linguistic representations from which the surface structures of a language are derived
  - Ambiguity: a surface language may represent more than one deep structure
- **Human modeling**: The process of representing something through language
  - Generalization: specific experiences that come to represent the entire category of which they are a member
  - Deletion: selected portions of the world are excluded from the representation created by an individual
  - Distortion: the relationship among the parts of the model which differ from the relationships they were supposed to represent

JOHN HATTIE'S THEORY OF SELF-CONCEPT

The major concepts of **Hattie's theory of self-concept** include:

- A cognitive appraisal consisting of beliefs about the self
- Expectations from self and others: High expectations can lead to low self-esteem and vice versa

Descriptions of oneself are:

- **Hierarchical**: From a description of simple or isolated characteristics to an all-inclusive description of the self
- **Multifaceted**: Having numerous dimensions

Methods of **integration** across dimensions include:

- **Self-verification**: Soliciting feedback to confirm the anticipated view of the self
- **Self-consistency**: Internal harmony among opinions, attitudes, and values
- **Self-complexity**: Viewing the self as complex and multifaceted
- **Self-enhancement**: Viewing the self's positive qualities as more important than the self's negative qualities

NEUROBIOLOGICAL THEORIES

The general features and findings foundational to **neurobiological theories** include:

- Cognitive and emotional dysfunctions may result from any insult that affects the brain's neurotransmitters, such as genetic anomalies, infection, and nutrition.
- Neurotransmitters, such as acetylcholine, are chemical substances found in the nervous system that carry messages from the axon of one neuron to the receptor site on another. In the brain, these neurotransmitters may affect cognitive, emotional, and behavioral functioning. After utilization, neurotransmitters are either inactivated by enzymatic degradation (such as a cholinesterase) or are drawn back into the presynaptic neuron.
- Psychotherapeutic drugs are prescribed to influence the process of neurotransmitter production and absorption in an attempt to establish a "normal" neurochemical balance.

THEORIES OF EMOTION

Cross-cultural research has distinguished six basic **universal human emotions**: Fear, anger, happiness, disgust, surprise, and sadness. The **James-Lange theory** of emotion asserts that emotions are the body's reaction to changes in the autonomic nervous system caused by external stimuli. This theory is supported by the fact that quadriplegics report feeling less-intense emotions. The **Cannon-Bard theory** of emotion proposes that the body and emotions react to stimuli based on thalamic stimulation of the cortex and peripheral nervous system. The **two-factor theory of Schachter and Singer** proposes that emotions are the result of arousal, the cognitive interpretation of that arousal, and the environment in which the arousal occurs.

CHANGE THEORIES
TRANSTHEORETICAL MODEL

The **transtheoretical model** focuses on changes in behavior based on the individual's decisions (not on society's decisions or others' decisions) and is used to develop strategies to promote changes in health behavior. This model outlines stages people go through when changing problem behavior and trying to have a positive attitude about change. Stages of change include the following:

- **Precontemplation**: The person is either unaware or under-informed about consequences of a problem behavior and has no intention of changing behavior within the next 6 months.
- **Contemplation**: The person is aware of costs and benefits of changing behavior and intends to change within the next 6 months but is procrastinating and not ready for action.
- **Preparation**: The person has a plan and intends to initiate change in the near future (≤1 month) and is ready for action plans.

- **Action:** The person is modifying behavior change occurs only if behavior meets a set criterion (such as complete abstinence from drinking).
- **Maintenance:** The person works to maintain changes and gains confidence that he or she will not relapse.

MOTIVATIONAL INTERVIEWING

Motivational interviewing (Miller, 1983) aims to help people identify and resolve issues regarding ambivalence about change and focuses on the role of motivation to bring about change. MI is a collaborative approach in which the interviewer assesses the individual's readiness to accept change and identifies strategies that may be effective with the individual.

Elements	Principles	Strategies
Collaboration rather than confrontation in resolving issues **Evocation** (drawing out) of the individual's ideas about change rather than imposition of the interviewer's ideas **Autonomy** of the individual in making changes	**Expression of empathy:** Showing understanding of individual's perceptions **Support of self-efficacy:** Helping individuals realize they are capable of change **Acceptance of resistance:** Avoiding struggles/conflicts with client **Examination of discrepancies:** Helping individuals see discrepancy between their behavior and goals	**Avoiding Yes/No questions:** Asking informational questions **Providing affirmations:** Indicating areas of strength **Providing reflective listening:** Responding to statements **Providing summaries:** Recapping important points of discussion **Encouraging change talk:** Including desire, ability, reason, and need

RESISTANCE TO ORGANIZATIONAL CHANGE

Performance improvement processes cannot occur without organizational change, and **resistance to change** is common for many people, so coordinating collaborative processes requires anticipating resistance and taking steps to achieve cooperation. Resistance often relates to concerns about job loss, increased responsibilities, and general denial or lack of understanding and frustration. Leaders can prepare others involved in the process of change by taking these steps:

- Be honest, informative, and tactful, giving people thorough information about anticipated changes and how the changes will affect them, including positives.
- Be patient in allowing people the time they need to contemplate changes and express anger or disagreement.
- Be empathetic in listening carefully to the concerns of others.
- Encourage participation, allowing staff to propose methods of implementing change so they feel some sense of ownership.
- Establish a climate in which all staff members are encouraged to identify the need for change on an ongoing basis.
- Present further ideas for change to management.

Copyright © Mometrix Media. You have been licensed one copy of this document for personal use only. Any other reproduction or redistribution is strictly prohibited. All rights reserved. This content is provided for test preparation purposes only and does not imply an endorsement by Mometrix of any particular political, scientific, or religious point of view.

Grief and Loss

GRIEF

Grief is an emotional response to a **loss** that begins at the time a loss is anticipated and continues on an individual timetable. While there are identifiable stages or tasks, it is not an orderly and predictable process. It involves overcoming anger, disbelief, guilt, and a myriad of related emotions. The grieving individual may move back and forth between stages or experience several emotions at any given time. Each person's grief response is unique to their own coping patterns, stress levels, age, gender, belief system, and previous experiences with loss.

KUBLER-ROSS'S FIVE STAGES OF GRIEF

Kubler-Ross taught the medical community that the dying patient and family welcomes open, honest discussion of the dying process and felt that there were certain **stages** that patients and family go through. The stages may not occur in order, but may vary or some may be skipped. Stages include:

- **Denial**: The person denies the diagnosis and tries to pretend it isn't true. During this time, the person may seek a second opinion or alternative therapies. They may use denial until they are better able to emotionally cope with the reality of the disease or changes that need to be made. Patients may also wish to save family and friends from pain and worry. Both patients and family may use denial as a coping mechanism when they feel overwhelmed by the reality of the disease and threatened losses.
- **Anger**: The person is angry about the situation and may focus that rage on anyone.
- **Bargaining**: The person attempts to make deals with a higher power to secure a better outcome to their situation.
- **Depression**: The person anticipates the loss and the changes it will bring with a sense of sadness and grief.
- **Acceptance**: The person accepts the impending death and is ready to face it as it approaches. The patient may begin to withdraw from interests and family.

> **Review Video: The Five Stages of Grief**
> Visit mometrix.com/academy and enter code: 648794

ANTICIPATORY GRIEF

Anticipatory grief is the mental, social, and somatic reactions of an individual as they prepare themselves for a **perceived future loss**. The individual experiences a process of intellectual, emotional, and behavioral responses in order to modify their self-concept, based on their perception of what the potential loss will mean in their life. This process often takes place ahead of the actual loss, from the time the loss is first perceived until it is resolved as a reality for the individual. This process can also blend with past loss experiences. It is associated with the individual's perception of how life will be affected by the particular diagnosis as well as the impending death. Acknowledging this anticipatory grief allows family members to begin looking toward a changed future. Suppressing this anticipatory process may inhibit relationships with the ill individual and contribute to a more difficult grieving process at a later time. However, appropriate anticipatory grieving does not take the place of grief during the actual time of death.

DISENFRANCHISED GRIEF

Disenfranchised grief occurs when the loss being experienced cannot be openly acknowledged, publicly mourned, or socially supported. Society and culture are partly responsible for an individual's response to a loss. There is a **social context** to grief; if a person incurring the loss will be putting himself or herself at risk if grief is expressed, disenfranchised grief occurs. The risk for disenfranchised grief is greatest among those whose relationship with the individual they lost was not known or regarded as significant. This is also the situation found among bereaved persons who are not recognized by society as capable of grief, such as young children, or needing to mourn, such as an ex-spouse or secret lover.

Grief vs. Depression

Normal grief is preoccupied with self-limiting to the loss itself. Emotional responses will vary and may include open expressions of anger. The individual may experience difficulty sleeping or vivid dreams, a lack of energy, and weight loss. Crying is evident and provides some relief of extreme emotions. The individual remains socially responsive and seeks reassurance from others.

Depression is marked by extensive periods of sadness and preoccupation often extending beyond 2 months. It is not limited to the single event. There is an absence of pleasure or anger and isolation from previous social support systems. The individual can experience extreme lethargy, weight loss, insomnia, or hypersomnia, and has no recollection of dreaming. Crying is absent or persistent and provides no relief of emotions. Professional intervention is required to relieve depression.

Loss

Loss is the blanket term used to denote the absence of a valued object, position, ability, attribute, or individual. The aspect of **loss** as it is associated with the death of an animal or person is a relatively new definition. Loss is an individualized and subjective experience depending on the **perceived attachment** between the individual and the missing aspect. This can range from little or no value of attachment to significant value. Loss also can be represented by the **withdrawal of a valued relationship** one had or would have had in the future. Depending on the unique and individual responses to the perception of loss and its significance, reactions to the loss will vary. Robinson and McKenna summarize the aspects of loss in three main attributes:

- Something has been removed.
- The item removed had value to that person.
- The response is individualized.

Mourning

Mourning is a public grief response for the death of a loved one. The various aspects of the mourning process are partially determined by **personal and cultural belief systems**. Kagawa-Singer defines mourning as "the social customs and cultural practices that follow a death." Durkheim expands this to include the following: "mourning is not a natural movement of private feelings wounded by a cruel loss; it is a duty imposed by the group." Mourning involves participation in religious and culturally appropriate customs and rituals designed to publicly acknowledge the loss. These rituals signify they are adjusting to the change in their relationships created by the loss, as well as mark the beginning of the reorganization and forward movement of their lives.

Bereavement

Bereavement is the emotional and mental state associated with having suffered a **personal loss**. It is the reactions of grief and sadness initiated by the loss of a loved one. Bereavement is a normal process of feeling deprived of something of value. The word bereave comes from the root "reave" meaning to plunder, spoil, or rob. It is recognized that the lost individual had value and a defining role in the surviving individual's life. Bereavement encompasses all the acts and emotions surrounding the feeling of loss for the individual. During this grieving period, there is an increased mortality risk. A **positive bereavement experience** means being able to recognize the significance of the loss while still recognizing the resilience and value of life.

Risk Factors Complicating Bereavement

The caregiver should assess for multiple **life crises** that take energy away from the grieving process. An important factor is the grieving individual's history with past grieving experiences. Assess for other recent, unresolved, or difficult losses that may need to be addressed before the individual can move toward resolution of the current loss. Age, mental health, substance abuse, extreme anger, anxiety, or dependence on the individual facing the end of life can add additional stressors and handicap natural coping mechanisms. Income strains, community support, outside and personal responsibilities, the absence of cultural and religious beliefs, the difficulty of the disease process, and age of the loved one lost can also present additional risk factors.

Counseling and Providing Emotional Support Regarding Grief and Loss to Children

The approach to counseling and providing emotional support regarding grief and loss to children is dependent on the age of the child. When available, children and family should be provided information about **peer support groups** (especially adolescents) and **bereavement art therapy groups** as these may be especially helpful. Healthcare professionals should use appropriate words (death, died) instead of euphemisms (passed on) when talking about the deceased and should encourage the child to ask questions. Children are often reluctant to express feelings directly, so it may be beneficial to encourage them to keep a journal about their feelings or draw pictures to express them. Parents should be encouraged to share their feelings of grief with their children rather than trying to hide their emotions and should be aware that children express grief in different ways and may regress or complain of physical ailments (stomach ache, headache) in response to grief. Children should be prepared for changes in routines or living situations, such as a stay-at-home parent having to take a job, which may occur as a result of a death or serious illness.

Signs of a Child Having Issues Managing Grief

Management of **grief** comes in stages for children as well as for adults. Grief may be complicated for a child who does not understand the significance of the situation, such as in the case of a parent's death, or for someone who does not have the necessary support systems in place, as in the case of a child who has a grieving parent who consequently becomes unavailable. **Signs that a child is not coping well with grief** include extended periods of sadness, lack of interest in regular activities, sleep disturbances, loss of appetite, statements of wishing for death or joining a person who has died, difficulties with concentration, problems taking direction at school, poor school performance, and fear of being alone.

Interventions for Patients and Family Experiencing Loss and Grief

Loss is painful and frightening. Loss can occur through death or loss of health, self-esteem, or relationships. Loss can also occur from threats, such as fire, flood, theft, or severe weather. The severity of the loss, preparation for it, and the maturity, stability, and coping mechanisms of the person all affect the grieving process. Multiple losses and substance abuse can complicate grief and recovery. Previous life experience and cultural and religious beliefs can help in resolution of grief. Many emotions are triggered, and if the loss is not acknowledged, the person may become depressed or develop health problems. **Interventions** for those experiencing grief and loss include:

- Teach patients to recognize symptoms, such as SOB, empty feelings in the chest or abdomen, deep sighing, lethargy, and weakness as signs of grief.
- Assist the patient and family to heal themselves by accepting the loss, recognizing the pain from it, making changes to adapt to and assimilate the loss, and moving toward new relationships and activity.
- Refer to groups or counseling for more intense support if needed.

Supporting Families and Patients as They Receive Bad News

It is often best if the patient can **receive bad news** while being **supported** by family, friends, physicians, nurses, support staff, social workers, and clergy if they so desire. However, the patient may not want family members or others to be present, and this too should be respected.

- Provide privacy and ensure that there will be no interruptions.
- Provide seating for all participants.
- Do not provide too much information at once, as the opening statement may be all that the patient can comprehend at one time.
- Allow time for reactions before providing more information.

- Wait for the patient to signal the need for more information and then provide an honest answer in layman's terms. Information may not be absorbed and may need to be repeated as the patient and family are ready for it later after the initial conference.
- Use techniques of therapeutic communication. People may need others to sit and listen and provide comforting empathy many times before having a conversation about problem solving.

SPIRITUALITY

Spirituality provides a connection of the self to a higher power and a way of finding meaning in life experiences. It provides guidance for behavior and can help to clarify one's purpose in life. It can offer hope to those who are ill or facing loss and grief and can give comfort, support, and guidance. **Spirituality** is not always connected to a religion and is highly individualized. A person may lose faith and confidence in his/her spiritual beliefs during trying times:

- Ask patients about their spiritual beliefs.
- Listen attentively and do not offer opinions about their beliefs or share your own unless invited.
- Show respect for their views and offer to obtain spiritual support by calling a spiritual leader or setting up a spiritual ritual that has meaning for them.

This support can help them to regain their beliefs and endure illness by helping them to rise above their suffering and find meaning in this experience.

PALLIATIVE AND HOSPICE CARE

Palliative care attempts to make the rest of the patient's life as comfortable as possible by treating distressing symptoms to keep them controlled. It does not attempt to cure but only to control discomfort caused by the disease. Palliative care does not require terminal illness/prognosis and can be implemented for any patient with chronic disease and suffering.

Hospice care uses palliative care as it supports the patient and family through the dying process. Hospice teams support the daily needs of the patient and family and provide needed equipment, medical expertise, and medications to control symptoms. They offer spiritual, psychological, and social support to the patient and family as needed and desired. Assistance with end-of-life planning is given to help the patient and family accomplish goals important to them. Bereavement support is also given. The team consists of the attending physician, hospice physician advisor, nurses, social worker, clergy, hospice aides, and volunteers. Hospice care is given in the home when the patient has family who are willing to assume care with the assistance of the hospice team. Hospice care also occurs in hospice facilities, hospitals, and extended care facilities. To qualify for Hospice care, the patient must be deemed terminal and given a 6-month or less life expectancy by two separate physicians. Should the patient survive 6 months in hospice, they can be extended for two 90-day periods, and then an unlimited number of 60-day periods per physician order.

Developmental Theories

MASLOW'S HIERARCHY OF NEEDS

In many cases, prioritizing nursing diagnoses and problems can be done by using **Maslow's hierarchy of needs.** Life-threatening needs and safety needs take priority over others, regardless of the prioritization method used.

- **Physiological** (Basic needs to sustain life—oxygen, food, fluids, sleep)
  - Risk for aspiration
  - Deficient fluid volume
  - Impaired spontaneous ventilation
- **Safety and security** (Physiological and psychological threats)
  - Verbal communication impaired
  - Latex allergy response
  - Death anxiety
- **Love/Belonging** (Support, caring, intimacy)
  - Risk for loneliness
  - Anxiety
  - Caregiver role strain
- **Self-esteem** (Sense of worth, respect, independence)
  - Defensive coping
  - Disturbed body image
  - Post-traumatic response
- **Self-actualization**
  - Health-seeking behaviors
  - Spiritual distress

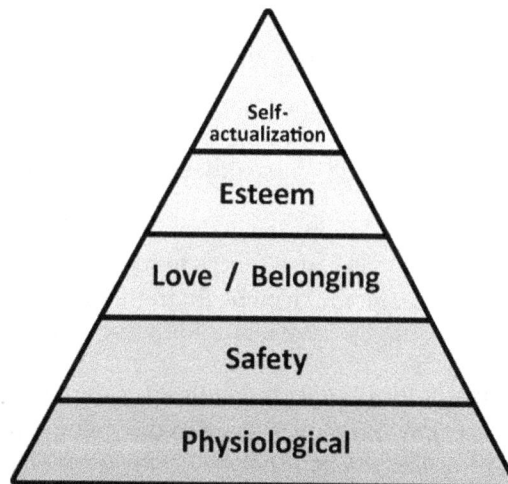

| Review Video: **Maslow's Hierarchy of Needs** |
| Visit mometrix.com/academy and enter code: 461825 |

ERIC ERIKSON'S THEORY OF HUMAN DEVELOPMENT

Eric Erikson's stages of psychosocial development include the following (with approximate age ranges):

- **Trust vs. Mistrust** (0-1.5 years): The infant develops trust in those who provide basic care and safety. Success leads to the virtue of hope.
- **Autonomy vs. Shame and Doubt** (1.5-3 years): Tasks are performed independently and there should be freedom to test independence. Success leads to confidence.
- **Initiative vs. Guilt** (3-5 years): More independence and initiative in decision-making develops. Success leads to security in actions.
- **Industry vs. Inferiority** (5-12 years): The peer group plays a larger role in self-esteem. There is confidence in achieving goals. Success leads to feeling competent.
- **Identity vs. Role Confusion** (12-18 years): The child is searching for self-identity and exploring who they want to be as an adult. Success leads to a positive self-esteem.
- **Intimacy vs. Isolation** (18-40 years): Committed relationships are formed. Success leads to security within a relationship.
- **Generativity vs. Stagnation** (40-65 years): Careers are established and there is giving back to society. Success leads to feelings of productivity.
- **Ego integrity vs. Despair** (65+ years): There is reflection on whether their active years have been productive. Success leads to not feeling guilty or unsuccessful with their life's work.

In order for an individual to psychosocially progress and mature functionally, Erikson believed that the previous stage had to be met. Dysfunction at any phase of development would then influence the individual's ability to successfully handle the more complex obstacles and stages of life.

Erikson also posited on the **stability of personality**, theorizing that an individual's personality remains consistent throughout life and that personality changes may be the result of physiological changes within the brain.

> **Review Video: Factors in Development**
> Visit mometrix.com/academy and enter code: 112169

PIAGET'S STAGES OF COGNITIVE DEVELOPMENT

Jean Piaget's **theory of cognitive development** proposes that **intelligence** is something that develops through a series of stages. He stated that children are not less intelligent than adults, but just think differently. He divided this development into four stages (with approximate age ranges):

- **The Sensorimotor Stage** (0-2 years): Infants learn their world through movements, sensations, and basic actions. They learn that actions can cause things to happen.
- **The Preoperational Stage** (2-7 years): Children begin to think symbolically and learn words and pictures. They tend to see things from their own point of view and find it hard to see someone else's perspective.
- **The Concrete Operational Stage** (7-11 years): Children begin to think logically and thoughts are more organized. Inductive logic, or reasoning, is used in the thought processes. They begin to understand that their thoughts are theirs and that others may not share these feelings.
- **The Formal Operational Stage** (12+ years): Thought is more abstract and there is reasoning about hypothetical problems. There is more thought about moral, ethical, social, and political issues that require abstract reasoning.

> **Review Video: Piaget's Cognitive Development Theory**
> Visit mometrix.com/academy and enter code: 100376

HARRY STACK SULLIVAN'S THEORY OF INTERPERSONAL DEVELOPMENT

The major concepts of **Sullivan's interpersonal theoretical model** include:

- **Self-esteem**: A concept built from a child's experiences, made up from the approval or disapproval of significant others.
- **The two basic drives that underlie behavior**: The drive for satisfaction—the basic physiological drives such as hunger. The drive for security—the need for a sense of wellbeing and belonging.
- **Anxiety**: Any painful feeling or emotion that arises from social insecurity or blocks satisfaction. The main disruptive force in interpersonal relations.
- **Security operations**: Measures taken by an individual to reduce anxiety and enhance security, such as selective inattention.
- **Self-system**: All the security operations an individual uses to protect against anxiety and ensure self-esteem.
- **Mental illness**: Wherein the self-system interferes with the ability to attend to the basic drives.

Therapy is based upon the belief that by experiencing a healthy relationship with the therapist, the patient can learn to build better relationships.

LAWRENCE KOHLBERG'S THEORY OF MORAL DEVELOPMENT

Kohlberg's **levels** in the **Theory of Moral Development** include:

- **Level I: Pre-Conventional Morality**: Morality is externally controlled.
  - **Stage 1**: The avoidance of punishment. The punishment or power of others determines what is right or wrong.
  - **Stage 2**: The desire for reward or benefit. Actions are based on getting something in return or in satisfying gratification. Though there is a sense of fairness, there is no sense of loyalty, gratitude, or justice.
- **Level II: Conventional Morality**: Conformity to social rules remains important.
  - **Stage 3**: Anticipation of disapproval of others with conformity to expectations of appropriate behavior.
  - **Stage 4**: Anticipation of dishonor with behavior oriented toward respecting authority, maintaining social order, and obeying social rules for their own good.
- **Level III: Post-Conventional Morality**: Morality is defined in terms of abstract principles and values that apply to all situations and societies.
  - **Stage 5**: Behavior is oriented toward the belief that justice flows from a social contract that assures equality for all. Behavior is geared toward rules and legalities.
  - **Stage 6**: Behavior is oriented toward universal, ethical principles.

THEORIES ASSOCIATED WITH AGING

The theories associated with aging are discussed below:

- **Biological programming theory**: This theory describes aging as being pre-programmed and irreversible. The life of the cell is pre-determined by the DNA and is on course with its destiny.
- **Cross-linkage theory**: This theory describes the increasing rigidity that occurs during aging. Flexibility decreases due to increased collagen bonds between many molecular structures within the body.
- **Error theory**: This theory describes aging in terms of malfunction and failures during protein synthesis that lead to errors within the cells. These mutated cells then multiply within the body.
- **Free radical theory**: Certain chemicals within the body, called free radicals, decrease the cell's life span by damaging the membrane around the cell. These cells accumulate leading to an overall declining physical status.
- **Gene theories**: These theories attribute the decline during aging to the activation of destructive genes that damage DNA, leading to unrepairable cellular decline. Some of these theories also consider the option that cells only divide a predetermined number of times.
- **Immunological theory**: This theory describes aging as a decline of the immune system. This decline can result in diminished ability to fight off disease and may become autoimmune in nature, causing the body to reject its own cells.
- **Stress adaptation theory**: This theory discusses the physiological effects of stress on the body. Stress decreases internal balance and leads to a decreased capacity to fight off illness or disease.
- **Wear and tear theory**: This theory discusses the cumulative effects that normal every day insults have on the cell over time. The body is machine-like and cells simply wear out from use over time.

SOCIOCULTURAL THEORIES OF THE AGING POPULATION

The **sociocultural theories** of disengagement, activity, family, and person-environment in the **aging population** are described below:

- **Disengagement theory**: This theory describes the withdrawal of the elderly person from engagement in society. This separation can be initiated by the person, society, or both and is considered the normal process.
- **Activity theory**: This theory describes the positive effects activity and involvement have for the aging population. The more involved and active they stay, the healthier both physically and mentally they will remain.
- **Family theories**: These theories place the family in the center of the aging population's wellbeing. Their ability to move through the generational cycles within the family is reflected in both their emotional and physical health.
- **Person-environment fit theory**: This theory emphasizes the relationship between the aging population and how well they fit in their environment. As they move from young-old to old-old they may no longer feel safe or competent within their environment.

Therapeutic Alliance Development and Management

THERAPEUTIC MILIEU

The **therapeutic milieu** is a stable environment provided by an organization to assist in a **treatment plan**. The main purposes of a milieu are to teach individuals certain social skills and to provide a **structured environment** that promotes interactions and personal growth along with attempting to control many types of deviant or destructive behaviors. There are **five main components** that the milieu should include in therapy. These components include containment, structure, support, involvement, and validation. Through the use of these components, the therapeutic milieu can help the individuals achieve their highest level of functioning.

CONTAINMENT COMPONENT

The **containment component** in a milieu involves the actual **physical safety** of the participants. It provides a **safe clean physical environment** as well as providing food and some medical care. The actual environment will often be very comfortable with colorful walls, pictures, and comfortable chairs and couches. Participants are allowed a certain freedom of movement throughout this environment. Many times, the participants will work to help maintain a clean and functioning environment. They may perform certain tasks or chores to help with the upkeep of the milieu. This containment will provide a feeling of safety and trust for the individual.

STRUCTURED COMPONENT

The **structured component** in the milieu lies hand in hand with **consistency**. The milieu provides a place with consistent staff members, consistent physical surroundings, and limits on behavior. This predictability allows the participants to feel safe and secure and to know what to expect. This environment also provides **structure** through providing an environment where the participants can interact with a purpose. These purposes can range from daily tasks and chores to the different roles they may assume within various meetings. Through acceptance of this consistent and structured environment, the individual can begin to achieve some level of self-responsibility and consequences for their actions.

SUPPORT COMPONENT

The **support component** in a milieu comes directly from the staff members involved in the milieu. Their goal is to help the participants have increased **self-esteem** through creating an environment of acceptance for all individuals. They provide a safe and comfortable atmosphere, therefore decreasing anxiety levels. Encouragement, empathy, nurturing, reassurance, and providing physical wellbeing for participants will help increase their feelings of self-worth. Consistency in attitudes and actions by all staff members are very important in the success of this setting. By providing this type of environment, the milieu will assist patients in their abilities to gain new healthy relationships and appropriate interactions with others.

INVOLVEMENT COMPONENT

The **involvement component** of the milieu is the development of a sense of **open involvement** for each patient from the staff members. The staff should convey their desire to be personally involved with each patient through both their actions and attitudes. They should encourage the patients to **communicate** with them openly about feelings and experiences. This sense of individual interest and involvement will help to increase the patient's sense of self-worth and self-esteem. The staff members should encourage patient involvement through encouraging patient-lead group sessions and activities. By becoming involved, the patients have opportunities to practice new social skills, such as working together with others, learning to compromise, and dealing with conflict. The hope of involvement is to achieve the goal of appropriate social interactions for each patient.

VALIDATION COMPONENT

The **validation component** of the milieu is the recognition of each patient as an **individual**. The staff members should convey **respect and consideration** for each and every patient. This respect and consideration should be shown through acts of kindness, empathy, nonjudgmental attitude, and acceptance of each individual for who they are. In a milieu, each patient contributes through responsibilities and involvement in many decision-making processes. Through these actions, the patients should begin to feel some self-responsibility and with this new sense of responsibility comes validation for their individuality and humanity.

CHARACTERISTICS OF A SUCCESSFUL MILIEU

The characteristics of a **successful milieu** include:

- Successful communication between and among staff and patients
- Standards that provide consistency and security
- Patient government using the democratic process
- Patient responsibility for his or her own treatment
- Encouraging self-perception and change
- Acknowledging and positively dealing with destructive behavior and poor judgment

The **nurse's role** in a successful milieu includes:

- The establishment and maintenance of the milieu
- Physical care and assurance of safety, including:
  - Promoting the patient's ability to perform ADLs
  - Evaluating for physical illness or medication effects
  - Assessing for detoxification effects in those chemically dependent
  - Assessing for self-destructive behavior
  - Medication administration and education

CONFLICT RESOLUTION

When attempting to **resolve conflict** between two or more individuals, the desired outcome is a feeling by each party of getting what they wanted out of the situation. Resolving conflict should include the following steps:

1. **Problem Identification**: The parties are each allowed their opportunity to discuss what they think is wrong. This portion of the resolution process may become emotional and involve angry outbursts.
2. **Ascertain Expectations**: Each party identifies exactly what they want. With the disclosure of these expectations, a sense of trust can begin to evolve. The nurse will need to remain objective and respectful to everyone involved during this phase.
3. **Identify Special Interest**: Determine if anyone has unspoken objectives or interests that could slow down the resolution progress. Everyone needs to be honest about what they want and need.
4. **Brainstorm Resolution Ideas**: Assist the parties with creating ideas to help resolve the conflict.
5. **Reach a Resolution**: Assist the parties in bringing together a situation where everyone can feel happy about the outcome.

PATIENT-PROVIDER RELATIONSHIP

INTRODUCTORY PHASE

The first thing the health care provider should do when meeting a patient is to find out **why** they are there. This **initial phase** provides a time for the provider and patient to get to know each other. There is no definite time frame and this phase can last for a few minutes to a few months. There are certain goals that should be accomplished during this time. The provider and patient should develop a mutual sense of trust, acceptance, and understanding. They may enter into a contract with each other. They will need to determine expectations, goals, boundaries, and ending criteria for the contract. This initial phase often involves obtaining the patient's history, his or her account of the problems, and developing a general understanding of the patient.

WORKING PHASE

The second phase of the patient-provider relationship is the **working phase**. During this time the patient will identify and evaluate specific problems through the development of insight and learn ways to effectively **adapt their behaviors**. The provider will assist the patient in working through feelings of fear and anxiety. They will also foster new levels of self-responsibility and coping mechanisms. The development of new and successful ways of approaching problems is the goal of this phase. The provider may often face resistance by the patient to move through this phase, and by utilizing different communication techniques may help to assist the patient in moving forward.

TERMINATION PHASE

The final stage of the patient-provider relationship is the **termination or resolution phase**. This phase begins from the time the problems are actually solved to the actual **ending of the relationship**. This phase can be very difficult for both the patient and the provider. The patient must now focus on continuing without the guiding assistance of the therapy. The patient will need to utilize their newfound approaches and behaviors. This time may be one of varying emotions for the patient and they may be reluctant to end the relationship. They may experience anxiety, anger, or sadness. The provider may need to guide the patient in utilizing their newfound strategies in dealing with their feelings about the termination of the relationship. Focus should be placed on the future.

THERAPEUTIC COMMUNICATION

VERBAL COMMUNICATION

Verbal communication is achieved through spoken or written words. This form of communication represents a very small fraction of communication as a whole. Much information achieved verbally may be **factual** in nature. Communication occurs along a two-way path between the nurse and the provider. One limitation of verbal communication can be **different meanings of words** in different ethnic and cultural populations. The meanings may differ in denotative, actual meaning, and/or connotative, implied meaning, of the words. The use of words may differ depending upon personal experiences. The patient may assume the provider understands their particular meaning of the word.

EMPATHY

Empathy is perhaps one of the most important concepts in establishing a therapeutic relationship with a patient, and it is associated with **positive patient outcomes**. It is the ability of one person to put themselves in the shoes of another. Empathy is more than just knowing what the other person means. The provider should seek to imagine the **feelings** associated with the other person's experience without having had this experience themselves and then communicate this understanding to the patient. Empathy should not be confused with sympathy, which is feeling sorry for someone. The provider should also be aware of any social or cultural differences that could inhibit the conveyance of empathy.

OPEN-ENDED STATEMENTS AND REFLECTION

Broad **open-ended statements** allow the patient the opportunity to expand on an idea or select a topic for discussion. This type of communication allows the patient to feel like the provider is actually listening and interested in what they have to say. It also helps the patient gain insight into his or her emotions or situations.

Reflection conveys interest and understanding to the patient. It can also allow for a time of validation so the provider can show that they are actually listening and understanding the shared information. It involves some minimal repetition of ideas or summing up a situation. These ideas or summaries are directed back to the patient often in the form of a question.

RESTATING AND CLARIFICATION

Restating and clarification are verbal communication techniques that the provider may use as part of therapeutic communication. **Restating** involves the repetition of the main points of what the patient expressed. Many times, the provider will not restate everything but narrow the focus to the main point. This technique can achieve both clarification of a point and confirmation that what the patient said was heard.

Clarification involves the provider attempting to understand and verbalize a vague situation. Many times, a patient's emotional explanations can be difficult to clearly understand and the provider must try to narrow down what the patient is trying to say.

SILENCE AND LISTENING

Silence and listening are very effective during verbal communication.

- **Silence** allows the patient time to think and formulate ideas and responses. It is an intentional lull in the conversation to give the patient time to reflect.
- **Listening** is more active in nature. When listening, the provider lends attention to what the patient is communicating. There are two different types of listening.
  - **Passive listening** allows the patient to speak without direction or guidance from the provider. This form of listening does not usually advance the patient's therapy.
  - **Active listening** occurs when the provider focuses on what is said in order to respond and then encourage a response from the patient.

RAPPORT AND VALIDATION

Communication between the health care provider and the patient can be improved by establishing rapport and validating certain information. **Establishing rapport** with a patient involves achieving a certain level of harmony between the provider and the patient. This is often achieved through the establishment of trust through conveying respect, nonbiased views, and understanding. By establishing rapport, the provider helps the patient feel more comfortable about sharing information.

Validation requires the provider to use the word "I" when talking with the patient. It evaluates one's own thoughts or observations against another person's and often requires feedback in the form of confirmation.

USE OF THERAPEUTIC COMMUNICATION WITH GROUPS

A **group** is a gathering of interactive individuals who have commonalities. Interventions through **group sessions** can provide an effective treatment opportunity to allow for growth and self-development of the patient. This setting allows the patients to interact with each other. This allows the patients to see the emotions of others, such as joy, sorrow, or anger, and to receive as well as participate in feedback from others in the group. The group can be very supportive and thrive in both inpatient and outpatient settings. The one thing the group cannot lack is definite **leadership and guidance** from the health care provider. The provider must guide the members of the group in facilitating therapeutic communications.

NONVERBAL COMMUNICATION IN THE THERAPEUTIC RELATIONSHIP

Nonverbal communication occurs in the form of expressions, gestures, body positioning or movement, voice levels, and information gathered from the five senses. The **nonverbal message** is usually more accurate in conveying the patient's feeling than the **verbal message**. Many patients will say something quite different than what their nonverbal communication indicates. Nonverbal communication may also vary by cultural influences. The health care provider must be aware of these cultural differences and respect their place within the therapy. The provider should utilize positive, respectful, non-threatening body language. A relaxed, slightly forward posture with uncrossed arms and legs may encourage communication.

VOCAL CUES, ACTION CUES, AND OBJECT CUES AS FORMS OF NONVERBAL BEHAVIORS

There are many different types of nonverbal behaviors. There are five main areas of **nonverbal communication**. They include vocal cues, action cues, object cues, space, and touch.

- **Vocal cues** can involve the qualities of speech, such as tone and rate. Laughing, groaning, or sounds of hesitation can also convey important communication.
- **Action cues** involve bodily movements. They can include things such as mannerisms, gestures, facial expressions, or any body movements. These types of movements can be good indicators of mood or emotion.
- **Object cues** include the use of objects. The patient may not even be aware that they are moving these objects. Other times the patient may choose a particular object to indicate a specific communication. This intentional use of an object can be less valuable than other forms of nonverbal communication.

Space and touch as nonverbal forms of communication can vary greatly depending upon social or cultural norms.

- **Space** can provide information about a relationship between the patient and someone else. Most people living in the United States have four different areas of space. **Intimate space** is less than 1.5 feet, **personal space** is 1.5-4 feet, **social-consultative space** is 9-12 feet, and **public space** is 12 feet or more. Observations concerning space and the patient's physical placement in a setting can give a great deal of insight into different interpersonal relationships.
- **Touch** includes personal or intimate space with an action involved. This fundamental form of communication can send very personal information and communicate feelings such as concern or caring.

NON-THERAPEUTIC COMMUNICATION

Techniques that are detrimental to establishing a trusting therapeutic relationship include giving advice, challenging the patient's communications, or indicating disapproval. **Giving advice** includes telling the patient what they should do in a particular situation. This does not allow the patient to develop the ability to solve their own problems and may not always be the right answer. **Challenging** occurs when the patient's thoughts are disputed by the provider. This communication only serves to lower the patient's self-esteem and create an environment of distrust between the patient and the health care provider. **Disapproval** occurs when the provider negatively judges the patient's beliefs or actions. This again serves to lower patient self-esteem and does not foster their ability to solve their own problems or create new coping abilities.

PATIENT SAFETY ISSUES

PROFESSIONAL ASSAULT RESPONSE

A protocol for a **professional assault response** should be established at all mental health facilities because statistics show that 75% of mental health staff experience a **physical assault**. Most injuries are incurred by nursing staff caring for violent patients. Assaults may occur in both psychiatric units and emergency departments, where security staff may also be assaulted. Additionally, patients may be victims. Common injuries include fractures, lacerations, contusions, and unconsciousness from head injuries. Victims are at risk for psychological distress and post-traumatic stress syndrome, so a prompt response is critical. The assault response should include the following:

- Routine assessment of patients for violent or aggressive tendencies
- Protocol for managing violent or aggressive patients
- Physical assessment and medical treatment as needed for injuries
- Completion of an incident report by those who were involved or who observed the incident

Psychological intervention, including individual counseling sessions and critical incident stress management, require a response team that includes staff members who are trained to deal with crisis intervention (e.g., psychologists, psychiatrists, nurses, peer counselors, social workers).

CONTRABAND AND UNSAFE ITEMS

State regulations identify **contraband and unsafe items** that are prohibited from mental health and correctional facilities; however, each facility must develop site-specific restrictions and protocols for responding to contraband and unsafe items. **Contraband** may include the following:

- Alcohol or products (mouthwash) that contain alcohol
- Drugs, including prescription, over-the-counter, and illicit drugs
- Poisonous and toxic substances
- Pornographic or sexually explicit material
- Food (hoarded or excessive)

Depending on the type of facility or patients, a wide range of items may be considered **unsafe**. These often include the following:

- Knives, scissors, sharp instruments, and razor blades
- Flammable materials, such as lighter fluid and matches
- Breakable items, such as glass and mirrors
- Dangerous materials (which might be used for a suicide attempt), such as belts (over 2 in wide), large buckles, rope, electrical cords (i.e., over 6 feet in length), and wire
- Potential weapons, such as pens (except felt point), pencils, and plastic bags
- Electrical equipment, such as fans and recording devices

PROFESSIONAL BOUNDARIES
GIFTS

Over time, patients may develop a bond with nurses they trust and may feel grateful to the nurse for the care provided and want to express thanks, but the nurse must make sure to maintain professional boundaries. Patients often offer **gifts** to nurses to show their appreciation, but some adults, especially those who are weak and ill or have cognitive impairment, may be taken advantage of easily. Patients may offer valuables and may sometimes be easily manipulated into giving large sums of money. Small tokens of appreciation that can be shared with other staff, such as a box of chocolates, are usually acceptable (depending upon the policy of the institution), but almost any other gifts (jewelry, money, clothes) should be declined: "I'm sorry, that's so kind of you, but nurses are not allowed to accept gifts from patients." Declining may relieve the patient of the feeling of obligation.

SEXUAL RELATIONS

When the boundary between the role of the professional nurse and the vulnerability of the patient is breached, a boundary violation occurs. Because the nurse is in the position of authority, the responsibility to maintain the boundary rests with the nurse; however, the line separating them is a continuum and sometimes not easily defined. It is inappropriate for nurses to engage in **sexual relations** with patients, and if the sexual behavior is coerced or the patient is cognitively impaired, it is **illegal**. However, more common violations with adults, particularly elderly patients, include exposing a patient unnecessarily, using sexually demeaning gestures or language (including off-color jokes), harassment, or inappropriate touching. Touching should be used with care, such as touching a hand or shoulder. Hugging may be misconstrued.

ATTENTION

Nursing is a giving profession, but the nurse must temper giving with recognition of professional boundaries. Patients have many needs. As acts of kindness, nurses (especially those involved in home care) often give certain patients extra attention and may offer to do **favors**, such as cooking or shopping. They may become overly invested in the patients' lives. While this may benefit a patient in the short term, it can establish a relationship of increasing **dependency** and **obligation** that does not resolve the long-term needs of the patient. Making referrals to the appropriate agencies or collaborating with family to find ways to provide services is more effective. Becoming overly invested may be evident by the nurse showing favoritism or spending too much time with the patient while neglecting other duties. On the other end of the spectrum are nurses who are disinterested and fail to provide adequate attention to the patient's detriment. Lack of adequate attention may lead to outright neglect.

COERCION

Power issues are inherent in matters associated with professional boundaries. Physical abuse is both unprofessional and illegal, but behavior can easily border on abusive without the patient being physically injured. Nurses can easily **intimidate** older adults and sick patients into having procedures or treatments they do not want. Regardless of age, patients have the right to choose and the right to refuse treatment. Difficulties arise with cognitive impairment, and in that case, another responsible adult (often the patient's child or spouse) is designated to make decisions, but every effort should be made to gain patient cooperation. Forcing the patient to do something against his or her will borders on abuse and can sometimes degenerate into actual abuse if physical coercion is involved.

PERSONAL INFORMATION

When pre-existing personal or business relationships exist, other nurses should be assigned care of the patient whenever possible, but this may be difficult in small communities. However, the nurse should strive to maintain a professional role separate from the personal role and respect professional boundaries. The nurse must respect and maintain the confidentiality of the patient and family members, but the nurse must also be very careful about **disclosing personal information** about him or herself because this establishes a social relationship that interferes with the professional role of the nurse and the boundary between the patient and the nurse. The nurse and patient should never share secrets. When the nurse divulges personal information, he or she may become vulnerable to the patient, a reversal of roles.

Ethical and Legal Principles

Patient's Bill of Rights

PATIENTS' RIGHTS

Patients' (and families') rights in relation to what they should expect from a healthcare organization are outlined in both standards of the Joint Commission and National Committee for Quality Assurance. **Rights include**:

- Respect for the patient, including personal dignity and psychosocial, spiritual, and cultural considerations
- Response to needs related to access and pain control
- Ability to make decisions about care, including informed consent, advance directives, and end-of-life care
- Knowledge of the procedure for registering complaints or grievances
- Protection of confidentiality and privacy
- Freedom from abuse or neglect
- Protection during research and information related to ethical issues of research
- Appraisal of outcomes, including unexpected outcomes
- Information about organization, services, and practitioners
- Appeal procedures for decisions regarding benefits and quality of care
- Organizational code of ethical behavior
- Procedures for donating and procuring organs/tissue

PATIENT RIGHTS IN PSYCHIATRIC CARE

A right is a fair claim that is due to an individual, established by policies or laws. Important **patient rights in psychiatric care** include:

- The right to **privacy**: No information will be shared with unauthorized people about the patient. Exceptions include:
  - Presence of suspected child abuse
  - Credible patient threats of physical harm to another (The potential victim must be alerted per "Tarasoff" regulations.)
  - During guardianship or involuntary commitment hearings
- The right to **treatment**: Patients have the right to participate in their treatment.
- The right to treatment in a **least restrictive setting**. Examples include:
  - Patients who pose no danger to themselves or others cannot be involuntarily hospitalized.
  - Patients who can function in an open ward cannot be held in a locked ward.
  - Clients who can live in the community and who have a support system must be treated in an outpatient setting.
  - Seclusion and restraint can only be utilized when it is in the patient's overriding best interest.
- The right to **informed consent**: Patients are to be made aware of any procedure to be performed and must give permission of their own accord. Only court-ordered commitment procedures give hospitals the right to involuntarily treat patients.
- The right to **refuse treatment**: Patients may not be forcibly medicated; however, legal guardians can give permission if a court order is obtained. Patients may be forcibly medicated if they could possibly cause harm to self or others.

- The right to **habeas corpus**: Committed patients must be brought before a judge or court and must be released if insufficient reasons for confinement exist.
- The right to **independent psychiatric examination**: Patients may demand an evaluation by a mental health specialist of their choice and must be released if it is determined that they are not mentally ill.

INFORMED CONSENT GUIDELINES

Patients or family must provide informed consent for all treatment the patient receives. This consent includes a thorough explanation of all procedures, treatments, and associated risks. Patients/family should be apprised of all options and allowed input on the type of treatments. Patients/family should be apprised of all reasonable risks and any complications that might be life threatening or increase morbidity. The American Medical Association has established **guidelines for informed consent**:

- Explanation of diagnosis
- Nature of, and reason for, treatment or procedure
- Risks and benefits
- Alternative options (regardless of cost or insurance coverage)
- Risks and benefits of alternative options
- Risks and benefits of not having a treatment or procedure
- Providing informed consent is a requirement of all states

ADVANCE DIRECTIVES, DNR, AND DURABLE POWER OF ATTORNEY

In accordance to Federal and state laws, individuals have the right to self-determination in health care, including decisions about end-of-life care through **advance directives** such as living wills and the right to assign a surrogate person to make decisions through a **durable power of attorney**. Patients should routinely be questioned about an advanced directive as they may present at a healthcare organization without the document. Patients who have indicated that they desire a **do-not-resuscitate (DNR) order** should not receive resuscitative treatments for terminal illness or conditions in which meaningful recovery cannot occur. Patients and families of those with terminal illnesses should be questioned as to whether the patients are currently hospice patients, in which case only comfort measures should be provided. For those with DNR requests or those withdrawing life support, staff should provide the patient palliative rather than curative measures, such as pain control and/or oxygen, and emotional support to the patient and family. Religious traditions and beliefs about death should be treated with respect.

INVOLUNTARY COMMITMENT OF PEDIATRIC PSYCHIATRIC PATIENTS

Involuntary commitment of pediatric psychiatric patients occurs in some instances. Assent is a productive and helpful aspect of treating pediatric patients. However, if the child does not assent, parents and guardians may still consent to therapy. **Involuntary mental holds** for 72 hours are sufficient to commence therapy. The legal premise behind these regulations is that parents act in good faith to ensure the wellbeing of their children. The legal guardian and healthcare provider are acting in place of the parents (*in loco parentis*). In most cases, the triage team on inpatient units has the option of deciding whether or not a patient should be admitted for evaluation or as protection for the patient's safety. For example, a teenager who attempts suicide may be placed on a 72-hour hold. Those healthcare professionals responsible for triage and treatment in the first 72 hours must act in the best interest of the patient and not under the influence of financial gain or parental desire.

PATIENT ADVOCACY AND ANA's DEFINITION OF NURSING

Patient advocacy is defined as the process of speaking on behalf of a patient to ensure that his or her rights are protected, and that he or she is provided with necessary information and services. The nurse frequently serves as patient advocate, although physicians, social workers, and other individuals in the health care industry may act on behalf of the patient as well.

The ANA includes patient advocacy as integral to the definition of nursing. It defines nursing as "the protection, promotion, and optimization of health and abilities, prevention of illness and injury, alleviation of suffering through the diagnosis and treatment of human response, and advocacy in the care of individuals, families, communities, and populations."

> **Review Video: Patient Advocacy**
> Visit mometrix.com/academy and enter code: 202160

FACILITATORS OF PATIENT ADVOCACY

Perhaps the greatest facilitator of patient advocacy is the **nurse-patient relationship**. If a strong relationship exists between the nurse and the patient, the nurse will be motivated to perform the duties of advocate. If the patient and nurse have a strained or limited relationship, advocacy can be difficult. **Recognizing the patient's needs** is another facilitator, one that goes hand in hand with a good nurse-patient relationship. If the nurse feels a sense of responsibility and accountability on behalf of the patient, he or she is more likely to serve as a good patient advocate, as conscience is a strong motivator. Another facilitator is if the **physician acts as a colleague of the nurses**, instead of as a superior. This strengthens the nurse-physician relationship, and the nurse feels that he or she can question the physician's judgment instead of constantly deferring. That being said, the greater the knowledge base and skill level of the nurse, the greater he or she will be as an advocate.

BARRIERS TO PATIENT ADVOCACY

Patient advocacy is often seen as both a moral obligation that the nurse must fulfill and a rewarding part of the nurse's job; however, patient advocacy can be difficult in certain situations. Various **barriers** exist in the practice of patient advocacy:

- A **feeling of powerlessness** on the part of the nurse, especially if the nurse has no support. (This general **lack of support** is an additional barrier to patient advocacy.)
- A **lack of knowledge of the law**, as certain laws may exist that provide obstacles when advocating for a patient
- A **lack of time, communication, or motivation** on the part of the nurse or the nurse's peers
- The **risks associated** with advocacy, such as disagreeing with other nurses and physicians, and a lack of legal support for the advocate

DECREASING THE STIGMA ASSOCIATED WITH MENTAL ILLNESS

Studies have shown that up to a third of Americans relate mental illness to defects of character. Negative beliefs about mental illness persist with people often fearing those who are mentally ill. Effective methods to **decrease the stigma** associated with mental illness include:

- **Educating people about mental illness**: People need to know factual information, including levels of violence associated with those who are mentally ill since this is a pervasive concern. People should be advised of the incidence of mental illness and available treatments.
- **Using words carefully**: Healthcare providers and others should choose words carefully, avoiding words such as "nuts" and "crazy," and remembering to put the person first by using terms such as "person with schizophrenia" rather than "schizophrenic."
- **Providing support services**: Helping those with mental illness find places to live and providing other necessary services may help to reduce substance abuse and homelessness, which increase stigma.
- **Increasing contact**: Integrating those with mental illness into the community through job placement and housing helps others become more familiar with those who are mentally ill.

Ethics in Clinical Decision Making

ETHICAL PRINCIPLES

Autonomy is the ethical principle that the individual has the right to make decisions about his or her own care. In the case of children or patients with dementia who cannot make autonomous decisions, parents or family members may serve as the legal decision maker. The nurse must keep the patient and/or family fully informed so that they can exercise their autonomy in informed decision-making.

Justice is the ethical principle that relates to the distribution of the limited resources of healthcare benefits to the members of society. These resources must be distributed fairly. This issue may arise if there is only one bed left and two sick patients. Justice comes into play in deciding which patient should stay and which should be transported or otherwise cared for. The decision should be made according to what is best or most just for the patients and not colored by personal bias.

Beneficence is an ethical principle that involves performing actions that are for the purpose of benefitting another person. In the care of a patient, any procedure or treatment should be done with the ultimate goal of benefitting the patient, and any actions that are not beneficial should be reconsidered. As conditions change, procedures need to be continually reevaluated to determine if they are still of benefit.

Nonmaleficence is an ethical principle that means healthcare workers should provide care in a manner that does not cause direct intentional harm to the patient:

- The actual act must be good or morally neutral.
- The intent must be only for a good effect.
- A bad effect cannot serve as the means to get to a good effect.
- A good effect must have more benefit than a bad effect has harm.

NURSING CODE OF ETHICS

There is more interest in the **ethics** involved in healthcare due to technological advances that have made the prolongation of life, organ transplants, prenatal manipulation, and saving of premature infants possible, sometimes with poor outcomes. Couple these with healthcare's limited resources, and **ethical dilemmas** abound. Ethics is the study of **morality** as the value that controls actions. The American Nurses Association Code of Ethics contains nine statements defining **principles** the nurse can use when faced with moral and ethical problems. Nurses must be knowledgeable about the many ethical issues in healthcare and about the field of ethics in general. The nurse must help a patient to reveal their values and morals to the health care team so that the patient, family, and team can resolve moral issues pertaining to the patient's care. As part of the healthcare team, the nurse has a right to express personal values and moral concerns about medical issues.

BIOETHICS

Bioethics is a branch of ethics that involves making sure that the medical treatment given is the most morally correct choice given the different options that might be available and the differences inherent in the varied levels of treatment. In the health care unit, if the patients, family members, and the staff are in agreement when it comes to values and decision-making, then no ethical dilemma exists; however, when there is a difference in value beliefs between the patients/family members and the staff, there is a bioethical dilemma that must be resolved. Sometimes, discussion and explanation can resolve differences, but at times the institution's ethics committee must be brought in to resolve the conflict. The primary goal of bioethics is to determine the most morally correct action using the set of circumstances given.

ETHICAL DECISION-MAKING MODEL

There are many ethical decision-making models. Some general guidelines to apply in using ethical decision-making models could be the following:

- Gather information about the identified problem
- State reasonable alternatives and solutions to the problem
- Utilize ethical resources (for example, clergy or ethics committees) to help determine the ethically important elements of each solution or alternative
- Suggest and attempt possible solutions
- Choose a solution to the problem

It is important to always consider the **ethical principles** of autonomy, beneficence, nonmaleficence, justice, and fidelity when attempting to facilitate ethical decision-making with family members, caregivers, and the healthcare team.

ETHICAL ASSESSMENT

While the terms *ethics* and *morals* are sometimes used interchangeably, ethics is a study of morals and encompasses concepts of right and wrong. When making **ethical assessments,** one must consider not only what people should do but also what they actually do, as these two things are sometimes at odds. Ethical issues can be difficult to assess because of personal bias, which is one of the reasons that sharing concerns with other internal sources and reaching consensus is so valuable. Issues of concern might include options for care, refusal of care, rights to privacy, adequate relief of suffering, and the right to self-determination. Internal sources might include the ethics committee, whose role is to make decisions regarding ethical issues. Risk management can provide guidance related to personal and institutional liability. External agencies might include government agencies, such as the public health department.

ETHICAL ANALYSIS OF A SITUATION

Assessment of the situation is done to reveal the ethical, legal, and professional **conflicts** that are present. Those who are involved are identified, including the patient, family, and healthcare personnel. The decision maker is determined if it is not the patient. Information about the situation is collected to determine medical facts about the disease and condition of the patient, options for treatment, and nursing diagnoses. Any pertinent legal information is included. The patient and family's cultural, religious, and moral values are determined. Possible courses of action are listed and compared in terms of outcomes for the patient using the utilitarian or deontological theory of ethics. Professional codes of ethics are also applied. A decision is made and evaluated as to whether it is the most morally correct action. Ethical arguments for and against the decision are given and responded to by the decision maker.

Scope and Standards of Practice

PSYCHIATRIC MENTAL HEALTH NURSING ORGANIZATIONS

Professional organizations provide nurses with the latest medical information, support meaningful legislation that encourages quality patient care through exceptional nursing care, and consist of a body of leadership to help guide the future of nursing. One of the best known and largest nursing organizations is the **American Nurses Association (ANA)**. ANA provides support to the mental health nursing field through advocacy at the national and state levels and also through collaboration with other psychiatric-mental health nursing organizations. The **American Psychiatric Nurses Association (APNA)** and the **International Society of Psychiatric-Mental Health Nurses (ISPN)** are two other well respected large organizations that support the mental health field of nursing.

APNA AND ISPN

The **American Psychiatric Nurses Association (APNA)** is the largest psychiatric nursing organization that focuses upon the advancement of nursing practice along with continued improvements in cultural diversity, families, groups, and communities. The **International Society of Psychiatric-Mental Health Nurses (ISPN)** is composed of three specialty divisions that include the Association of Child and Adolescent Psychiatric Nurses, the International Society of Psychiatric Consultation Liaison Nurses, and the Society for Education and Research in Psychiatric-Mental Health Nursing. The main goal of ISPN is to bring together all psychiatric-mental health nurses and to advance quality care available for both the individual and the family unit. Many of these organizations have annual meetings where the newest information on the forefront of mental health nursing is presented. There are membership fees to join these associations.

ACCREDITATION OF MENTAL HEALTH CARE DELIVERY SYSTEMS

Mental health care facilities are highly regulated and evaluated by several different accrediting bodies. The process of **accreditation** occurs when a facility is determined to be providing acceptable quality care based upon certain established standards. Nursing is vital in meeting **agency accreditation standards**, and therefore is critically evaluated during the accreditation process. When a facility is accredited, this information is made public so that the consumer will be aware of which institutions meet the acceptable standards of care. It is also necessary for a facility to maintain to receive third party reimbursement for services.

ACCREDITING BODIES FOR MENTAL HEALTH CARE DELIVERY SYSTEMS

There are many different organizations that provide accreditation to mental health care delivery systems. One of the most important accrediting bodies is the **Joint Commission (TJC)**. This is the accrediting body for hospitals throughout the United States. The accrediting body of the Centers for Medicare and Medicaid Services (CMS) determines accreditation standards for facilities seeking Medicare or Medicaid reimbursement. Community mental health facilities do not seek accreditation from TJC or CMS. These outpatient facilities seek accreditation from the Commission on Accreditation of Rehabilitation Facilities.

PROFESSIONAL PERFORMANCE AND DEVELOPMENT

All professional psychiatric nurses are expected to achieve and maintain competent nursing practice as identified by the standards of professional performance found in the **Scope and Standards of Psychiatric-Mental Health Nursing** by the American Nurses Association. The defined standards of practice include quality of care, performance appraisal, education, collegiality, ethics, collaboration, research, and resource utilization. The nurse is evaluated against each of these standards of care, with the achievement of becoming and remaining competent being each nurse's own professional responsibility.

PERFORMANCE APPRAISALS

A performance appraisal is one in which the nurse evaluates their own psychiatric mental health nursing practice in regard to standards of practice, statutes, and regulations that are relevant to their field of practice. There are two types of performance appraisals, the administrative performance appraisal and the clinical performance appraisal.

- The **administrative performance appraisal** reviews the nurse's performance against role expectations. It should identify areas needing improvement and areas in which the nurse has achieved competency.
- The **clinical performance appraisal** provides guidance through clinical supervision with a mentor. The mentor will have greater clinical experience, skill, and education. The purpose of this relationship is to provide the nurse with a support mechanism. They can share clinical, developmental, and emotional information with their confidant in order to gain knowledge and grow within their field of practice. This appraisal reviews clinical care and also functions as a support role.

LEVELS OF NURSING PRACTICE IN PSYCHIATRIC MENTAL HEALTH FIELD

BASIC LEVEL

There are two main levels of nursing practice within the psychiatric mental health field. There is the basic level of practice and then the advanced level of practice. Nurses that practice under the **basic level** belong to one of two subgroups.

- The first subgroup includes registered nurses that function in the role of a general staff nurse in a mental health facility, case managers, nurse managers, or other various nursing roles.
- The second subgroup includes the psychiatric-mental health nurse (RN-PMH), which is a baccalaureate prepared registered nurse that has practiced in the mental health field for at least two years.

The functions of a nurse practicing at the basic level may include health promotion, education, intake admission screening and evaluation, case management, milieu therapy, promotion of self-care, psychobiologic interventions, counseling, crisis care, and rehabilitation.

ADVANCED LEVEL

The advanced level of nursing practice within the psychiatric mental health field is the second level of practice. This registered nurse has a **master's level degree** and is licensed as an **advanced registered nurse practitioner psychiatric-mental health (ARNP-PMH)** and functions as a clinical specialist or a nurse practitioner. The ARNP-PMH is nationally certified as a psychiatric mental health specialist by the **American Nurses Credentialing Center (ANCC)**. The advanced level of practice also includes nurses who have earned a doctorate in nursing (DNS, DNSc) or a doctorate of philosophy (PhD). Nurses functioning at this level can provide complete delivery of direct primary mental health services. They are able to diagnose, order, evaluate, or interpret diagnostic information. They are also able to conduct psychotherapy, pharmacotherapy, and monitor the patient's progress in regards to both types of intervention.

DEVELOPMENT OF COMMUNITY MENTAL HEALTH CENTERS (CMHCS)

In 1963, Congress passed the **CMHC Act**, which started the process of decentralizing mental health centers in all fifty states—from public hospitals to flexible community care settings—based on the principle that people with mental illness have a right to treatment in the least restrictive environment. In 1965, Congress legislated that five essential services were to be provided by the CMHCs. These services were inpatient, outpatient, partial hospitalization, consultation, and education. Initially, federal funding was provided to communities for the construction and staffing of CMHCs. This funding would eventually cease, and the state would take-up the responsibility for operating the facilities. CMHCs were originally designed to serve the entire community, creating a mental health safety net. Ultimately, a "priority population" was defined, which included adults with severe, persistent mental illness and severely emotionally disturbed children. Over time, an increasing proportion of the CMHCs resources were allocated to these populations.

Since **deinstitutionalization** began in the 1970s, the number of patients in mental health hospitals has declined significantly; however, the type of patients that have been admitted since tend to be younger and more violent.

The intent of deinstitutionalization was to allow the patient to return home as soon as possible, thereby avoiding the negative effects of a lengthy hospital stay. The aim was to have these patients followed-up by community-support networks. This intention led to many families assuming the burden of care for numerous patients with mental health problems, and failed community-support networks have resulted in many of these patients becoming homeless street people.

In 1975, Congress mandated that several other services were to be added. These services were: children's services, geriatric services, aftercare, drug abuse treatment, alcohol abuse treatment, transitional housing, and prescreening for admission to a state hospital. After patients were discharged from the public mental hospital, they were to continue with their follow-up care within the CMHC system.

Many **unanticipated problem**s arose with this concept. Many discharged patients found it difficult to adjust to independent community living because they needed a slow, gradual introduction to becoming self-sufficient. Many mental health patients, particularly those that became homeless, had difficulties keeping appointments and complying with medication schedules.

Some of the successes of the CMHC concept include working with chronic patients by using crisis intervention, community outreach programs, supportive living arrangements and work programs.

TESTIFYING AS AN EXPERT WITNESS
PREPARATION
Nurse preparation for offering expert testimony should include:

- Reviewing all relevant medical information in the case. The witness should then testify to its content fairly, honestly, and in a balanced manner.
- The expert witness should be prepared to distinguish between actual negligence (substandard medical care that results in harm) and an unfortunate medical outcome (recognizing complications may occur as a result of medical uncertainty).
- The expert witness should be prepared to state the basis of his or her testimony or opinion and whether it is based on personal experience, specific clinical references, evidence-based guidelines, or a generally accepted opinion in the specialty.
- The expert witness should be knowledgeable of important alternate methods and views and be prepared to discuss them.
- The expert witness should review the standards of practice prevailing at the time and under the circumstances of the alleged occurrence.

An expert witness has specialized knowledge of a subject that may help a judge or jury make decisions. An expert witness is authorized to express his or her opinion on a subject for which he or she is an expert, while a non-expert witness is not allowed to express an opinion. Non-expert witnesses are permitted to only testify on facts that they have observed.

REQUIRED EXPERIENCE
The experience required to be considered an expert witness includes:

- Educational accomplishments and licensure
- Specialized training in the area for which testimony is offered
- An adequate percentage of time treating children and adolescents (if acting as an expert witness for that age group)
- Knowledge of professional literature

- Knowledge of the standards of care about which testimony is offered
- Memberships in professional organizations
- Publications
- Professional recognition and awards

RISK MANAGEMENT

Risk management is an organized and formal method of decreasing liability, financial loss, and risk or harm to patients, staff, or others by doing an assessment of risk and introducing risk-management strategies. Much of risk management has been driven by the insurance industry in order to minimize costs, but quality management utilizes risk management as a method to ensure quality health care and process improvement. An organization's risk management program usually comprises a manager and staff with a number of **responsibilities**:

- **Risk identification** begins with an assessment of processes to identify and prioritize those that require further study to determine risk exposure.
- **Risk analysis** requires a careful documenting of the process and utilizing flow charts, with each step in the process assessed for potential risks. This may utilize root cause analysis methods.
- **Risk prevention** involves instituting corrective or preventive processes. Responsible individuals or teams are identified and trained.
- **Assessment/evaluation** of corrective and preventive processes is ongoing to determine if they are effective or require modification.

MALPRACTICE

Malpractice is the improper or negligent treatment of a person under a medical professional's care that results in injury or death, as judged by national standards of care and by other members of the same medical profession. Many **malpractice suits** stem from angry patients who had higher expectations of treatment outcomes than they obtained.

Malpractice suits involving nurses usually involve the administration of medications or the treatment of patients. Most malpractice suits are filed under the law of "tort", which is a private civil wrong committed by one individual against another for which monetary damages are collected by the injured party from the wrongdoer.

NEGLIGENCE

Risk management must attempt to determine the burden of proof for acts of **negligence**, including compliance with duty, breaches in procedures, degree of harm, and cause. Negligence indicates that proper care has not been provided, based on established standards. Reasonable care uses rationale for decision-making in relation to providing care. State regulations regarding negligence may vary but all have some statutes of limitation. There are a number of different types of negligence:

- **Negligent conduct** indicates that an individual failed to provide reasonable care or to protect/assist another, based on standards and expertise.
- **Gross negligence** is willfully providing inadequate care while disregarding the safety and security of another.

- **Contributory negligence** involves the injured party contributing to his or her own harm.
- **Comparative negligence** attempts to determine what percentage of negligence is attributed to each individual involved.

Review Video: **Medical Negligence**
Visit mometrix.com/academy and enter code: 928405

BATTERY AND ASSAULT

Differences between battery and assault include:

- **Battery** is defined as the physical touching of a person without their consent. To be considered a crime, the contact must be intentional and cause harm. Unintentional or non-deliberate physical contact is not considered battery. An example of battery is touching a patient inappropriately without their permission; by contrast, accidentally tripping and falling on a patient is considered "unintentional harmful conduct" and is not considered battery.
- **Assault** is a threat of causing bodily harm coupled with the ability to cause the harm. Physical contact is not necessary for an action to be considered an assault. A simple verbal threat to harm is not an assault; however, combining this verbal threat with a raised hand or fist could be considered an assault if the patient feels threatened.

Standards of Advanced Practice

ADVANCED PRACTICE REGISTERED NURSING (APRN)

An **APRN**, according to the NCSBN, is a registered nurse who has gained additional specialized knowledge, skills, and experience and is licensed to perform advanced practice nursing. This nurse has an RN license and has completed and received a diploma from graduate school in an APRN program that has been accredited from a nationwide accrediting body. This nurse has up-to-date certification from a nationwide certification board, such as the American Nurses Credentialing Center (ANCC), to work in the proper APRN area. Being an APRN defines the nurse as someone that has more **responsibility**, which may or may not come with higher compensation for the nurse.

Some responsibilities include:

- Provide professional education and leadership
- Handle patient and medical center leadership
- Support the patient and local area by keeping the ideal concerns for the patient or community
- Assess the results of interventions and how well these interventions are working
- Collaborate with patients, patient relatives, and colleagues
- Employ research; seek and use new information and equipment
- Educate others regarding APRN

There are four types of APRNs: nurse practitioner (NP), certified nurse midwife (CNM), clinical nurse specialist (CNS), and certified registered nurse anesthetist (CRNA).

STANDARDS OF ADVANCE PRACTICE

The nurse practitioner (NP), and all APRNs, must practice within the **standards of advance practice** and the individual's scope of practice, which is directly related to the individual's educational preparation and certification. An NP must have 2 types of licenses/certificates: a registered nurse (RN) license and an advanced practice certificate. The NP must function legally under the Nurse Practice Act of the state in which the NP practices. In some cases, an NP license/certification in 1 state is automatically recognized in other states through a compact agreement. Educational experience and scope of practice must relate to patient population in terms of age, disease, diagnosis, and treatment.

The **standards of advance practice** provide the framework for practice and describe the NP's responsibilities, related to the values and priorities of the profession:

- **Care process**: In assessing, diagnosing, developing, and implementing a plan of care, as well as evaluating the patient's response, the NP must use scientific method and national standards as the basis for care.
- **Establishing priorities**: Providing education and encouraging the patient/family to take an active role in self-care is of primary concern. The NP must ensure that the patient can make informed decisions. The NP must assist the patient through all aspects of health care to ensure patient safety and optimal care.
- **Collaboration**: The NP is a member of the interdisciplinary health team and consults with others when appropriate and refers the patient to specialists as needed. When collaboration is mandated by law, the NP complies with all requirements.
- **Documentation**: The NP keeps accurate, legal, and legible records and also maintains patient confidentiality. The NP ensures that the patient signs a release before providing medical records to other parties.
- **Patient advocacy**: The NP advocates for the individual patient in the process of care but also advocates for patients at the state and national level in order to facilitate patient access to care and improve the quality of care.

- **Continuous quality improvement**: The NP recognizes the need for constant learning, evaluation, and reevaluation and participates in quality review, continuing education while maintaining certification, and utilizing clinical guidelines and standards of care.
- **Research and education**: The NP initiates, participates in, and utilizes the results of research in clinical practice.

SCOPE OF PRACTICE FOR APRN

The **scope of practice for the APRN** is dependent on each state and what the APRN in this position can do according to the Nurse Practice Act for that state. The scope provides guidelines instead of particular directives. There is a wide range of responsibilities that an APRN may manage, depending on the state's regulations. Many times, the scope is founded on what is allowed legally both in the state and in the country.

A complete list of the state nursing practice acts can be found on the NCSBN website (http://www.ncsbn.org). An authorizing board of nursing is available in every state to lead statutes with regard to licenses for an RN. They have responsibility for how titles are used, scope of work, and how to handle discipline cases. Nurse practice acts come out of statutory law.

Depending upon the state's nurse practice act, **NP privileges** vary:

- NPs may be able to practice **independently** or in **collaboration/agreement** with a physician, podiatrist, or chiropractor. The type of physician oversight and collaboration required varies considerably. Currently, 21 states and the District of Columbia have no collaboration requirement, allowing NPs to work autonomously.
- NPs can be **reimbursed** by Medicare, Medicaid, the Civilian Health and Medical Program of the Uniformed Services (CHAMPUS), and private insurance. Currently, governmental reimbursement for NPs is at the rate of 85% of the customary physician reimbursement. However, a billing rate of 100% is allowed with "incident to" billing that allows the physician to charge for services that are incident to practice as though he or she performed the service.
- **Prescriptive authority** varies from state to state. Many states require physician oversight for all or some prescriptions. There are often limits to the types of treatments/drugs that can be prescribed. Currently, 22 states and the District of Columbia allow NPs to be completely independent (hold full prescriptive authority) in prescribing medication.

PRESCRIPTION MEDICATION AND DIAGNOSTIC TESTS

Both **prescribing** medications and treatment and ordering **diagnostic** tests are within the scope of practice of the NP but, as with other aspects of practice, each state establishes how that will be carried out. Additionally, insurance reimbursement varies from one area to another and must be considered.

- **Prescription**: Terminology varies from state to state with NPs allowed to "furnish" or "prescribe" some types of medications. In some states they may do so independently; in others, they must be "supervised" by a physician under whose auspices they provide care to patients. The NP should maintain a list of medications and consider cost-effectiveness when ordering medications.
- **Diagnostics**: NPs can order laboratory, electrocardiogram, and radiographic tests for routine screening and health assessment as well as make a diagnosis based on assessment. There are limitations, depending upon the individual state nursing practice act.

CONSULTATION, REFERRAL, AND COORDINATION

As part of the **scope of practice**, the NP is able to provide and augment primary care to patients/families through a number of different services:

- **Consultation services** may include a variety of services, such as an assessment of growth, development, and risk factors, providing interventions such as diet and exercise programs, and educating patients/families.
- **Referral services** include referring patients to physicians, such as specialists, and to organizations or agencies, such as drug rehabilitation programs.
- **Coordination services**, with the NP maintaining contact and receiving reports from referrals in order to provide an integrated plan of care, serves as a valuable service to patients/families, who often must deal with many different healthcare providers who have little or no contact with each other. This type of service can prevent unnecessary duplications of service but also ensure that findings are not overlooked.

DELEGATION OF TASKS TO UNLICENSED ASSISTIVE PERSONNEL

The scope of nursing practice includes **delegation of tasks** to unlicensed assistive personnel, providing those personnel have adequate training and knowledge to carry out the tasks. Delegation should be used to manage the workload and to provide adequate and safe care. The NP who delegates remains accountable for patient outcomes and for supervision of the person to whom the task was delegated, so the NP must consider the following:

- Whether knowledge, skills, and training of the unlicensed assistive personnel provides the ability to perform the delegated task
- Whether the patient's condition and needs have been properly evaluated and assessed
- Whether the NP is able to provide ongoing supervision

Delegation should be done in a manner that **reduces liability** by providing adequate communication. This includes specific directions about the task, including what needs to be done, when, and for how long. Expectations related to consultation, reporting, and completion of tasks should be clearly defined. The NP should be available to assist if necessary.

ROLES OF THE PMHNP

The **roles** of the psychiatric and mental health NP (PMHNP) can be quite varied depending on the setting and job description but can include providing direct care and treatment; consulting; educating patients, families, and staff members; supervising; administering; carrying out independent practice; and conducting research. The PMHNP may also be actively engaged in needs identification and planning, implementing, and evaluating change. The PMHNP is often the primary advocate for the patient and, as such, must often work to ensure that all patients have access to needed treatment. The PHMNP works collaboratively with other members of the healthcare team. As an advocate for the role of the PMHNP, the NP serves as a role model for the profession by upholding the highest standards and sharing expertise with other healthcare providers. The PMHNP should be actively engaged in political efforts to expand the scope of practice of the PMHNP and should address organizations and community groups about the role of the PMHNP.

CONSULTANT

The mental health professional often serves as a **consultant** to others, especially during discharge planning, to ensure that patients receive the continued care and services that they need. The NP may serve as an **educational consultant**, providing general information about the needs of those with psychiatric or mental health issues, or may specifically deal with the needs of a particular patient, in which case the NP must be sure that proper release forms have been signed and issues of privacy are respected. Areas of consultation include:

- **Schools**: The school nurse or educators may require information on dealing with behavioral or treatment issues.
- **Housing**: If a patient is placed in housing such as board-and-care homes or supervised apartments, authorities need to understand the patient's condition and needs.
- **Social Services**: The NP may provide consultation services to social workers. If a child is placed in foster care, the foster parents should be provided information necessary to provide care and support to the child.

INDEPENDENT CONTRACTOR

A nurse practitioner working as an **independent contractor** may sign a contract for services, which is a legal financial agreement that outlines the conditions of service. Typically, a contract includes:

- The name of the NP and the client, outlining the qualifications, appropriate licensure, and certification
- The purpose of the service agreement
- The extent of the contract period, including beginning date and ending date of the contract
- Compensation, including daily, weekly, or hourly rate of payment
- Expenses, such as travel pay or money for office support, equipment, or training and methods of submitting invoices
- Performance description outlining the type of services that the independent contractor will perform, including any limitations and legal responsibilities
- Disclaimers

Laws and Regulations

OLDER AMERICANS ACT

The Older Americans Act (OAA) (Title III) of 1965 (amended in 2006 and reauthorized through fiscal year 2024) provides improved access to services for older adults and Native Americans, including community services (meals, transportation, home health care, adult day care, legal assistance, and home repair). The OAA provides funding to local **area agencies on aging (AAA)**, state, or tribal agencies, which administer funding. These local agencies can assess community needs and contract for services. One of the programs commonly supported with funds from the OAA is meals-on-wheels. Low-cost adult day care is also offered in some communities. The OAA includes the **National Family Caregivers Support Act**, which provides services for caregivers of older adults. The OAA also provides grants for programs that combat violence against older adults and others to provide computer training for older adults. Additionally, the OAA mandates that each state must have an ombudsman program. Ombudsmen provide services to residents of nursing homes and other facilities to ensure that care meets state standards.

OBRA AND THE NURSING HOME REFORM AMENDMENTS

The **Omnibus Budget Reconciliation Act (OBRA)** of 1987 was a groundbreaking revision of nursing home federal standards and was amended in 1990 to include the **Nursing Home Reform Amendments (NHRA)**. These amendments establish guidelines for nursing facilities (such as long-term care facilities). Provisions include:

- Complete physical and mental assessment of each patient on admission, annually, and with change of condition
- Requirement for 24-hour nursing care with registered nurses (RNs) on duty for at least 1 shift
- Mandated nurse aide training and regular in-service and state registry of trained/qualified aides
- Required availability of rehabilitative services
- Requirement for physician/physician's assistant/NP to visit every 30 days for the first 3 months and then every 90 days
- Outlawing/discouraging Medicaid discrimination
- Requirement for independent monitoring of psychopharmacologic drugs
- Recognition of patients' rights
- Survey protocols to assess patient care and patient outcomes
- State sanctions to enforce nursing home regulations

EMTALA

The Emergency Medical Treatment and Active Labor Act (EMTALA) is designed to prevent patient "dumping" from emergency departments (EDs) and is an issue of concern for risk management, requiring staff training for compliance. **EMTALA guidelines concerning the transfer of an ED patient** include:

- Transfers from the ED may be intrahospital or to another facility.
- Stabilization of the patient with emergency conditions or active labor must be done in the ED prior to transfer, and initial screening must be given prior to inquiring about insurance or ability to pay.
- Stabilization requires treatment for emergency conditions and reasonable belief that, although the emergency condition may not be completely resolved, the patient's condition will not deteriorate during transfer.
- Women in the ED in active labor should deliver both the child and placenta before transfer.
- The receiving department or facility should be capable of treating the patient and dealing with complications that might occur.
- Transfer to another facility is indicated if the patient requires specialized services not available intrahospital, such as to burn centers.

AMERICANS WITH DISABILITIES ACT

The 1990 Americans with Disabilities Act (ADA) is civil rights legislation that provides the disabled, including those with mental impairment, access to employment and the community. While employers must make reasonable accommodations for the **disabled**, the provisions related to the community apply more directly to **older Americans**. The ADA covers not only obvious disabilities but also disorders such as arthritis, seizure disorders, psychiatric disorders, cardiovascular, and respiratory disorders. Communities must provide transportation services for the disabled, including accommodation for wheelchairs. Public facilities (schools, museums, physician's offices, post offices, restaurants) must be accessible with ramps and elevators as needed. Telecommunications must also be accessible through devices or accommodations for the deaf and blind. **Compliance** is not yet complete because older buildings are required to provide access that is possible without "undue hardship," but newer construction of public facilities must meet ADA regulations.

PATIENT SELF-DETERMINATION ACT

The Patient Self-Determination Act (1990), an amendment to the Omnibus Budget Reconciliation Act, allows a mental health patient to develop an **advance psychiatric directive (APD)** during a period when a professional mental healthcare provider certifies the person is of sound mind. The APD allows the patient to determine in advance the types of treatment that are acceptable and those that are not. The patient can also designate another person, such as a family member, to make decisions if the patient is unable to do so. State regulations regarding APDs may vary somewhat. The APD is particularly valuable to those who have severe chronic psychiatric illnesses, such as schizophrenia, and may face involuntary commitment. A patient may outline preferences regarding specific treatments and interventions, such as medications, seclusion, restraint, and electroshock therapy.

FAMILY MEDICAL LEAVE ACT

The Family and Medical Leave Act (FMLA) (1993) is a federal law that requires employers (such as hospitals and rehabilitation centers) with 50 or more employees to provide unpaid leave and job-protected time off up to 12 weeks during any 12-month period for medical and family reasons to fulltime and part-time employees who have worked more than 1250 hours within the previous year. During leave time, the employer must continue the same benefits and insurance coverage and must maintain the position or provide another that is approximately equal in salary, benefits, and area of responsibility. Leave may be used to care for a newborn, adopted, or fostered child, to care for a sick spouse, child, or parent, and for adverse health conditions that prevent the employee from carrying out work functions. FMLA allows extended leave up of up to 26 workweeks in a 12-month period to care for a service member's seriously ill or injured spouse, parent, or child.

Transition and Continuum of Care

DISCHARGE PLANNING

Discharge planning should begin on admission and must be a joint effort so that the **transfer and discharge documents** provide the information that the individual or staff at transfer facilities/home need. Information should include:

- Contact telephone numbers, email addresses, and street addresses for the nurse practitioner (NP) (to contact patient for discharge surveillance) and patient or transfer facility staff (to contact the NP if problems arise)
- Information sheets outlining signs for all risk factors, especially if the patient is discharged to their home without nursing care
- Follow-up appointment dates, with physicians, labs, or the other practitioners
- Specific directions for medication or treatments, including side effects
- Information about 12-step/self-help/community-assistance programs

Patients who are **homeless** require further assistance with discharge, as compliance with treatment and follow-up appointments is poor in the homeless population. Homeless patients should receive:

- Lists of safe shelters and places they can go to bathe, eat, and get mail
- Assistance in applying for welfare assistance or Social Security

CONTINUUM OF CARE

The **continuum of care** can move from inpatient treatments to various outpatient treatments and support systems. This allows for varying **levels of intensity** throughout the patient treatment program. It allows for treatment to be coordinated in many different environmental settings, care levels, by different health care providers, and by a variety of different services. This continuum of care occurs over a long period of time and includes the involvement of many different services. Its purpose is to meet the comprehensive needs of the patient through the **coordination of interdisciplinary care and services**.

SERVICES THAT MAY PARTICIPATE IN THE CONTINUUM OF CARE

The continuum of care occurs throughout the course of treatment for the individual patient. This may begin with acute crisis intervention and stabilization in the hospital setting and may then move to partial hospitalization allowing for the patient to leave for periods of time or go home at night. **Residential services** are included in this continuum and may provide a place for patients to stay at any time during the day or night. Services provided here can include medical treatments, nursing care, psychosocial care, vocational training, or recreational diversion. **Respite care** can provide short-term relief housing and care for psychiatric patients living at home with their family. **Outpatient treatment programs** as well as **supportive employment programs** also participate in the provision of the continuum of care.

ALTERNATIVE HOUSING ARRANGEMENTS AND RESIDENTIAL SERVICES

The need for **adequate housing** is an ongoing problem with psychiatric patients. Many of these patients are **homeless** and once released from inpatient care services do not have anywhere to live. A safe and affordable option is vital to the success of their treatment. Many of these patients have a relapse of their mental illness or suffer from medical illnesses, incarceration, or abuse by others. The most common housing available includes group homes, such as personal care homes or board and care homes; therapeutic foster care; and supervised apartments. Many of these provide some type of rehabilitation and/or support services such as group therapy, job training, and counseling to help the patient make the transition from the treatment facility to the home environment and to learn to manage self-care.

PERSONAL CARE HOMES AND BOARD-AND-CARE HOMES

Personal care homes are located in homes in residential communities. These homes can usually provide supervised care for up to approximately 10 individuals. Services often include supervision of medication regimens, provision for transportation needs, meals, and assistance with activities of daily living. Many of these patients are elderly or suffer mild intellectual disability or psychiatric illness.

Board-and-care homes are similar to personal care homes; however, there is little assistance with activities of daily living. Many of these patients can provide their own self-care with little supervision. These homes are usually larger in size and accommodate up to 150 individuals. Both of these residential services are licensed by the state.

THERAPEUTIC FOSTER CARE HOMES AND SUPERVISED APARTMENTS

Therapeutic foster care provides for the patient in a home setting with a family that is trained to care for high needs patients. This training includes medication education, crisis management, and disease education. The **foster family** supervises all aspects of the patient's care and incorporates them into the structure of the home. Many times, the patients will share household work and may attend daytime care programs. This level of care is available for both children and adults.

Supervised apartments provide each patient with their own apartment. Patients may either live alone or share the apartment with a roommate. They are responsible for the upkeep of the apartment and are independent in their self-care needs. The apartment is supervised by staff members that regularly check on the residents to ensure that they are doing well and following prescribed medication regimens.

CARE SYSTEM SUPPORTS AVAILABLE TO PSYCHIATRIC PATIENTS

RESPITE CARE

Respite care is a service available for family members of psychiatric patients who are providing the majority of one-on-one care for the patient. The toll that this responsibility can take on a person is immense and respite care is available to provide a "break" from those responsibilities. This can allow family members to attend appointments, make social engagements, and have some time to themselves in order to maintain their own health and wellbeing. There are some respite care services that may be available over night, as well.

TRANSPORTATION

Many community-based mental health service companies offer **transportation** to help get psychiatric patients to their appointments. This helps by taking some of the responsibility off family members who may not always be available to drive them, and also ensures that they will receive the important medical follow up visits they need.

ADULT DAY CARE

Adult day care is available to engage mental health patients in a safe environment while their regular caregivers are working or fulfilling other obligations. There are organized programs that offer social time, group therapies, and craft projects to entertain mental health patients who need assistance.

RESILIENCY IN THE ROAD TO RECOVERY

Resiliency is the ability to cope with risk factors and tragedies, such as poverty and disasters, and to remain emotionally healthy. Resiliency is a critical element in recovery. One of the current trends is to aid patients in developing resiliency by providing a safe and supportive environment. Promoting resiliency also includes identifying problems early and taking steps to deal with them before they become ingrained, as well as providing aid for severe or long-term problems. Holding patients to high expectations and supporting them in attaining goals helps to build self-confidence and coping skills. Patients who are resilient have the ability to regulate their emotions and to avoid self-defeating thoughts and actions. Resilience does not mean that patients remain unaffected by stressful events but rather that they are able to recognize that which is causing stress and find ways to deal with it and learn. Researchers have found that experience in coping with stress helps people to deal with later stressful events.

SAMHSA's Recovery to Practice

Substance Abuse and Mental Health Services Administration (SAMHSA)'s Recovery to Practice program promotes expanding recovery-oriented mental health care and provides educational and training materials, such as webinars and other resources, with curricula developed by a number of different mental health organizations, including the APA, APNA, AACP, INAPS, CSWE, and NAADAC. Recovery to Practice is based on **4 dimensions** that support a life in recovery: home, health, community, and purpose. There are also **10 guiding principles** of recovery: Recovery emerges from hope, is person-driven, occurs via many pathways, is holistic, is supported by peers, through relationships and social networks, is culturally-based and influenced, supported by addressing trauma, involves individual, family, and community strengths and responsibility, and is based on respect. Recovery to practice is centered on the **needs of the patient** who should be an active participant along with clinicians, psychiatrist, case manager, and rehabilitation staff in setting goals and working toward recovery. Recovery to practice stresses the importance of community resources and encourages patients to build their own network of support. Recovery-oriented care is person-centered and individualized but includes the family and allies as well as community resources and peer recovery support programs and is responsive to culture and personal beliefs.

Interdisciplinary Collaboration

INTERDISCIPLINARY COLLABORATION

Interdisciplinary collaboration is absolutely critical to nursing practice if the needs and best interests of the patients and their families are central. Interdisciplinary practice begins with the nurse and physician but extends to pharmacists, social workers, occupational and physical therapists, nutritionists, and a wide range of allied health care providers, all of whom cooperate in diagnosis and treatment; however, state regulations determine to some degree how much autonomy a nurse can have in diagnosing and treating patients. While nurses have increasingly gained more legal rights, they are also dependent on **collaboration** with others for their expertise and for referrals if the patient's needs extend beyond the nurse's ability to provide assistance. Additionally, the prescriptive ability of nurses varies from state to state, with some states requiring direct supervision by physicians while others require other types of supervisory arrangements.

COORDINATION OF INTRA- AND INTERDISCIPLINARY TEAMS FOR PATIENT CARE

There are a number of skills that are needed to lead and facilitate the **coordination of intradisciplinary teams** (those consisting of individuals from the same specialty) and **interdisciplinary teams** (those consisting of individuals across multiple specialties) for patient care, which are listed below:

- Communicating openly is essential, with all members encouraged to participate as valued members of a cooperative team.
- It is important to avoid interrupting or interpreting the point another is trying to make to allow a free flow of ideas.
- It is important to avoid jumping to conclusions, which can effectively shut off communication.
- Active listening requires that health care professions pay attention and ask questions for clarification rather than challenging the ideas of other health care professionals.
- Respecting the opinions and ideas of others, even when they are opposed to one's own, is absolutely essential.
- Reacting and responding to facts rather than feelings allows one to avoid angry confrontations or diffuse anger.
- Clarifying information or opinions stated can help avoid misunderstandings.
- Keeping unsolicited advice out of the conversation shows respect for other professionals, allowing them to solicit advice without feeling pressured.

PROBLEMS ASSOCIATED WITH UTILIZING AN INTERDISCIPLINARY APPROACH

Many times, the **collaborative process** between the different disciplines involved in caring for the psychiatric patient does not proceed without some difficulties, as the roles and functions of the team members may overlap. This can lead to **confusion** of exactly what each team member is to contribute to the patient outcome. For the collaborative process to work smoothly, team members should agree upon a common philosophy, respect each other's input, clearly define each member's role and responsibility, specify a hierarchy of decision-making, and communicate on a regular basis.

PROMOTING COLLABORATION

Promoting collaboration and assisting others to understand and use the resources and expertise of others requires a commitment in terms of time and effort. Examples of promoting collaboration include:

- Coaching others on methods of collaboration, which can include providing information in the form of **handouts** about effective communication strategies and, in turn, **modeling** this type of communication with the staff being coached.
- **Team meetings** are commonly held on nursing units and provide an opportunity to model collaboration and suggest the need for outside expertise to help with planning patient care plans. The mentoring nurse can initiate discussions about resources that are available in the facility or the community.
- Selecting a **diverse group** for teams or inviting those with expertise in various areas to join the team when needed can help team members to appreciate and understand how to use the input of other resources.

COLLABORATION WITH EXTERNAL AGENCIES

The nurse must initiate and facilitate collaboration with external agencies because many have direct impacts on patient care and needs:

- **Industry** can include other facilities sharing interests in patient care or pharmaceutical companies. It's important for nursing to have a dialog with drug companies about their products and how they are used in specific populations because many medications are prescribed to women, children, or the aged without validating studies for dose or efficacy.
- **Payors** have a vested interest in containing health care costs, so providing information and representing the interests of the patient is important.
- **Community groups** may provide resources for patients and families, both in terms of information and financial or other assistance.
- **Political agencies** are increasingly important as new laws are considered about nurse-patient ratios and infection control in many states.
- **Public health agencies** are partners in health care with other facilities and must be included, especially in issues related to communicable disease.

CONFLICT RESOLUTION

Conflict is an almost inevitable product of collaboration with the patient, and the nurse must assume responsibility for **conflict resolution**. While conflicts can be disruptive, they can produce positive outcomes by forcing people to listen to different perspectives and opening dialogue. The nurse should make a plan for dealing with conflict resolution. The best time for conflict resolution is when differences emerge but before open conflict and hardening of positions occur. It is beneficial to pay close attention to the people and problems involved, listen carefully, and reassure those involved that their points of view are understood. Steps of conflict resolution include:

1. Allow both sides to present their side of conflict without bias, maintaining a focus on opinions rather than individuals.
2. Encourage cooperation through negotiation and compromise.
3. Maintain the focus, providing guidance to keep the discussions on track, and avoid arguments.
4. Evaluate the need for renegotiation, formal resolution process, or third party.
5. Utilize humor and empathy to diffuse escalating tensions.
6. Summarize the issues, outlining key arguments.
7. Avoid forcing resolution if possible.

LEADERSHIP STYLES

Leadership styles often influence the perception of leadership values and commitment to collaboration. There are a number of different leadership styles:

- **Charismatic**: Depends upon personal charisma to influence people and may be very persuasive, but this type leader may engage "followers" and relate to one group rather than the organization at large, limiting effectiveness.
- **Bureaucratic**: Follows the organization's rules exactly and expects everyone else to do so. This is most effective in handling cash flow or managing work in dangerous work environments. This type of leadership may engender respect but may not be conducive to change.
- **Autocratic**: Makes decisions independently and strictly enforces rules, but team members often feel left out of process and may not be supportive. This type of leadership is most effective in crisis situations, but may have difficulty gaining commitment of staff.
- **Consultative**: Presents a decision and welcomes input and questions although decisions rarely change. This type of leadership is most effective when gaining the support of staff is critical to the success of proposed changes.
- **Participatory**: Presents a potential decision and then makes final decision based on input from staff or teams. This type of leadership is time-consuming and may result in compromises that are not wholly satisfactory to management or staff, but this process is motivating to staff who feel their expertise is valued.
- **Democratic**: Presents a problem and asks staff or teams to arrive at a solution although the leader usually makes the final decision. This type of leadership may delay decision-making, but staff and teams are often more committed to the solutions because of their input.
- **Laissez-faire (free rein)**: Exerts little direct control but allows employees/teams to make decisions with little interference. This may be effective leadership if teams are highly skilled and motivated, but in many cases, this type of leadership is the product of poor management skills and little is accomplished because of the lack of direct leadership.

NETWORKING

Networking is the act of meeting others in order to make mutually beneficial connections. The nurse should attend local, state, and national conferences. **Conferences** offer the opportunity to network, build skills, and refresh an organization's style. An essential aspect of business is networking. Effective networking involves speaking with others and learning about their services and ideas. Sharing contact information is a must when networking. Conferences also offer nurses the opportunity to learn new skills and approaches to various situations and to comply with national standards. Conferences offer nurses opportunities for personal professional development, so that he or she will be more knowledgeable. Conferences also allow the nurses an opportunity to gain recognition for his or her research and the institution he or she represents.

SCHOOL RESOURCES

School resources vary widely. Most colleges and universities provide **mental health services** to students. Some have mental health clinics or other counseling services available, and these services can provide valuable support for students with psychiatric or mental health concerns. K-12 schools are more limited in the mental health services that they provide. In some cases, the school nurse or academic counselors may provide some mental health counseling or referrals, but mental health professionals are usually not available on site. Children who are receiving mental health care and/or medications may need support in the school environment, so the nurse and family may need to discuss the needs with the school administration to determine what services the school is able to provide. **SchoolMentalHealth.org**, a feature of the Baltimore School Mental Health Technical Assistance and Training Initiative, provides resources for students, healthcare providers, and educators with protocols for management of different types of behavioral problems, such as anger management.

SAMHSA AND NMHIC

The Substance Abuse and Mental Health Services Administration's (SAMHSA's) National Mental Health Information Center (NMHIC) provides information about opportunities for grants and application forms as well as a number of resources for mental health professionals. SAMHSA provides grants in a wide range of areas, including supportive housing, suicide prevention, family intervention, jail diversion, traumatic stress, and substance abuse prevention. The NMHIC provides fact sheets and brochures, which can be ordered for distribution, on all aspects of mental illness. Training guides are also available free of charge. NMHIC also provides state resource guides for each state. Many fact sheet and reports are available for download directly from the website. SAMHSA provides a newsroom that lists all press announcements, including information about available grants and recent awards.

NAMI

The National Alliance on Mental Illness (NAMI) is an invaluable community resource for those with mental illness and their families. Programs include:

- **Family-to-Family**: Free 12-week course intended to help family members or caregivers of those with severe psychiatric disorders (such as schizophrenia or bipolar disorder).
- **In Our Own Voice**: People living with mental illness speak about their experiences and recovery.
- **NAMI Connection**: Weekly support groups for those with mental illness.
- **Parents and Teachers as Allies**: Two-hour in-service program for teachers about early signs of mental illness, interventions, and dealing with families.
- **Peer-to-Peer**: Nine 2-hour courses taught by trained mentors with a history of mental illness, teaching participants to better manage their mental illness and avoid relapses.
- **NAMI Provider Education**: Ten-week course taught by a panel of 5 (2 family members, 2 mental health patients, and a mental health professional) for staff working directly with people with mental illness.

Cultural and Spiritual Competence

CULTURAL VIEWS ON PHYSICAL AND MENTAL ILLNESS

Many cultures have specific traditional beliefs regarding the **source and meaning** of illnesses. For instance, some cultures may believe that illness is the result of an imbalance between a person's body and spirit or that it is a punishment for actions taken earlier in life. **Mental illnesses** are particularly subject to these types of beliefs. Even in cultures where beliefs are not primarily based on superstition, mental illness frequently has a stigma attached to it. Many Eastern cultures value conformity to social norms and emotional control, and mental illness directly interferes with a person's ability to achieve these things. In Western cultures, mental illness is still often misunderstood and stigmatized, seen by many as a sign of a weak mind or simply a lack of willpower on the part of those affected.

The nurse should be aware that the client's **cultural background** may significantly impact how the client receives a diagnosis of mental illness and what information, support, and resources they will require. Beliefs held by the **client's family**, regardless of whether they are shared by the client, can directly affect the client. If the client has a strong negative reaction to a psychiatric diagnosis, the nurse should attempt to determine the source of the distress and address it appropriately, including offering reassurance that the client will not be forced to receive any treatment he or she does not wish to receive.

ISSUES RELATED TO GAY, LESBIAN, BISEXUAL, AND TRANSGENDER PATIENTS

Gay, lesbian, bisexual, and transgender patients often experience **hostility and discrimination** because of their sexual identification. Some experience anxiety and stress when coming to terms with their sexuality or when "coming out" to family or friends. Increasingly, adolescents are self-identifying as homosexual, some as early as age 12, and they may face intense pressure from family and peers. Homosexual or transgender military personnel must deal with the fear of being identified and losing their careers. Hate crimes against homosexual or transgender individuals continue. Children of gay or lesbian parents may face discrimination as well. While some religious groups and therapists recommend "reparation" therapy to convert homosexuals to heterosexuals, the American Psychiatric Association opposes such therapy, and evidence suggests that it is virtually never successful and can be damaging psychologically. The nurse must respect the individual's sexual identification, remain supportive, and should be knowledgeable about issues that are important to gay, lesbian, bisexual, and transgender patients. The rights and needs of partners should also be respected.

ISSUES RELATED TO POVERTY AND ACCESS TO CARE

Poverty often **limits access** to care. Many patients with psychiatric and mental health problems are **ineligible** for Medicaid, lack other health insurance, or do not have the financial resources to pay for care. Free clinics and mental health programs are sometimes available, especially in urban areas, but many people do not have access to or money for public **transportation** to go to medical visits, especially in rural areas, and cannot afford medications. Additionally, rates of depression are higher among those with low income, and depression often prevents people from seeking help. Employers may not allow people to take time off from work when practices are open to provide care, or patients cannot afford to lose income; thus, most medical care is provided by emergency departments when a crisis arises.

ISSUES RELATED TO HOMELESSNESS AND ACCESS TO CARE

The homeless population has **disproportionate** rates of **serious mental illness**, estimated at about 40–45%, such as schizophrenia and bipolar disorder, complicated by substance abuse. The need for **adequate housing** is an ongoing problem with homeless patients. Once released from inpatient care services, the homeless often return directly to the streets or to shelters. They often are victimized by others, suffer relapses, or engage in substance abuse in an attempt to self-medicate. The homeless often resist treatment (sometimes not believing they are ill), fail to keep appointments, or lack a reliable means of transportation. They may have no money for medication, not qualify for assistance, or be reluctant to deal with government agencies to gain assistance.

DIFFERENCES IN COMMUNICATION AMONG CULTURES

According to a study conducted by **Srebalus and Brown**, American Indians and Asian Americans typically regard self-control, soft-spoken voices, and uninterrupted speech as acceptable. They can handle pauses well that other cultures find awkward. Their speech uses less direct methods than other cultures. A firm handshake grasp is not acceptable to them; use a softer handshake instead. Smiles and nods are not forms of communication that achieve the desired results in these cultures. Some Asian Americans may offer a nod or two to indicate that they have an interest in something being said. Direct eye contact is not usually the norm, except for African Americans and European Americans. Many cultures like to keep a distance of about 3 feet or more from each other, except for Hispanics and Arabs, who usually can tolerate closer spaces.

DEVELOPING CULTURAL COMPETENCE

The linear tool used to help a health care provider gain cultural competence is the **Multicultural Awareness Continuum**. The provider cannot expect to achieve mastery, as the continuum is designed to be on-going and revisited throughout the career of the provider. Progression allows the provider to go on to the next level, but if the provider is confronted by a deficiency in his or her awareness when treating a culturally diverse person, then the provider returns to the previous level for insight into that aspect of the culture.

LEVEL 1

The first level of the Multicultural Awareness Continuum is a **high level of self-awareness**. This component is essential for the provider to understand why he or she feels a certain way, and to identify biases in his or her own thinking. It is imperative for a provider to understand how he or she interacts with others. Likewise, the provider needs to examine his or her beliefs, attitudes, opinions, and values. A multicultural health care provider must spend time in introspection to determine areas in which he or she may have cultural biases.

LEVEL 2

The second level has to do with an **awareness of one's own culture**. Certain cultures may place values upon a person's name, its origin and cultural significance. Other cultures may place values upon birth order. Some cultures have naming ceremonies for infants. Language and its use can also play a significant part in the values placed upon a person through his or her culture.

LEVEL 3

The third level on the Multicultural Awareness Continuum is **awareness of racism, sexism, and poverty bias**. Providers discover this awareness by looking closely at their own personal belief system. Sexism and racism are an entrenched part of cultural beliefs. Some providers and clients may not have biases against token minority individuals whom they know personally, but may think of smaller cultures folded into the American melting pot as subtly inferior. Poverty touches everyone to some extent. Many have either experienced poverty directly, or have simply seen shocking evidence of its existence. The mental health care provider must determine his or her own bias before helping others gain insights into a cultural belief system.

LEVEL 4

The provider must not generalize any culture too much. This lends itself to the fourth and fifth levels of multicultural awareness. The fourth level is an **awareness of individual differences**. Over-generalization leads to misconceptions founded on observations of only a few members of a culture. To avoid misconceptions, treat the client first and foremost as an individual with his or her own set of unique needs, and then as a member of his or her specific culture. Understand that the individual has to function both as a member of his or her own culture, and in American society at large. Avoid projecting personal cultural beliefs on the client.

LEVEL 5

The fifth level is an **awareness of other cultures**. This begins with the client's language. A multicultural provider does not need to learn a foreign language in its entirety, but just certain words that have significant meanings. Multicultural clients in the U.S. will predominantly be: African Americans, Native American Indians, Hispanics (Latinos or Chicanos), and Asian Americans.

In 1980, **Hofstede** researched 40 countries to determine identifiable differentiations in their various cultures. He determined the following characteristics are the most identifiable:

- Power distance
- Uncertainty avoidance
- Masculinity/femininity
- Individualism/collectivism

In 1961, **Kluckhohn** and **Strodtbeck** determined the following characteristics are the most identifiable:

- Time
- View of human nature
- Importance of relationships
- Human activity
- View of the supernatural

LEVEL 6

Professor Don Locke is known for his contributions to the field of counseling, particularly relating to culture and diversity. He created the Multicultural Awareness Continuum in 1986, which still contributes to the discussion of multicultural counseling today. The sixth level of awareness in this continuum is the awareness of diversity, which begins with a grasp of just how erroneous the idea is that America's cultures have joined to become one super-culture. There are marked differences in the cultures of African Americans, White Anglo-Saxon Protestants, Native American Indians, Hispanics (Latinos or Chicanos), Asian Americans, and various religious groups and sexual orientations within races. In melting pot theory, the differences in these cultures went undervalued and unrecognized. Immigrants and the poor were encouraged to buy into the values, beliefs, and attitudes of mainstream America. Melting pot theory is being replaced by mosaic theory, and the terms "salad bowl" or "rainbow coalition." The salad bowl idea suggests a mix of ingredients that are best when the flavors are allowed to stand out and complement each other.

LEVEL 7

The final level on the multicultural awareness continuum is the **necessary skills and techniques required to counsel diverse populations**. A prerequisite for beginning the multicultural process is the provider's general competence in counseling. The provider is required to complete each level of study successfully, and satisfy internship requirements, to achieve general competency. The provider should be thoroughly educated in theories, standards, and applications. The historical significance of the theory must be understood in context of the time period in which the theory was framed. The theorist's own cultural belief system should be noted, in conjunction with the theory he or she developed. By studying the theory in context, the provider can better understand how to maintain the integrity of the theory when applying it to cultural groups. A provider should perform within his or her own cultural sub-group before attempting to perform those same duties with clients of other cultural groups. There is no replacement for basic counseling/nursing skills.

DETERMINING PERSONAL STANCE ON ISSUES OF POVERTY, SEXISM, AND RACISM

The mental health care provider may choose to use a **systems approach** in exploring differences between **personal prejudices**, which determine how an individual acts, and **organizational prejudices**, which determine how an organization or institution acts. For example, discrepancies in behavior result when:

- The worker's personal beliefs conflict with official policies in the workplace.
- The congregation's beliefs do not follow the church's official policy.
- The electorate does not agree with government policy on sexism, racism, and poverty.

Therefore, the provider must determine what beliefs and attitudes are promoted by those organizations in which the provider is a member. A mental health care provider may wish to apply a systems approach to his or her place of employment to find out if there are institutional prejudices present within.

FRAMEWORK FOR CULTURAL UNDERSTANDING

The framework for cultural understanding is based on the diverse cultural backgrounds that exist between a client and provider. Personal experiences shape the provider's and the client's worldview and impact the behaviors of both. Areas in which different points of view surface are: *historical perspectives*, *social perspectives*, *economical perspectives*, and *political perspectives*. Likewise, socialization and life experiences change the client's and provider's worldviews and behaviors. Counseling and therapy sessions are impacted by differences between the provider and the client because they can cause a lack of empathy and understanding in the client/provider relationship. Prejudices and biases are detrimental to the client/provider relationship. If considering becoming a mental health care provider, one should expect to their own belief system scrutinized, and to establish an operations framework where commonalities are first identified to achieve empathy and understanding.

CONTENT OF CULTURAL AWARENESS FRAMEWORK

The content of the framework for multicultural counseling is communicative, collaborative, open to alteration or exchange, and open to quality improvement according to the client's needs. Consider the client's existing issues and incorporate up-to-date research that impacts these issues. Some core structures are needed to provide consistency of care. The **essentials** are:

- Communication styles that involve an exchange of ideas and information
- Beliefs, opinions, and attitudes about psychological problems or issues
- Strategies or devised plans of actions for handling and solving problems
- Counseling/therapy expectations of conduct and performance levels
- Racial identity development (the way someone absorbs cultural behavior and societal thinking from birth)
- The way the provider sees people, events, and happenings in relation to their world view

Following this framework will help the provider meet the needs of the client.

ISSUE OF TRUST IN BUILDING A THERAPEUTIC RELATIONSHIP

Some cultures have specific viewpoints regarding how a personal problem must be dealt with in the scope of the family structure. African Americans and Asian cultures have firm beliefs that the person should solve the problem with the help of family members. However, to seek help outside of the family is unthinkable. This may be a roadblock that stops mental health care providers from being trusted, especially when the provider belongs to a dominant culture or may be perceived as one who does not understand the person's cultural background. This initial distrustful perception needs to be changed. The provider must communicate genuineness, empathy and understanding of the client's needs, and build **trust within the relationship**. Trust is built when the driving force behind the client's expectations and conduct is seen as one that supports a therapeutic and beneficial relationship.

COMMUNICATION STYLES ESSENTIAL TO THE FRAMEWORK

Communication incorporates a wide range of verbal and nonverbal patterns. The mental health care provider must be aware of the different **viewpoints** and **perspectives** from which two races or cultures approach the communication process. For example, a study was conducted involving black and white college students, which asked each population to make comments about the other. The African Americans used these descriptors for communication efforts made by the white students: insistent and demanding, manipulative and scheming, organized and structured, rude and disrespectful, and critical and disparaging. The Caucasians used the following descriptors for communication efforts made by the black students: loud-mouthed, exhibited a showy or vulgar display designed to impress people, a readiness to attack or do harm to others, active, and a tendency to make excessively proud comments. The two groups held perceptions that need to be remediated before fruitful interactions can be made with members of the opposite group.

SHARED VIEW IN MULTICULTURAL COUNSELING FRAMEWORK

In 2001, Gelso and Fretz exhibited a series of dimensions to describe the differences they found between ethnic groups and Caucasian groups within American society. Gelso and Fretz described five areas:

- Family relationships, and how the person perceived himself in relation to family
- Value of self over value of family
- Value of individual success or value of combined success of the family
- Importance of the past versus importance of the present or future
- Concepts regarding focus of control over one's life choices and events

In each of these five areas, the mental health care provider must be able to understand and identify exactly what viewpoint the client holds. Out of this understanding, the provider can give explanations regarding the nature of the client's stress that will initiate a more trusted, **shared view**.

MULTICULTURAL COUNSELING

The United States of America has a populace derived from a variety of different countries and cultures. The Association of Multicultural Counseling and Development publishes a guide to the culture, ethnicity, and race of individual groups of people served by mental health providers. The foundation for the publication was laid by civil rights groups of the 1950s and 1960s, renowned for their social justice reforms that addressed racial problems, discrimination issues, subtle biases, and segregation in schools and public places. **Multicultural counseling** promotes cultural competence as an ongoing training effort for counselors working in other disciplines. **Cultural awareness outlines** are used during multicultural counseling. Multicultural counselors must receive appropriate training and preparation that includes preventive care.

> **Review Video: Multicultural Counseling**
> Visit mometrix.com/academy and enter code: 965442

ESSENTIAL ELEMENTS

In 1990, Don C. Locke defined these **four elements** of the ever-changing role of multicultural counseling:

1. Multicultural counseling is aware of the cultural background, values, and world view of the client and the therapist.
2. Multicultural counseling makes note of socialization aspects in regard to race, ethnicity, and culture of the client.
3. Multicultural counseling makes every effort to see the individual within the group of people that he or she belongs.
4. Multicultural counseling does not label the person as deficient, but acknowledges that there can be a difference between the person as an individual and his or her group.

The differences in a person may need to be addressed to help the person come to terms with his or her own self-identity. The individual is also encouraged to value the racial or ethnic group of which he or she is a member.

SYSTEMS APPROACH USED IN MULTICULTURAL COUNSELING MODELS

The multicultural mental health care provider uses his or her progressive insights and creativity to produce a positive result in helping clients. Different systems are incorporated within this task. Social justice and equity issues are a part of the lifestyle of the provider. The provider is willing to take preventive actions to make a difference for the client. The provider works hard to gain cultural awareness and understanding by learning through experience, study, and training to acquire needed skills. A **systems approach** makes note of the following parameters:

- The client and existing issues
- Societal surroundings attributed to the existing issues
- The way that the person relates to issues within his or her surroundings

The provider makes an initial assessment to determine the client's overall mental health status and how that is impacted by the issues at hand.

PREVENTION AS PART OF MULTICULTURAL COUNSELING MODEL

Prevention is any practice that eliminates client suffering from psychological, emotional, and social distress. The Surgeon General reports one out of five Americans has a mental disorder but only a small portion seek out mental health services. *The Culture, Race, and Ethnicity Supplement* of the U.S. Department of Health and Human Services reports persons of diverse ethnic and racial backgrounds are highly unlikely to access needed mental health services. Statistics would improve if multicultural health care was available in areas not currently serviced. Ideally, at-risk groups should receive preventive care through schools, employers, social policy, vocational programs, and women and infant medical facilities. Communities can promote preventive care models through advocacy, outreach, psychoeducational interventions, and self-help groups.

SOCIAL JUSTICE AS PART OF THE MULTICULTURAL COUNSELING MODEL

Social justice is equated with problematic issues in racial conflicts, sexism, and sexual preferences. Discrimination and prejudice negatively impact quality of life for both individuals and groups. Changing discriminatory practices and prejudicial viewpoints is preventive mental health. Domestic violence, sexual attacks, child abuse, discriminatory educational and suspension practices, discriminatory employment and promotion procedures, culturally insensitive managers and contemporaries are just some possible areas where **social justice** should be applied. The counselor instructs the client in coping or empowerment skills that assist the client to overcome the detrimental effects of the social injustice experience. The multicultural counselor works to change organizational, institutional, and societal thought patterns and actions of social injustice which have an adverse impact on a client's mental health status and general feeling of wellbeing.

MULTICULTURAL COUNSELING MOVEMENT

In recent years, the African-American population has grown, and a large portion of this population has moved to suburban areas and more lucrative socioeconomic positions. The Latino population has also grown and may outnumber the African-American population in the next few years. This anticipated growth will elevate the Latino population to the largest minority group in America. Native Americans are the smallest minority group in America. However, this small group has had a lucrative experience in the operation of reservation-based casinos and other service-oriented businesses. The Native American population has made economic gains from construction and retail. The mental health care provider needs to be aware and cognizant of the **diverse mental health needs of the minority groups in America**. Competence in these areas include: Self-awareness about one's own prejudices and cultural backgrounds; knowledge about diverse populations; and skills in treating diverse populations.

COMPONENTS THAT CAN IMPROVE MULTICULTURAL EDUCATIONAL COURSES

Multicultural educational courses can be improved with a broader scope on diverse populations. America has a diverse populace of African-Americans, Latinos, Asians, and Native American groups. The Asian population should be revamped to include those of Middle Eastern descent. Currently, multicultural programs only look at the cultures of Japan, China, and Korea. The world is becoming one of mixed cultures. The mental health care provider should be apprised of issues that might arise in multiracial or multiethnic families. Educational courses include: Religious factors, spiritual factors, gender factors, sexual orientation, disability issues, socioeconomic statures, age factors, and immigrant issues. The multicultural element may be introduced across the curriculum in all areas of study. Counselor educators can promote multicultural competencies in educational courses. These competencies will influence the care the minority client receives by ensuring that the counselor is skilled in consultation, outreach, and advocacy.

NP Practice Test #1

Want to take this practice test in an online interactive format?
Check out the online resources page, which includes interactive practice questions
and much more: **mometrix.com/resources719/nppmh-27810**

1. If the psychiatric and mental health nurse practitioner (PMHNP) notes that therapists are using a variety of treatment modalities for patients with depression and believes that cognitive behavioral therapy (CBT) is the most effective and takes less time than many other therapies, the best course of action is to:

    a. Ask the administration to mandate the use of CBT.
    b. Tell the therapists that CBT is the best approach to treatment.
    c. Carry out evidence-based research and present his or her findings.
    d. Recognize that a PMHNP cannot influence therapists.

2. Mike Brown has completed gender reassignment surgery (male-to-female) and is now legally Mikaela Brown. Mikaela states that she is still attracted to females and not males. The PMHNP should classify Mikaela's sexual orientation as:

    a. Lesbian
    b. Heterosexual
    c. Gay
    d. Bisexual

3. A 14-year-old states that she has occasional episodes of sleep paralysis at the onset of sleep, especially after staying up late to study. She is taking no medications and has no other symptoms. The most appropriate initial intervention is:

    a. Sleep medications
    b. Reassurance
    c. Testing for narcolepsy
    d. Testing for epilepsy

4. When serving as an agent of change in quality improvement, the PMHNP recognizes that innovation adopters who won't bring forth an innovation but are willing to readily adopt it when proposed by others are classified as:

    a. Early adopters
    b. Early majority
    c. Late majority
    d. Laggards

5. A patient scheduled for electroshock therapy tells the PMHNP, "I'm so afraid of how much this will hurt." The most appropriate response is:

    a. "Don't worry, you won't feel a thing."
    b. "I'm sure your doctor explained this treatment."
    c. "Tell me what you think is going to happen."
    d. "Electroshock therapy is a common treatment."

6. The PMHNP is aware that environmental, social, physiological, and psychological stressors may all impact the quality of care. An example of a social stressor is:

    a. Negative thoughts
    b. Noise
    c. Inadequate sleep
    d. Deadlines

7. As unit supervisor, the PMHNP uses disciplinary action to control the behavior of a staff member. The type of power the PMHNP is using is:

    a. Expert
    b. Coercive
    c. Legitimate
    d. Referent

8. If a PMHNP tells a patient, "If you don't stop yelling, we're going to hold you down, put you in restraints, and give you an injection," this could be considered as:

    a. An assault
    b. A battery
    c. Negligence
    d. Malpractice

9. When assessing the relationship between a patient and her 10-month-old infant, the PMHNP notes that the infant showed no distress when the mother briefly left the room and did not acknowledge the mother on her return. The PMHNP classifies this attachment style as:

    a. Secure
    b. Ambivalent
    c. Disorganized
    d. Avoidant

10. In managing a conflict among staff on the psychiatric unit, the PMHNP helped those in disagreement to reach a compromise with each side giving up something and each side gaining something. One disadvantage of compromise is:

    a. One side is a winner and one side a loser.
    b. It may lead staff members to believe that conflict is not tolerated.
    c. The conflict may arise again because of the losses.
    d. The parties to the conflict may feel taken advantage of.

11. A 45-year-old patient is undergoing alcohol withdrawal. Which of the following medications are NOT appropriate for the PMHNP to prescribe to relieve symptoms?

    a. Haloperidol (Haldol Decanoate)
    b. Chlordiazepoxide (Librium)
    c. Lorazepam (Ativan)
    d. Oxazepam (Serax)

12. The PMHNP is assessing a patient with the Controlled Oral Word Association Test (COWAT) and has asked the patient to name as many items as possible starting with the letter "D," but the patient is only able to name two items. This suggests brain damage to the:

    a. Frontal lobe
    b. Parietal lobe
    c. Temporal lobe
    d. Occipital lobe

13. The area of psychology that involves the study of the mental process involved in attention, memory, and perception and how these processes affect behavior is:

    a. Social psychology
    b. Psychoanalysis
    c. Cognitive psychology
    d. Gestalt psychology

14. If the PMHNP is applying the STAR approach to patient safety, the letter T represents:

    a. Teach the patient
    b. Think about the task
    c. Test understanding
    d. Track patient needs

15. When the PMHNP is communicating with colleagues about a problem in an email, the most appropriate message is:

    a. "ATTENTION!! MEETING AT 3 PM TO DISCUSS PROBLEMS WITH STAFFING."
    b. "Critical meeting at 3 p.m. to discuss requests for time off."
    c. "Meeting for all staff members scheduled for 3 p.m. this afternoon."
    d. "Please attend a 15-minute meeting at 3 p.m. to discuss coordinating time-off requests."

16. According to the National Center for Complementary and Integrative Health (NCCIH—previously called the National Center for Complementary and Alternative Medicine [NCCAM]), which of the following is an example of a whole medical system?

    a. Acupuncture
    b. Meditation
    c. Vitamin therapy
    d. Massage

17. During an interview with a 76-year-old patient with moderate cognitive impairment, the patient gets up abruptly and states that she is going for a walk. The best intervention of the PMHNP is to:

    a. Direct the patient to stay seated until the interview is over.
    b. Ask to accompany the patient on the walk.
    c. Reschedule the interview.
    d. Conclude the interview with the patient's spouse.

18. When conducting observational research of patients in a group therapy setting, the PMHNP notes that patients seem to behave as they believe they should in the group setting but that this behavior does not carry over into interactions in the unit. The patients are likely responding to:

    a. Groupthink
    b. Fear of authority
    c. Learned behaviors
    d. Demand characteristics

19. An outpatient with generalized anxiety disorder (GAD) has as an emotional support animal (a cat) and wants to take the cat to work with her when she returns to her job. The PMHNP should advise the patient that, according to Title II and Title III of the Americans with Disabilities Act (ADA), an emotional comfort animal:

    a. Does not qualify as a service animal
    b. Must be accommodated by employers as a service animal
    c. Can be certified as a service animal only if it is a dog
    d. Is certified as a service animal only on special request

20. Cocaine and amphetamine may produce symptoms similar to schizophrenia primarily because they:

a. Inhibit dopamine receptors
b. Stimulate dopamine receptors
c. Inhibit serotonin receptors
d. Stimulate serotonin receptors

21. According to Piaget, during which stage would a child be expected to first understand conservation of physical properties?

a. Sensorimotor
b. Preoperational
c. Concrete operational
d. Formal operational

22. As the supervisor, the PMHNP carried out a time study that showed that the nursing staff members spent only 25% of their time in direct patient care, 30% of their time documenting, and 45% of their time on other activities. The next step is to:

a. Tell staff members they must increase time spent in direct patient care.
b. Review documentation procedures.
c. Closely review the "other activities" that require 45% of their time.
d. Hire more staff to assist with direct patient care.

23. A 24-year-old patient with autism spectrum disorder, level 1, cannot judge the intention behind commands and often becomes distraught over simple directions, such as "eat your lunch now," and ignores important directions, such as "leave by the fire exit." The PMHNP would classify this type of deficit as:

a. Impaired social interaction
b. Mind blindness
c. Meltdown
d. Stereotypy

24. Based on research of best practices, the PMHNP has recommended a number of best practice guidelines to improve patient safety and patient outcomes. The type of best practice that the PMHNP should generally attempt to institute first is a practice that:

a. Requires new equipment
b. Involves the entire staff
c. Requires organizational change
d. Requires simple changes in procedure

25. A 12-year-old child dying of leukemia tells the PMHNP that she is worried about how her parents will cope after she dies. The most appropriate response is:

a. "Just think about getting better, and don't worry about your parents."
b. "I'll let your parents know that you are worried about them."
c. "Perhaps you can tell your parents what your hopes are for them."
d. "It's not your job to worry about taking care of your parents."

26. The psychiatric unit is changing from a primary care nursing model with all registered nurses or advance practice nurses to a team nursing model that includes LPNs and psychiatric technicians. To help combat resistance, the PMHNP should focus on the:

   a. Benefits of working in a team
   b. Cost savings that will result
   c. Challenges to be faced
   d. Need to cooperate

27. A 35-year-old recently widowed patient was a happily married stay-at-home mom but has experienced severe anxiety and panic attacks since her husband's death left her with few employable skills, little money, and three children to raise. Considering Maslow's hierarchy of needs, the patient's primary need at this time is likely to be:

   a. Physiological
   b. Love/belonging
   c. Esteem
   d. Safety/security

28. When conducting psychoeducation for a patient and family members, the initial action of the PMHNP is to:

   a. Evaluate current knowledge
   b. Develop written materials
   c. Identify and mitigate barriers to learning
   d. Plan lessons from simple to complex

29. A patient is admitted for an extended stay in a rehabilitation facility for drug and alcohol addiction. The patient's 8-year-old child asks the PMHNP if his mother will be able to come home soon. The most appropriate response is:

   a. "You should talk about that with your father."
   b. "Not soon because your mom needs to get well first."
   c. "Why do you want to know that?"
   d. "Just take one day at a time and try not to worry."

30. The evidence-based therapy that the PMHNP recommends for adolescents with anorexia nervosa is:

   a. Family-based therapy
   b. Cognitive behavioral therapy (CBT)
   c. Reality-based therapy
   d. Psychoanalysis

31. The three steps in the process of valuing are (1) choosing, (2) prizing, and (3) _____

   a. Confirming
   b. Collaborating
   c. Sharing
   d. Acting

32. An example of secondary prevention used by the PMHNP for an at-risk adolescent is:

   a. Refer to Alateen if the parents are alcoholics.
   b. Refer to a support group for children of divorce.
   c. Work with the patient to modify negative behaviors.
   d. Provide sex education courses.

33. If a patient states, "I don't understand! My daughter said that she had to leave town," an appropriate clarifying question for the PMHNP to ask would be:

   a. "Your daughter said that she had to leave town?"
   b. "Are you confused because you don't know why she had to leave town?"
   c. "Did she say anything else about it?"
   d. "Why don't you call her and ask for more information?"

34. A 9-year-old girl has vaginal tearing, bruising, and scarring, which the mother claims occurred as a result of horseback riding. The child seems emotionally stable and repeats that she hurt herself riding, but the PMHNP suspects sexual abuse. The most appropriate action is to:

   a. Assume that the mother is correct about the injuries.
   b. Ask for further assessment and a second opinion.
   c. Ask to do follow-up visits with the child.
   d. Report the suspected abuse to the appropriate authorities.

35. When working with a 28-year-old female patient with bulimia nervosa, the PMHNP finds a container of laxatives hidden in the patient's bed linens. The best response is to:

   a. Tell the patient about finding the laxatives.
   b. Reprimand the patient for having the laxatives.
   c. Ignore the finding and say nothing about it.
   d. Ask the psychiatrist what action to take.

36. Memory (immediate, remote, and recent) can be assessed in a young child beginning at about:

   a. 2 years of age
   b. 3 years of age
   c. 4 years of age
   d. 5 years of age

37. A patient who has received long-term treatment with haloperidol as an antipsychotic agent has developed repetitive behaviors, including tongue thrusting, lip smacking, and hair pulling. The most likely cause is:

   a. Pseudoparkinsonism
   b. Serotonin syndrome
   c. Neuroleptic malignant syndrome
   d. Tardive dyskinesia

38. The PMHNP overhears a nurse telling a disruptive patient, "Shut up, stop acting stupid, and go to your room." The best response to the nurse is:

   a. "You were very rude to that patient."
   b. "I heard you tell the patient to shut up, stop acting stupid, and go to her room."
   c. "Your behavior was completely inappropriate."
   d. "It's understandable that the patient would upset you."

39. If the PMHNP is gathering data about a patient, a tertiary source of information is:

   a. Medical records
   b. Patient statements
   c. Family statements
   d. Personal observation

40. As the supervisor of the psychiatric unit of a large hospital, the PMHNP carries out an assessment of patient satisfaction and then devises a strategy to reduce patient complaints regarding the time required for staff members to respond to patient needs. The competency skill that he or she is exhibiting is:

    a. Technical
    b. Conceptual
    c. Interpersonal
    d. Functional

41. The PMHNP has prescribed chlorpromazine hydrochloride (Thorazine) for a patient with psychosis, and the patient is to continue on the oral medication after discharge from the psychiatric unit. As part of educating the patient about the medication, the PMHNP should advise him or her to avoid:

    a. Exercise
    b. Milk products
    c. Tobacco products
    d. Sun exposure

42. The parents of an 11-year-old boy are concerned that their son no longer wants to be involved in family activities. The PMHNP points out that, according to Erikson's stages of human development, the key event during the stage of adolescence (12 to 18 years) is:

    a. School
    b. Love relationships
    c. Peer relationships
    d. Independence

43. With rational emotive behavior therapy (REBT), the ABCDE model suggests that adversity (A—the activating event) and consequences (C) are strongly influenced by _____ (B)

    a. Beliefs about the event
    b. Behavior associated with the event
    c. Background leading to the event
    d. Behavior of others

44. As part of evidence-based research, the PMHNP finds that one instrument produces the same results whenever it is used to measure a similar behavior, suggesting that the instrument has:

    a. Reliability
    b. Validity
    c. Sensitivity
    d. Variability

45. A patient experiencing auditory hallucinations tells the PMHNP that he hears voices warning him of danger, "Don't you hear them?" The most therapeutic response is:

    a. "There are no voices. You are hallucinating."
    b. "I know the voices seem real to you, but I don't hear them."
    c. "I can't make them out. What are they saying?"
    d. "Try to stay focused on what's real. There are no voices."

46. The PMHNP is concerned that the state's nurse practice act needs revision to more accurately reflect the competencies of PMHNPs. The best means of promoting revision of the act is to:

a. Encourage the administration to lobby the state.
b. Survey other PMHNPs in the area.
c. Write to the state legislature.
d. Become active in a state nursing organization.

47. Which of the following statements by a patient is most likely to indicate suicidal ideation and risk for suicide?

a. "My children would be better off without me."
b. "I can't stop crying when I think about my mother's death."
c. "My brother thinks he is so much better than I am."
d. "Sometimes I think this therapy is totally pointless."

48. A patient believes that messages are being sent to her in newspapers, magazines, radio, and television and that she must decipher them. This type of delusion is a:

a. Delusion of persecution
b. Delusion of control
c. Delusion of reference
d. Delusion of grandeur

49. When conducting evidence-based research, the PMHNP observes that a natural correlation appears to exist between two variables. Based on this, the PMHNP considers that:

a. One variable is the cause, and the other is the effect.
b. There may be a third-variable correlation.
c. The correlation is valid, and either may be the cause.
d. The research procedures were likely inadequate.

50. When using clinical pathways, patient progress is measured in relation to:

a. Length of stay.
b. Cost of care.
c. Actual outcomes.
d. Expected outcome.

51. In establishing a therapeutic relationship with a patient, the PMHNP's goal for the patient at the end of the orientation phase is for the patient to:

a. Exhibit alternating periods of effort and resistance
b. Be able to sustain change
c. Develop trust in the PMHNP
d. Express feelings of sadness or anger

52. A patient whose partner has left him for someone else and who spends an hour discussing all of the positive aspects of being single is probably using the ego defense mechanism of:

a. Displacement
b. Intellectualism
c. Denial
d. Rationalization

53. The four essential elements of informed consent before a patient can make a decision about care are:

    a. Competence, disclosure, options, and voluntarism
    b. Competence, comprehension, noncoercion, and disclosure
    c. Voluntarism, competence, noncoercion, and disclosure
    d. Voluntarism, competence, disclosure, and comprehension

54. The PMHNP is interviewing a 20-year-old patient who has a four-year history of cyclothymia but is currently asymptomatic. Based on this diagnosis, the maximum period of time during which the PMHNP expects the patient to remain asymptomatic is:

    a. One month
    b. Two months
    c. Three months
    d. Four months

55. According to Maslow's hierarchy of needs, which of the following nursing diagnoses would have priority?

    a. Risk for injury
    b. Ineffective coping
    c. Sleep deprivation
    d. Social isolation

56. A patient with obsessive-compulsive disorder (OCD) will begin medication to control symptoms. An FDA-approved drug for OCD that the PMHNP may prescribe is:

    a. Nefazodone
    b. Imipramine (Tofranil)
    c. Amitriptyline (Elavil)
    d. Fluoxetine (Prozac)

57. According to Peplau's interpersonal relations theory, a patient who is miserly, suspicious, and envious of others has likely failed to complete developmental tasks associated with the stage of:

    a. Infancy (learning to count on others)
    b. Toddlerhood (learning to delay satisfaction)
    c. Early childhood (identifying oneself)
    d. Late childhood (developing participatory skills)

58. As leader of an interdisciplinary team, the PMHNP notes that one team member who has worked on the unit for more than 20 years frequently criticizes younger and less experienced nurses. The best initial approach to resolving this is to:

    a. Ask the experienced nurse to serve as a mentor.
    b. Ask the experienced nurse to be more patient and supportive.
    c. Tell the experienced nurse that the behavior is detrimental to the team.
    d. Suggest that the experienced nurse transfer to a different team.

59. The structure in the brain that plays a role in emotional memories is the:

    a. Hippocampus
    b. Thalamus
    c. Amygdala
    d. Basal ganglia

60. The PMHNP is conducting a smoking cessation class for a group of patients, and two patients are adamant in stating that they plan to resume smoking after discharge from the psychiatric facility. The best solution is to:

   a. Exclude the two patients from the group.
   b. Warn the patients that smoking could endanger their lives.
   c. Arrange for the two patients to meet a person with lung cancer from smoking.
   d. Provide information about symptoms of concern, such as increased cough.

61. The PMHNP is observing a patient whose behavior is aggressive. The behavior that would differentiate aggression from anger is:

   a. Passive-aggressive behavior.
   b. Holding clenched fists.
   c. Yelling and shouting.
   d. Verbal threats.

62. Under provisions of the Americans with Disabilities Act (ADA) related to people with psychiatric disabilities, employers are required to:

   a. Provide reasonable accommodations.
   b. Hire a person with psychiatric disabilities.
   c. Provide any work accommodations that the person requests.
   d. Hold the person's position indefinitely until the person can return to work.

63. During a severe storm, four psychiatric unit staff members are unable to report for duty, leaving the unit understaffed. The PMHNP should proceed by:

   a. Working from one room to another in order.
   b. Prioritizing patient care needs.
   c. Demanding more staff from the administration.
   d. Asking responsible patients to assist with routine tasks.

64. A 28-year-old female patient who experienced sexual abuse as a child expresses distorted feelings of guilt and shame, blaming herself for the abuse and exhibiting low self-esteem. The most effective therapeutic approach is likely:

   a. Therapeutic milieu
   b. Psychoanalysis
   c. Cognitive behavioral therapy (CBT)
   d. Eye movement desensitization and reprocessing (EMDR)

65. A patient with a right-sided above-elbow (AE) amputation has become increasingly depressed because of persistent severe phantom limb pain. The PMHNP suggests the use of a mirror box to create the illusion that the limb has been restored. This therapeutic treatment is based on:

   a. Biofeedback
   b. Self-hypnosis
   c. Cognitive behavioral therapy (CBT)
   d. Neuroplasticity

66. If a patient who has been using heroin is admitted to the psychiatric unit, the PMHNP will advise the staff that after the last dose of heroin the patient is likely to exhibit withdrawal symptoms within:

   a. 6 to 12 hours
   b. 12 to 24 hours
   c. 24 to 48 hours
   d. 48 to 74 hours

67. **A patient with antisocial personality disorder tells the PMHNP (who is sensitive about her weight) that other staff members are making fun of her appearance and state that she is "fat and lazy." The PMHNP should:**

    a. Confront the other staff members.
    b. Report this to the department head.
    c. Advise the patient that he is lying.
    d. Advise the patient that his comments are inappropriate.

68. **The most appropriate documentation regarding an incident with a disturbed patient is:**

    a. "Patient threw a plate at his father, grabbed him by the shirt, and threw him onto the floor."
    b. "Patient became very upset with his father during their visit."
    c. "Patient exhibited violent behavior during his father's visit."
    d. "Patient required intervention to control aggressive behavior."

69. **A patient in CBT for major depressive disorder is experiencing negative thoughts. The statement by the patient that indicates that she is applying principles learned in therapy is:**

    a. "I know I need to change because I feel so worthless all the time."
    b. "I can't fix this situation, so I'm going to think about being on a vacation."
    c. "I should have known better than to think I could fix this situation."
    d. "I want to feel better about this situation."

70. **The PMHNP notes during a patient interview that the patient consistently expresses surprise at information of which the PMHNP knows that he is already aware. The display rule that this behavior exemplifies is:**

    a. Intensification
    b. Deintensification
    c. Masking
    d. Neutralizing

71. **For a patient taking lithium to control bipolar disorder, the serum level for maintenance should be:**

    a. 0.5 to 1.5 mEq/L
    b. 1.5 to 2.0 mEq/L
    c. 2 to 3 mEq/L
    d. 3 to 4 mEq/L

72. **If a patient has an intellectual disability and an IQ of 45, a realistic maximal expectation is that he or she may:**

    a. Develop minimal self-help skills
    b. Be able to acquire vocational skills
    c. Be capable of working in a sheltered workshop
    d. Benefit from systematic habit training

73. **A Southeast Asian patient is admitted to the psychiatric unit with major depressive episode. On physical examination, the PMHNP notes a symmetrical pattern of bruising and petechiae up and down her back, chest, and shoulders, and across the forehead. The PMHNP recognizes this as:**

    a. Coining
    b. Cupping
    c. Sadistic/masochistic ritual
    d. Physical abuse

74. When prescribing lithium for a patient with bipolar disorder, the PMHNP reviews the patient's list of medications and identifies a drug that may increase the risk of lithium toxicity. The medication that the PMHNP recognizes should not be taken concurrently with lithium is:

    a. Oral contraceptive (Ortho-Novum)
    b. Hydrochlorothiazide
    c. Levothyroxine
    d. Amoxicillin

75. An example of feedback that is directed at an action/state that the patient cannot modify is:

    a. "Your comment is inappropriate."
    b. "You seem angry at your therapist."
    c. "You have memory problems because of your alcohol abuse."
    d. "I noticed that you didn't make eye contact with your son."

76. According to CBT, the type of automatic thought exemplified when a patient states, "My mother thinks I'm a failure" is:

    a. Personalizing
    b. All-or-nothing thinking
    c. Discounting positives
    d. Mind reading

77. In a group process, the three major types of roles that group members assume within the group are (1) completing group tasks, (2) supporting the group process, and (3) _____

    a. Fulfilling personal needs
    b. Controlling the group
    c. Challenging the group
    d. Providing moral guidance

78. The daughter of a 68-year-old patient with Alzheimer's disease states that the patient, who had exhibited only mild symptoms on rivastigmine (Exelon), has suddenly had a marked increase in confusion. In reviewing the patient's medications, the PMHNP recognizes that one of the patient's drugs that may increase confusion when taken with rivastigmine is:

    a. Clopidogrel (Plavix)
    b. Atorvastatin (Lipitor)
    c. Budesonide/formoterol (Symbicort) per nebulizer
    d. Oxybutynin

79. A patient with dementia related to Alzheimer's disease has severe confusion and agitation. The PMHNP recognizes that the most appropriate intervention is:

    a. A selective serotonin reuptake inhibitor (SSRI)
    b. An antipsychotic
    c. An anticonvulsant
    d. Nonpharmacological measures

80. A new member of a team on the psychiatric unit failed to follow unit safety protocols when a patient became aggressive and, as a result, sustained injuries when attacked by the patient. In a just culture model, the appropriate response would be:

    a. Consolation/support
    b. Punitive action
    c. Coaching/additional training
    d. No action because of the injuries

81. The PMHNP is caring for a patient who has been experiencing blackouts associated with drinking alcohol, which he often sneaks and denies drinking. According to the four phases of alcoholic drinking behavior (Jellinek), the blackouts and other behaviors are a characteristic of:

    a. Phase I, prealcoholic
    b. Phase II, early alcoholic
    c. Phase III, crucial alcoholic
    d. Phase IV, chronic alcoholic

82. When conducting an outreach program to screen homeless people for mental health and/or substance abuse disorders, the best method for the PMHNP to use to encourage participation is to:

    a. Offer free food, water, and hygiene products.
    b. Advertise on TV and radio and in local newspapers.
    c. Ask the police department to refer homeless people.
    d. Advertise through community volunteers.

83. A patient is undergoing opioid withdrawal. The medication that the PMHNP prescribes to relieve symptoms is:

    a. Phenobarbital
    b. Clonidine (Catapres)
    c. Naloxone (Narcan)
    d. Diazepam (Valium)

84. If a patient who was voluntarily committed to a psychiatric facility wants to leave and is restrained from doing so by the PMHNP, this may constitute:

    a. Assault and battery
    b. Intentional tort
    c. Negligence
    d. False imprisonment

85. The PMHNP is caring for a patient admitted to the hospital with schizophrenia and polydipsia, drinking water excessively and becoming increasing confused and psychotic. The electrolyte imbalance of most concern to the PMHNP is:

    a. Hyponatremia
    b. Hypernatremia
    c. Hypocalcemia
    d. Hypercalcemia

86. A 55-year-old patient complains of increasing memory loss. When reviewing the patient's list of medications, the PMHNP notes one drug that may induce memory impairment. The drug of concern is:

    a. Levothyroxine
    b. Calcitonin
    c. Atorvastatin (Lipitor)
    d. Docusate (DSS)

87. During a patient interview, the PMHNP notes that the patient is rubbing her hands together, sitting tensely, answering abruptly, and avoiding eye contact. The PMHNP tells the patient, "I can see that you are upset." This therapeutic technique is:

    a. Clarifying
    b. Observing
    c. Restating
    d. Empathizing

88. After an automobile accident resulted in the death of his wife months earlier, a Mexican immigrant has become very depressed and relates multiple health complaints, including headache, stomachache, insomnia, nausea, and diarrhea. The patient agrees to take an antidepressant but insists that he needs to also receive treatment by a *curandero* for *susto* (loss of soul). The best response is to:
   a. Tell the patient that a *curandero* cannot help.
   b. Caution the patient that the *curandero* ritual may interfere with treatment.
   c. Tell the patient that he must choose between the *curandero* or Western medicine.
   d. Be supportive and facilitate *curandero* treatment.

89. A patient with bulimia nervosa is very angry at the PMHNP because of the restrictions that the PMHNP has prescribed after meals to prevent the patient from purging. However, the patient denies she is angry and accuses the PMHNP of being angry with her. This is an example of:
   a. Suppression
   b. Denial
   c. Projection
   d. Repression

90. During assessment and problem identification for a newly admitted patient with multiple physicians, if inconsistencies in medical data are found, the PMHNP should first:
   a. Consult with the client.
   b. Accept the latest information as being the most accurate.
   c. Consult with the source(s) of inconsistent data.
   d. Ask for a medical review of the patient's care.

91. Which of the following tests used to assess cognitive abilities for a patient with dementia includes remembering and later repeating the names of three common objects and drawing the face of a clock with all 12 numbers and with the hands indicating a specified time?
   a. Mini-Mental State Exam (MMSE)
   b. Mini-Cog test
   c. Instrumental Activities of Daily Living (IADLs)
   d. Confusion Assessment Method

92. The PMHNP is the manager of the unit and has hired two new graduate nurses to work on the unit. The PMHNP expects that the nurses will likely need the most guidance related to:
   a. Acting professionally
   b. Documenting correctly
   c. Maintaining ethical standards
   d. Delegating tasks

93. The PMHNP has discovered that Medicare and Medicaid are routinely being charged for services that patients have not received and records are being falsified. The most appropriate action is for the PMHNP to:
   a. Confront the administration
   b. Contact the local district attorney
   c. File a *qui tam* lawsuit
   d. Notify a local newspaper

94. A patient is diagnosed with psychogenic nonepileptic seizure (pseudoseizure). The most appropriate treatment approach includes:

    a. Antianxiety medication and psychological counseling
    b. An anticonvulsant drug
    c. No treatment is necessary
    d. Anticonvulsant and antianxiety drugs

95. A 17-year-old girl with a history of anorexia and depression is taking topiramate (Topamax) to control generalized tonic-clonic seizures. The adverse effect associated with topiramate that is of most concern is:

    a. Initial sedation
    b. Anorexia/weight loss
    c. Increased appetite/weight gain
    d. Dulling of cognition

96. According to the theory of cognitive dissonance (Festinger), which of the following is most likely to change if dissonance occurs?

    a. Beliefs
    b. Behaviors
    c. Actions
    d. Emotions

97. The PMHNP should monitor adolescents taking atypical antipsychotics, such as olanzapine and risperidone, for:

    a. Drug-induced anemia
    b. Hypertension
    c. Weight gain
    d. Acne

98. The PMHNP prescribes antipsychotic medications for patients even though the PMHNP is aware that the medications have numerous adverse effects that may impair overall health, basing treatment on the ethical principle of:

    a. Nonmaleficence
    b. Beneficence
    c. Fidelity
    d. Justice

99. A 45-year-old female patient visits the PMHNP with complaints of increasing depression. The patient reports increasing lethargy, weight gain, hair loss, dry skin, and sensitivity to cold. Her BP is 110/68 and her pulse is 58. The initial diagnostic test(s) indicated to determine potential causes for the depression include(s) which one of the following:

    a. Kidney function tests
    b. Liver function tests
    c. Magnetic resonance imaging (MRI) of the brain
    d. Thyroid function tests

100. If the PMHNP is basing her leadership style on expectancy theory (Vroom), then she is expected to focus on:

    a. Positive reinforcement
    b. Working conditions and salary
    c. Safety and security
    d. Feedback from staff

101. If a PMHNP is interested in becoming a leader in healthcare reform and the role of the PMHNP, his first step is to:

a. Join a number of organizations promoting healthcare reform.
b. Begin to write to politicians expressing opinions about health care.
c. Become knowledgeable about the current healthcare system.
d. Ask other leaders what topics to focus on for activism.

102. The ethnic group with the highest rates of suicide in the United States is:

a. Caucasian
b. African American
c. Native American
d. Asian

103. As a nurse manager, the PMHNP has informational, decisional, and interpersonal responsibilities. An example of a decisional responsibility is:

a. Disseminating policies
b. Conflict negotiations
c. Serving as a spokesperson
d. Allocation of resources

104. The PMHNP is the project manager for a quality improvement project that requires multiple activities and stages of development over a 12-month period. The best method of illustrating the sequence of tasks is by developing a:

a. Q & A report
b. Program evaluation and review technique (PERT) flowchart
c. Narrative explanation
d. Decision-making grid

105. A patient being treated for antisocial personality disorder became very agitated and refused to participate in activities. The PMHNP best engages in reflective thinking by:

a. Telling the patient several positive reasons for participating
b. Asking the patient why he doesn't want to participate
c. Reviewing interactions to determine how to better deal with the patient
d. Describing the event to other nursing staff and asking for input

106. The type of organizational structure in which the PMHNP would likely need to report to more than one manager is:

a. Matrix
b. Flat
c. Tall
d. Product line

107. The PMHNP is considering how to use technology in therapy. The PMHNP recognizes that virtual reality programs may best be used as part of:

a. CBT
b. Therapeutic milieu
c. Family therapy
d. Exposure therapy

108. The PMHNP discovers that a coworker has posted information on a social media site about a patient who is well known in the community, giving the person's name and diagnosis and describing the patient's condition. The PMHNP should:

    a. Tell the coworker to remove the information.
    b. Tell the patient what the coworker has done.
    c. Notify the administration of a breach in confidentiality.
    d. Advise the coworker that this is a Health Insurance Portability and Accountability Act of 1996 (HIPAA) violation.

109. If the PMHNP has been offered a leadership position but feels unprepared, the best solution is to:

    a. Study books on leadership.
    b. Ask subordinates for guidance.
    c. Find a mentor.
    d. Turn down the position.

110. A 16-year-old patient with diabetes mellitus, type 1, since age 4 has been hospitalized twice recently for elevated serum glucose and once for diabetic ketoacidosis. In all three cases, the patient was with friends and failed to follow dietary and medication protocols because of peer pressure to conform. The PMHNP recommends:

    a. Assertiveness training
    b. Diabetes education
    c. Separation from peers
    d. Parental disciplinary actions

111. The PMHNP can withhold bad news about a patient's diagnosis from the patient if:

    a. The family of an adult patient requests that the nurse withhold the information.
    b. The patient is depressed, and bad news may worsen the patient's condition.
    c. The PMHNP believes doing so is in the best interest of the patient.
    d. The patient requests that the nurse not tell the truth about negative results.

112. Under the legal doctrine of *respondeat superior*, if the PMHNP is in private practice and directs a nurse employed by the practice to give a patient a half dose of medication but the nurse gives a double dose and the patient has a severe reaction, then the PMHNP is:

    a. Exempt from liability because the nurse made the error
    b. Liable only if aware of the dose the nurse was administering
    c. Liable for the employee's negligence
    d. Exempt from liability because the order was correct

113. A patient complains to the PMHNP that she is exhausted because the unit is so noisy in the daytime and she is awakened repeatedly during the night. The response that shows the best collaborative response to the patient's needs is:

    a. "I'll talk about this with staff members."
    b. "Let's talk about ways to allow you to get more rest."
    c. "We can provide you with a sedative at night to help you sleep better."
    d. "I understand your concerns, but there is little that can be done."

114. Which element of malpractice is violated if the PMHNP gives a patient a sedative and fails to monitor the patient's response?

    a. Foreseeability
    b. Causation
    c. Breach of duty owed
    d. Duty owed to the patient

115. In communicating with an interdisciplinary group, the PMHNP is aware that the most critical skill is:

a. Listening
b. Making eye contract
c. Verbal tracking
d. Using body language

116. The organization has flattened the chain of command and widened the span of control. As a supervisor, the PMHNP expects that this will mean:

a. Decreased authority to make decisions
b. Increased numbers of managers to report to
c. Increased numbers of staff to manage
d. Decreased numbers of staff to manage

117. An 8-year-old boy has been sleeping poorly, complaining of stomachaches, crying frequently, and refusing to go to school. A complete physical examination ruled out a physical ailment. As part of an assessment for anxiety, the simplest assessment tool to use with a child is the:

a. Hamilton Anxiety Scale (HAS)
b. Beck Anxiety Inventory (BAI)
c. Beck Depression Inventory (BDI)
d. Revised Children's Manifest Anxiety Scale (RCMAS)

118. The PMHNP is using SWOT analysis as part of a quality improvement process. The S represents *strength*, the W *weaknesses*, and the O *opportunities*. What does the T represent?

a. Time
b. Threats
c. Targets
d. Testing

119. According to Rogers' Innovation–Decision Process, individuals can bring about personal change and accept innovations in five stages that begin with:

a. Confirmation
b. Decision
c. Knowledge
d. Persuasion

120. An observant Muslim patient is hospitalized during the month of Ramadan. When advising staff members about the patient's needs, the PMHNP points out that they should expect the patient to:

a. Refuse treatment during the month
b. Refuse to eat or drink from sunup to sundown
c. Insist on staying separate from non-Muslims
d. Pray 10 times a day

121. In a recovery-oriented system of care, a patient who is discharged after treatment for drug or alcohol addiction should expect:

a. Referral to community resources
b. To need no further treatment
c. To be provided a sheltered living situation
d. To receive disability payments

122. When helping individuals to resolve conflicts, the PMHNP realizes that the most difficult conflicts to resolve are:
 a. Goal based
 b. Fact based
 c. Approach based
 d. Value based

123. The administration has asked the PMHNP for guidance in eliminating lateral violence (bullying among coworkers) from the workplace. The initial recommendation should be to:
 a. Conduct an anonymous survey.
 b. Publish a zero-tolerance policy.
 c. Interview key personnel.
 d. Discuss the issue at staff meetings.

124. The PMHNP using the STAMP acronym as a guide to identify behaviors that pose the risk of violence knows that the "S" stands for:
 a. Scowling
 b. Sarcasm
 c. Staring
 d. Speech change

125. A patient who looks at a picture of red roses and perceives a monster dripping blood from its mouth is experiencing:
 a. An illusion
 b. A delusion
 c. A hallucination
 d. Magical thinking

126. Which of the following is NOT true about the epidemiology and risk factors of violent behavior?
 a. More than 50% of people who commit criminal homicides and who engage in assaultive behavior have imbibed significant amounts of alcohol immediately beforehand.
 b. For aggression classified as homicide, battery, assault with a weapon, or rape, the frequency among males clearly exceeds that among females.
 c. Most adults with and without mental disorders who commit aggressive acts do so against people they do not know, that is, strangers.
 d. For domestic violence, in which one partner hurts another, the frequency among men and women is about equal.

127. A client is a 14-year-old girl brought in by her parents for evaluation because of episodes of defiance over curfews and of staying out late with friends. The initial approach to her situation is which of the following?
 a. Meet with the family and tell the parents that such separation-individuation behavior is healthy and normal.
 b. Meet with the girl alone and explain that her behavior is exposing her to many high-risk behaviors, including substance abuse, delinquency, unprotected sex, pregnancy, and sexually transmitted diseases.
 c. Arrange for a separate therapist for the girl, a separate therapist for the parents, and yourself as the family counselor.
 d. Assess the family situation, assess the level of communication in the family, and attempt to identify specific stressors or situations that could be aggravating a normal development stage in order to address them.

128. A PMHNP is working in a substance-abuse treatment clinic where the clients are subject to random, mandatory drug screening as a part of their probation for substance abuse–related offenses. If a client has a negative urine test result, the NP can be confident that the client has not abused any of the following drugs in the past 2 to 3 days EXCEPT:

a. Heroin
b. Toluene
c. Cocaine
d. Marijuana

129. A client is a 34-year-old Hispanic American farm worker who was diagnosed last year with bipolar disorder and who has been prescribed lithium carbonate. He came to the United States from Nicaragua 18 months ago. The PMHNP is meeting him for the first time, after he has had 4 hospitalizations for his disorder and during which his lithium levels ranged from "undetectable" to 2.1 mEq/liter. What is the first step that the NP would take to assess his "health literacy" concerning his disorder?

a. Determine whether he speaks English well enough to understand explanations and directions in English or whether he needs a translator.
b. Ask him whether he was given information on bipolar disorder during and after his hospitalizations.
c. Ask him to describe in his own words what his illness is and what he must do to manage it.
d. Find out how much formal schooling he has had.

130. Which of the following is true about the heredity of bipolar disorder?

a. The risk of one identical (monozygotic) twin having bipolar I disorder if the other twin has it is 75%.
b. First-degree relatives of someone with bipolar disorder have a risk of developing bipolar disorder that is 4 to 6 times that of the general population.
c. The risk of one fraternal (dizygotic) twin having bipolar I disorder if the other twin has it is 25%.
d. If unipolar depression and bipolar I disorder are considered, then a co-twin has an even higher risk of affective illness if the index twin has bipolar I disorder, namely 100% for monozygotic twins and 50% for dizygotic twins.

131. The pathophysiology of major depressive disorder includes which of the following biochemical abnormalities?

a. Cortisol secretion following administration of 1 mg of dexamethasone will be suppressed after 12 hours in 75% of patients with clinical signs and symptoms sufficient to diagnose major depressive disorder.
b. Secretion of TSH following administration of TRH is suppressed in a significant proportion of patients with major depressive disorder relative to normal subjects.
c. CSF levels of 5HIAA are elevated in the majority of patients with major depressive disorder who commit suicide.
d. MHPG (3-methoxy-4-hydroxyphenylglycol), a metabolite of norepinephrine, is lower in the urine of patients with delusional depression than in patients with nondelusional depression.

132. Which of the following is required for the diagnosis of major depressive disorder?

a. At least 1 week of persistently depressed mood.
b. Suicidal ideation.
c. The symptoms cause clinically significant distress or impairment of function.
d. At least 4 of the following symptoms (depressed mood, loss of pleasure or interest, appetite or weight change, sleep disturbance, psychomotor agitation or retardation, fatigue, worthlessness or guilt, decreased concentration, and suicidal ideation) are present during most of 2 weeks and represent a change from the preceding 2 weeks.

133. A 25-year-old woman is brought by her family to the emergency room after complaining of having seizures again. She had been evaluated fairly recently for this same complaint, according to the family, but no medication was prescribed. The patient states that she doesn't like the neurologist and doesn't want him involved. The NP suspects that she is having pseudoseizures with a psychogenic etiology. What clinical observations or symptoms would help to confirm this possibility?

    a. Her seizures involve bilateral tonic/clonic movements during which she remains conscious and verbal.
    b. The patient holds her breath and becomes slightly cyanotic during an observed seizure in the ER.
    c. She reports having the olfactory hallucination of burning rubber just before the seizures.
    d. The patient and the family report that she is sometimes incontinent during the seizures.

134. A family brings in an elderly grandmother who is 87 years of age and who has been living with them. They express concern that she needs nursing home level of care. The patient's primary care physician evaluated her independently from the family and did not find a level of impairment or risk adequate to justify admission. The PMHNP is called in to consult on the situation. Which of the following should be prominent in the differential diagnosis?

    a. Munchausen syndrome by proxy
    b. Malingering
    c. Substance abuse
    d. "granny dumping"

135. Which one of the following disorders requires the presence of an overall disregard for the rights and feelings of others as a diagnostic criterion?

    a. Borderline Personality Disorder
    b. Obsessive Compulsive Personality Disorder
    c. Schizoid Personality Disorder
    d. Antisocial Personality Disorder

136. A 32-year-old woman with Borderline Personality Disorder sees a PMHNP in her private practice for medication management every 2 weeks. When the NP responded to a phone message while on call, she obtained her cell phone number and now calls the NP up to 5 times a day for crises. The PMHNP should:

    a. Change her cell phone number and make sure that she blocks her number when returning calls to her in the future.
    b. Arrange to terminate services with her and refer her for more comprehensive treatment at a mental health clinic or group practice that has a DBT or other specialized approach to these patients.
    c. Set limits on her phone calls, telling her that she may only leave messages on the business phone line (no more than once a day) and that she will return her calls at her discretion.
    d. Tell her that the NP contract with her is for office visits every 2 weeks and that she will not speak with her in between appointments.

137. The PMHNP has obtained a position as a psychiatric nurse at a maximum-security corrections facility. Many of his clients—who are men incarcerated for serious, violent crimes—complain of anxiety or insomnia and frequently request medication for help with these symptoms. The NP's response is to:

    a. Counsel them about progressive relaxation techniques—a non-medical approach to their symptoms.
    b. Assume that they are attempting to manipulate the NP to obtain drugs that will give them some kind of "high."
    c. Prescribe low-dose benzodiazepine medications that will be dispensed by the nurse on duty on an as-needed basis.
    d. Prescribe SSRI medications, which have no abuse potential and may help with anxiety symptoms.

138. A PMHNP receives a notice from the pharmacy management service of her patient's insurance plan that he has been obtaining benzodiazepine medication from three other practitioners besides herself, violating her agreement with him that she would prescribe these medications only if she was the sole provider. The NP decides that she will terminate treatment with this individual. The NP is concerned that he may become abusive, violent, or threatening if confronted with this directly. The best course of action is which of the following?

    a. Leave him a phone message telling him that she is canceling his next appointment, not refilling any more prescriptions for him, and terminating services as his clinician.

    b. At the next appointment, have a security guard or policeman present as she discusses the notice with him, give him a chance to respond to it, state that she believes that he is abusing these medications and may be dependent on them or addicted to them, suggest in-patient detoxification and substance abuse treatment, and inform him that she has decided that she can no longer treat him and will cease to be available as his clinician after 1 month, which will give him time to find another practitioner.

    c. Send him a registered letter (return receipt requested), in which she informs him of her decision to terminate with him as his clinician, cancel his next appointment, and tell him that she will be available for emergencies only for the next month, during which time he can seek alternative sources of treatment.

    d. Speak with him directly by phone to discuss the notice and its implications, give him a chance to respond to it, inform him of her decision to terminate with him as his clinician, suggest possibilities for in-patient detoxification and substance abuse treatment, and offer to be available by phone only for emergencies for 1 month while he seeks alternative treatment. Document the conversation fully in the medical record.

139. A challenging patient with a paranoid personality disorder has gone to an emergency room with some physical complaints. The emergency room physician notices from his medical record who the patient's psychiatric nurse is, but the patient refuses to grant permission for the ER doctor to speak with him. The ER doctor calls the PMHNP nonetheless, citing the Health Insurance Portability and Accountability Act (HIPAA), which states that clinicians may share information about patients for clinical purposes, and requests that the NP "fill him in" on the patient. What is the best response?

    a. Ask whether there is a life-threatening emergency that makes such a request legitimate under the laws of the state. If there is not, the NP should reply that he is unable to tell him anything about the patient because of confidentiality.

    b. Even though the ER physician is correct, the PMHNP should appreciate that there is a good chance that the patient will find out about the conversation, which would risk disrupting the therapeutic alliance, given his diagnosis.

    c. Because there will be nothing in writing and it's just between the doctor and the NP, provide some information to the ER doctor that will be helpful in managing the patient while he is in the ER in an effort to optimize his medical care.

    d. Ask the physician to put the patient on the phone and attempt to convince the patient that he should give permission to speak with the ER doctor.

140. A 70-year-old recently widowed patient complains of initial insomnia as she works through her bereavement and requests something from her PMHNP to help her with sleep. The best medication option is:

    a. Flurazepam

    b. Diazepam

    c. Temazepam

    d. Eszopiclone

141. In initiating and monitoring pharmacotherapy with lithium carbonate, which of the following should be performed or measured every 6 to 12 months?

    a. Electrocardiogram (ECG)
    b. BUN and creatinine
    c. Serum parathyroid hormone (PTH) level
    d. Dermatology consultation for psoriasis

142. Of the commonly prescribed antipsychotic medications for treatment of schizophrenia, which pair of the following drugs are most likely (first member of pair) and least likely (second member of pair) to cause weight gain, increased appetite, and abnormal glucose metabolism?

    a. Olanzapine (Zyprexa) and aripiprazole (Abilify)
    b. Quetiapine (Seroquel) and clozapine (Clozaril)
    c. Risperidone (Risperdal) and paliperidone (Invega)
    d. Perphenazine (Trilafon) and chlorpromazine (Thorazine)

143. A 25-year-old man complains of progressive symptoms of recurrent and persistent thoughts about germs and contamination experienced as intrusive and upsetting as well as feeling driven to perform repetitive hand washing, which has left his skin very dry and chapped. In addition to prescribing a selective serotonin reuptake inhibitor antidepressant, the PMHNP recommends referral to a practitioner that specializes in:

    a. Psychoanalysis
    b. Therapeutic massage
    c. Cognitive-behavioral therapy
    d. Interpersonal psychotherapy (IPT)

144. The ethics manual of the American Psychological Association explicitly requires informed consent for psychotherapy, whereas informed consent for psychiatrists practicing psychotherapy is implicitly required in The Principles of Medical Ethics with Annotations Especially Applicable to Psychiatry. The advantages of obtaining informed consent from a patient before embarking on a course of psychotherapy include all of the following EXCEPT:

    a. Informed consent ensures that the patient has been informed about the risks and benefits of psychotherapy and about available alternative treatments, which increases the ability of patients to help themselves and feel empowered in decision-making.
    b. Informed consent lessens the risk of regressive dependency by deemphasizing any tendency for the patient to see the therapist as "special" or uniquely empowered to help the patient, making the patient an equal partner in the undertaking.
    c. Informed consent acknowledges the uncertainty of outcomes in psychotherapy, making both the patient and therapist partners in the task of obtaining a positive result and allowing the therapist to have a more realistic role in the treatment process.
    d. Informed consent, by interposing a more formal and legally based discussion between the therapist and the patient, tempers the formation of the therapeutic alliance and injects an element of doubt or negative perspective into the patient's hope for benefit.

145. The nurse-in-charge of an in-patient psychiatric unit is present when staff must intervene to forcibly restrain a 35-year-old man recently admitted with mania who has assaulted his brother, who was visiting him. The charge nurse makes the decision to place the patient in physical restraints so that he can be medicated and prevented from injuring others or himself. What is true about situations of this type?

a. Clients in restraints must be assessed every 30 minutes for circulation, respiration, nutrition, hydration, and elimination.

b. As soon as possible, but no longer than 1 hour after the initiation of restraint or seclusion, a qualified staff member must notify the physician of the patient's condition and obtain a verbal or written order for the restraint or seclusion.

c. Orders for restraints or seclusion of adults must be reissued by a physician every 8 hours.

d. A physician must evaluate the patient while in restraints every 24 hours.

146. A 56-year-old man whose wife died 1 year ago and who was recently diagnosed with inoperable lung cancer is brought to a PMHNP's clinic by his 32-year-old son, who expresses concern about his father's depressed mood. The NP concludes from her assessment that he has signs and symptoms sufficient to qualify for a diagnosis of major depressive disorder: 10-lb. weight loss, anhedonia, anergy, and some self-neglect of hygiene and clothing. He is lucid and competent, adamantly insists that he is not suicidal, does not have guns at home, is not at risk of injuring himself, and refuses recommended psychiatric hospitalization. He accepts a prescription for an antidepressant and an appointment for the next week. Two days later he dies of a self-inflicted gunshot wound. The son files a lawsuit for failure to diagnose and treat. Which of the following is true?

a. If he deliberately concealed suicidal ideation and intent while competent and able to cooperate in a psychiatric examination, there is no liability.

b. He should have been committed involuntarily to a psychiatric hospital for his safety because he had many risk factors for suicide.

c. The son should have been instructed to determine whether his father had any firearms in the house and, if so, to remove them.

d. Because he had lost 10 lbs. and was disheveled, he should have been committed involuntarily because of his inability to care for himself by reason of mental illness.

147. Which of the following organizations is responsible for the evaluation of standards for institutional healthcare?

a. The Centers for Disease Control and Prevention (CDC)

b. The National Center for Health Statistics (NCHS)

c. The Joint Commission

d. The Agency for Healthcare Research and Quality (AHRQ)

148. The American Nurses' Association (ANA), in collaboration with the American Psychiatric Nurses Association (APNA) and the International Society of Psychiatric-Mental Health Nurses (ISPN), has outlined a set of standards of practice that includes which of the following components of the nursing process?

a. Coordination of Care; Health Teaching and Health Promotion; Milieu Therapy; Pharmacological, Biological, and Integrative Therapies; Prescriptive Authority and Treatment; Psychotherapy; and Consultation

b. General Information, Predisposing Factors, Precipitating Event, Client's Perception of the Stressor, Adaptation Responses, Summary of Initial Psychosocial/Physical Assessment including Knowledge Deficits, and Nursing Diagnoses

c. Assessment, Diagnosis, Outcome Identification, Planning, Implementation, and Evaluation

d. Subjective Data, Objective Data, Assessment, Plan, Intervention, and Evaluation

149. A PMHNP is meeting in his office with a 24-year-old man and his mother. His working diagnosis is schizophrenia, but he has become very depressed and is almost mute. His therapist and his mother agree that he should be hospitalized, but the mother would like him to be at the university hospital psychiatric unit, which will not have a bed available until the next day. The local community hospital psychiatric unit has a bed available immediately. Although he mumbles "no" to questions about suicidality, the NP feels that he should be hospitalized immediately because he is psychotic and unpredictable. The NP's supervisor is unavailable for consultation. What is the safest course of action?

    a. Allow the mother to take him home until tomorrow because she has agreed to take responsibility for monitoring him.

    b. Explain that there is no choice but to hospitalize him immediately, given his assessment, and instruct the mother to take him to the community hospital for admission.

    c. Ask the patient and his mother to sit in the waiting area while making arrangements and then call the police and the ambulance service, fill out an involuntary commitment form, and wait for the police to arrive.

    d. Outline the recommendation that the patient be admitted immediately. State that he will arrange for him to be taken to the community hospital by ambulance and that he will assist with the transfer to the university hospital psychiatric unit the next day, if possible. Explain that he would prefer to avoid an involuntary commitment action but that he is willing to do so if the family does not agree to the plan.

150. A PMHNP has noticed that her clients who take a multivitamin daily seem to suffer less from upper respiratory infections and have less trouble with depression. She decides to perform a small study to determine whether the vitamin C and vitamin D content of the multivitamins is a factor. She obtains funding; obtains IRB approval; arranges for the preparation of identical capsules containing placebo, vitamin D, vitamin C, or both vitamins; and arranges for patients, as they come for their appointments, to be randomly assigned into the treatment groups. The contents of the capsules given to a particular patient will be unknown to her, the clinicians, and the patients. This type of clinical trial is called:

    a. A double-blind, placebo-controlled clinical trial

    b. A case-control study

    c. A single-blind, placebo-controlled clinical trial

    d. A cross-sectional study

151. Which of the following statements are true about risk of suicide?

    a. Suicide risk declines with age, reaching its lowest level among persons 65 years of age and older.

    b. Of all racial groups, African Americans have the highest suicide risk.

    c. Women have a higher risk of completed suicide per attempt than do men.

    d. Suicide risk is elevated by a history of suicide in a first-degree relative, especially the same-sex parent.

152. Motivational interviewing for reduction of high-risk behaviors includes which of the following components?

    a. Vigorous confrontation of resistance to change

    b. Maintenance of a detached, impersonal attitude

    c. Encouragement of the client to accept the therapist as authoritative and to foster dependency

    d. Developing discrepancy by helping the client to see how their day-to-day behavior deviates from their ideals

153. Which of the following situations does NOT correlate with an increased risk of vulnerability to unhealthy levels of stress?

    a. Working more than 48 hours per week

    b. Having been divorced or separated in the past year

    c. Having a network of friends and acquaintances

    d. Drinking alcohol, smoking, or using drugs to relax

154. All of the following are questions included in the CAGE screening test for alcohol problems EXCEPT:

a. Have you ever felt you should cut down on your drinking?
b. Have you ever annoyed people by your drinking?
c. Have you ever felt bad or guilty about your drinking?
d. Have you ever had a drink first thing in the morning to steady your nerves or to get rid of a hangover (eye opener)?

155. The following prevalence rates for schizophrenia in specific populations are accurate EXCEPT:

a. General population   1%
b. Non-twin sibling of a schizophrenic patient   16%
c. Child with one schizophrenic parent   12%
d. Child of two schizophrenic parents   40%

156. A 23-year-old man presents to the emergency room requesting referral for opiate detoxification and complaining of withdrawal symptoms. On physical examination, the PMHNP finds all of the following signs and symptoms EXCEPT:

a. Rhinorrhea and lacrimation
b. Constricted pupils (miosis)
c. Profuse diarrhea
d. Piloerection (gooseflesh)

157. A 17-year-old adolescent girl is brought to a PMHNP by her parents, who complain that she doesn't eat and is very thin. On examination it is determined that her body weight is less than 85% of normal, she has not had a menstrual period in 6 months, she worries about being overweight, and she complains that she is "too fat." Which of the following additional features allows the NP to confidently diagnose Anorexia Nervosa, Binge-Eating/Purging Type as a single diagnosis rather than Bulimia Nervosa additionally?

a. Binging and purging occur only during episodes of anorexia nervosa.
b. Episodes of binge eating are recurrent.
c. Inappropriate compensatory behavior to prevent weight gain—such as self-induced vomiting, use of diuretics or laxatives, fasting, or excessive exercise—is recurrent.
d. Binge eating and inappropriate compensatory behaviors have both been occurring, on average, at least twice per week for 3 months.

158. Which of the following features distinguishes malingering from factitious disorder?

a. Medical history, physical examination, and laboratory evaluations do not identify specific abnormalities.
b. The patient's symptoms have necessitated his being kept in the hospital rather than returning to prison to continue serving his sentence.
c. The patient's symptoms are vague, ill-defined, at times overdramatized, and not in accordance with known clinical conditions.
d. The patient has a long history of previous hospitalizations, during which his symptoms have been severe but little pathologic evidence has been identified.

159. Which of the following is the most helpful in distinguishing a syndrome of dementia from one of delirium?

a. The patient has a fluctuating level of consciousness.
b. The patient is disoriented to person, place, and time.
c. The patient is unable to remember more than 1 of 3 objects at 3 minutes.
d. The patient keeps asking of the whereabouts of his spouse, who died last year.

160. A PMHNP is conducting an assessment of a 37-year-old unmarried mother of 4 who works as a unit clerk at the local community hospital. In reviewing her level of functioning in various areas, which of the following stands out as needing attention and exploration?

    a. Her children attend school regularly, earn above-average marks, have friends, and receive positive reports from their teachers.

    b. She is financially stable, making ends meet with her salary and with some help from extended family for occasional childcare needs.

    c. She obtained restraining orders, through Legal Aid services, on two former boyfriends who became abusive and exploitative.

    d. Despite having to take time away from work to help her youngest child get treatment for severe asthma, she negotiated with her employer to use vacation and sick time from the coming year and took minimal unpaid leave under the Family Medical Leave Act (FMLA).

161. Which of the following is a warning sign that a nurse is in danger of crossing the professional boundary of the nurse-client relationship?

    a. A married patient with whom the NP has worked for several years through several crises brings him a small box of candy as a gift just before the Christmas holidays.

    b. The NP finds herself anticipating appointments with an attractive single patient, paying special attention to how she dresses and wondering if the patient finds her attractive.

    c. A patient who is a parent confides her distress over the serious illness of one of her children, and the NP mentions that one of his children had been similarly ill in the distant past and that he can understand some of what she must be going through.

    d. A patient shares with the NP that his parent died unexpectedly last week and he spends much of the session grieving and tearful. After the session, the patient embraces the NP in appreciation, and she reciprocates, hugging the patient for a few seconds before he departs.

162. A married Italian man in his 60s has a history of treatment-resistant depression. The PMHNP consults with the patient's psychiatrist, and the recommendation is to initiate treatment with an MAO inhibitor antidepressant. What is the most important reason to meet with the patient's family when prescribing this medication?

    a. MAO inhibitors can cause orthostatic hypotension, which may be worse on arising; therefore, family members need to be watchful.

    b. MAO inhibitors can cause sexual dysfunction; therefore, the patient's spouse should be informed so as to anticipate this possibility.

    c. MAO inhibitors can interact with certain foods and over-the-counter medications and cause an abrupt increase in blood pressure, which can be harmful.

    d. MAO inhibitors can disrupt the sleep-wake cycle, which can result in daytime somnolence and nighttime insomnia.

163. Evidence-based treatment approaches to Attention-Deficit Hyperactivity Disorder (ADHD) include all of the following EXCEPT:

    a. Progressive relaxation techniques and meditation

    b. Stimulant medication and monitoring of heart rate and blood pressure

    c. Behavioral parent training (BPT) and behavioral classroom management (BCM)

    d. Intensive peer-focused behavioral interventions implemented in recreational settings (e.g., summer programs)

164. All of the following medication interventions would be reasonable as a next step in the treatment of Major Depressive Disorder when the patient has only partially improved after 6 to 8 weeks in response to an adequate dose of a standard SSRI antidepressant (e.g., fluoxetine, sertraline, fluvoxamine, paroxetine, citalopram, or escitalopram) EXCEPT:

a. A second SSRI
b. The switch to an MAO inhibitor antidepressant
c. A tricyclic antidepressant, such as nortriptyline or desipramine
d. The addition of lithium carbonate

165. Which of the following is NOT an important reason for monitoring lithium therapy with periodic blood tests?

a. Long-term use of lithium may be associated with a decline in renal function, as indicated by elevations in BUN and creatinine levels.
b. Lithium may exacerbate psoriasis.
c. Lithium has been associated with elevated levels of parathyroid hormone and hypercalcemia in some patients.
d. Lithium can cause elevations in thyrotropin (TSH) and subclinical or clinical hypothyroidism, much more frequently in females than in males.

166. All of the following situations support the use of psychotherapy EXCEPT:

a. The therapist maintains a neutral demeanor as a "blank canvas" to facilitate transference.
b. The objective of the therapist is to reinforce the patient's healthy and adaptive patterns of thought and behavior.
c. The therapist engages in a fully emotional, encouraging, and supportive relationship with the patient.
d. One aim of the treatment is to strengthen healthy defense mechanisms, especially in the context of interpersonal relationships.

167. Which of the following statements is true concerning the use of phototherapy for Seasonal Affective Disorders?

a. Light therapy must be used to extend the period of daylight artificially by exposure before sunrise or after sunset.
b. The optimum time of day for treatment is during the evening.
c. A session must last at least 2 hours for any positive effect to occur.
d. Evidence indicates that the wavelengths of light in the blue-green end of the visual spectrum are as effective as white light.

168. Which of the following statements is NOT true about informed consent?

a. Adult patients are assumed to have the right to consent to or refuse treatment.
b. Sufficient information about the diagnosis, the prognosis, and the risks and benefits of the proposed treatment must be provided.
c. The provider is not required to inform the patient of the risks and benefits of possible alternative treatments, including no treatment at all.
d. A procedure performed without informed consent is considered battery and may be malpractice as well.

169. Nurses are mandated to report abuse or neglect in all of the following situations EXCEPT:

a. A 12-year-old boy being seen for ADHD medication appears malnourished and has visible bruises on his forearms.

b. A 35-year-old woman complains that her boyfriend often forces her to have sex when she is unwilling and that she is distressed by this and unsure of what to do about it.

c. An 82-year-woman who lives with her son and daughter-in-law recounts that she doesn't know what happens to her Social Security check every month and that her family refuses to discuss it with her, telling her "it's taken care of."

d. An 8-year-old girl tells the NP that she dislikes being left at her grandfather's house because he cajoles her into playing games during which they dress and undress in front of each other and then wrestle on the floor.

170. A 42-year-old married man brought to the hospital by police is agitated, claims not to have slept for 3 days, believes that God has revealed a special mission to him to meet with the President of the United States and confront him directly about the budget deficit, and says he will pursue this or die trying. He was found wandering on the street in his underwear in mid-January in New England, and his wife states that he has not been eating. All of the following are reasons for which he may be involuntarily committed for psychiatric care by reason of mental illness EXCEPT:

a. He presents a danger to others, specifically to the President of the United States.

b. He is a danger to himself because his behavior, if unchecked, would certainly cause security personnel to stop him from approaching the President of the United States, with deadly force if necessary.

c. His lack of sleep, being underdressed for the weather, and not eating suggest that he is unable to care for himself in his current state.

d. His wife reports that he has been spending money irresponsibly, risking financial ruin for the family.

171. Which of the following is an example of 1 of the 4 stages of cognitive development identified by Piaget?

a. Formal Operations (12-15+ years)

b. Preconventional Level (ages 4-10 years)

c. Toddlerhood (learning to delay satisfaction)

d. The Symbiotic Phase (ages 1-5 months)

172. Which of the following is NOT considered Personal Health Information (PHI) under the Health Insurance Portability and Accountability Act (HIPAA)?

a. Biometric identifiers, including finger and voice prints

b. The name of the patient's attending physician

c. Device identifiers and serial numbers

d. Internet Protocol (IP) address numbers

173. The family of an elderly patient with a recent diagnosis of terminal cancer takes his PMHNP aside and requests that the NP not inform the patient of the diagnosis because it would be too upsetting for them. The NP conducts an assessment and finds that the patient is competent and rational. The patient asks his NP to discuss the doctor's findings, and the NP focuses on the patient's mild chronic history of asthmatic bronchitis. Which ethical principle has been violated?

a. Beneficence

b. Justice

c. Veracity

d. Nonmaleficence

276

174. Which is the best reason for obtaining a consultation?

  a. The possibility exists that a diagnosis might be incorrect and obtaining a second opinion will provide greater protection from a lawsuit.

  b. The patient's condition is complex and interesting, and the NP knows that the consulting psychiatrist will consider the case of interest in teaching nurses and medical students.

  c. The NP's supervisor has encouraged him to obtain consultations more frequently because he doesn't seem to ask for help often enough and he or she is concerned that the NP might be overlooking subtleties or ignoring complexities.

  d. The patient's situation is complicated by many psychosocial and medical issues and the NP is not certain which course of treatment will be most advantageous; the NP believes that proper care demands additional expertise.

175. The following are 4 of the criteria used to evaluate qualitative research. Which of them is incorrectly defined?

  a. Descriptive Vividness – The researcher describes the data gathering process in sufficient detail that the reader can personally experience it. The data collected, often in the form of personal statements, should be quoted directly and extensively, because this is the raw data from the study.

  b. Methodological Congruence – The researcher presents the philosophical and methodological approach used and cites references to support their approach. The subjects, sampling method, data-gathering and data-analysis strategies, and processes for informed consent are clearly and concisely described.

  c. Analytical Precision – The methods used to determine statistical significance, study size, the number of subjects needed, and the precision and accuracy of the instruments used to measure the data are described in detail.

  d. Theoretical Connectedness – Any theory developed from the study is clearly stated, logically consistent, reflective of the data, and in accord with other available knowledge.

Answer Key and Explanations for Test #1

1. C: If the psychiatric and mental health nurse practitioner (PMHNP) notes that therapists are using a variety of treatment modalities for patients with depression and believes that cognitive behavioral therapy (CBT) is the most effective and takes less time than many other therapies, the best course of action is to carry out evidence-based research and present his or her findings. The PMHNP should present his or her findings to administrators as well as the therapists because administrators may be in a position to influence the choice of therapy, especially if it reduces costs.

2. A: Once a person completes gender reassignment surgery and legally changes genders, that person is then considered the reassigned gender; thus, Mikaela is considered female, so her attraction to other females would result in her sexual orientation being a lesbian. If she were attracted to males, she would be heterosexual. Although she could be classified as gay by some definitions, this term is more commonly used for males attracted to the same gender, and she is no longer considered a male. She does not report a bisexual attraction to both genders.

3. B: Up to 40% of people experience sleep paralysis, most often during adolescence, so the teen should be reassured. The associated muscle atonia occurs during the onset of sleep (hypnagogic) or upon waking (hypnopompic), and the person is unable to move for seconds to minutes. In some cases, sleep paralysis is associated with sleep-related visual, auditory, or tactile hallucinations. If both symptoms are present along with daytime somnolence, then testing for narcolepsy is appropriate. Occasional sleep paralysis by itself does not warrant testing for epilepsy. Sleep paralysis may be triggered by lack of adequate rest or by stress.

4. B: Characteristics of innovation adopters include the following:

- Innovators: Actively seek innovation, visionaries.
- Early adopters: Apply innovations that they learn about, opinion leaders.
- Early majority: Won't bring forth an innovation but are willing to readily adopt it when proposed by others
- Late majority: Adopt innovations only under pressure.
- Laggards: Prefer the status quo and fail-safe innovations only.

5. C: If a patient scheduled for electroshock therapy tells the PMHNP, "I'm so afraid of how much this will hurt," the most appropriate response is, "Tell me what you think is going to happen." It's important to get clarifying information to determine what the patient's misconception is in order to alleviate the patient's concerns. For example, the patient may be concerned about pain during the procedure or after the procedure.

6. D: Deadlines. The following four different types of stressors may impact a patient's quality of care:

- Environmental: Noise, pollen, traffic, temperature, and weather.
- Social: Deadlines, time demands, interactions with others, and financial concerns.
- Physiological: Aging, pain, injuries, lack of sleep, poor nutrition, and illness.
- Psychological: Negative thoughts, worries, and anxiety.

7. B: If, as unit supervisor, the PMHNP uses disciplinary action to control the behavior of a staff member, the type of power the PMHNP is using is **coercive**, which is the power to punish others. **Expert** power derives from knowledge and expertise. **Legitimate** power derives from educational degrees and job title. **Referent** power derives from affiliating with others who hold power in the organization.

8. A: If a PMHNP tells a patient, "If you don't stop yelling, we're going to hold you down, place you in restraints, and give you an injection," this could be considered an assault, which includes threats to cause harm. If the PMHNP actually carries through with the threat against the patient's will, then this action could be considered battery. Patients should be made aware in advance of consequences of behavior, but the patient should not be reminded of them in a threatening manner.

9. D: If, when assessing the relationship between a patient and her 10-month-old infant, the PMHNP notes that the infant showed no distress when the mother briefly left the room and did not acknowledge the mother on her return, this exemplifies the avoidant attachment style. Attachment is the emotional bond between the child and a caregiver. The avoidant attachment style often indicates that the child has learned that the mother will not respond to the child.

10. C: If, in managing a conflict among staff on the psychiatric unit, the PMHNP helped those in disagreement to reach a compromise with each side giving up something and each side gaining something, the conflict may arise again because of the losses. In some cases, that which is lost becomes more important to people on reflection than that which is gained, leading to an additional conflict.

11. A: If a 45-year-old patient is undergoing alcohol withdrawal, guidelines recommend that the PMHNP prescribe a benzodiazepine such as chlordiazepoxide (Librium), lorazepam (Ativan), diazepam (Valium), or oxazepam (Serax) to relieve symptoms. Antipsychotics such as haloperidol are contraindicated in the context of alcohol withdrawal because they lower the seizure threshold, thereby increasing risks for this dangerous complication. For alcoholism, the medication is usually administered IM or IV every 2 to 4 hours. The dose is reduced over a 5- to 7-day period.

12. A: If a patient taking the Controlled Oral Word Association Test (COWAT) test is only able to name a few items when asked to name as many items as possible starting with a particular letter, such as "D," this suggests brain damage to the frontal lobe. The COWAT is the test most frequently used to assess injury to the frontal cortex. Other tests include those that measure the patient's ability to sequence events according to time or another logical manner, to reason, and to behave spontaneously.

13. C: The area of psychology that involves the study of the mental process involved in attention, memory, and perception and how these processes affect behavior is cognitive psychology. Cognitive psychology views the functions of the mind as being similar to those of a computer with input, processing, and output. Attention aids in filtering input to allow processing. Memory involves both short- and long-term memory. Perception involves interpreting sensory input (smells, sights, touch, taste, sounds, and position).

14. B: The STAR approach to patient safety is used when delivering patient care to ensure that no mistakes are made. The components of the STAR approach include the following:

- S: Stop to concentrate on the task at hand, eliminating distractions when possible.
- T: Think about the task, what the nurse is doing, and the purpose.
- A: Act to carry out the task, ensuring it is done correctly.
- R: Review how well the task was completed and if the outcomes are as predicted.

15. D: When the PMHNP is communicating with colleagues about a problem in an email, the most appropriate message is "Please attend a 15-minute meeting at 3 p.m. to discuss coordinating time-off requests." This relays the purpose of the meeting and the expected duration, and it is neutral in tone. Using all capital letters should be avoided because this is the digital equivalent of shouting. Including the word "problems" in the message sets a negative tone.

16. A: **Whole medical systems** include homeopathic medicine, naturopathic medicine, acupuncture, and Chinese herbal medication. **Mind–body medicine** includes support groups, meditation, music, art, or dance therapy. **Biologically based practices** include the use of food, vitamins, or nutrition for healing. Manipulative/body-based programs include massage or other types of manipulation, such as chiropractic treatment. **Energy therapies** may include biofield therapies intended to affect the aura (energy field) that some believe surrounds all living things. These therapies also include therapeutic touch and Reiki. **Bioelectromagnetic-based** therapies use a variety of magnetic fields to heal.

17. B: Patients with cognitive impairment may get up and move away or go for a walk during therapy, and the PMHNP should not try to restrain the patient but should ask if he or she can walk with the person. Communicating with patients with cognitive impairment can be challenging, and patients may have very different and individual responses, so observation of the patient must serve as a guide. If responses are unclear or inappropriate, the PMHNP can say, "I didn't understand that," but he or she should not laugh or indicate frustration. The PMHNP should face the patient and maintain eye contact to help the patient stay focused.

18. D: If, when conducting observational research of patients in a group therapy setting, the PMHNP notes that patients seem to behave as they believe they should in the group setting but that this behavior does not carry over into interactions in the unit, the patients are likely responding to demand characteristics. Demand characteristics are aspects of the environment (including expectations) that affect behavior. Demand characteristics are a concern when patients are aware that they are being observed because this may cause them to change their behavior.

19. A: According to Title II and Title III of the Americans with Disabilities Act (ADA), an emotional comfort animal does not qualify as a service animal. Service animals must actually provide some type of active service and must be canine, although special requests can be made to qualify miniature horses. Psychiatric service dogs, for example, are qualified to and may be trained to identify oncoming psychiatric episodes, remind the patient to take medications, interrupt self-injurious behavior, or protect disoriented patients from danger.

20. B: Cocaine and amphetamine may produce symptoms similar to schizophrenia because they stimulate dopamine receptors, increasing the level of dopamine. Antipsychotic drugs control symptoms of schizophrenia by inhibiting these receptors. Cocaine and amphetamine cause a buildup of dopamine at the receptor sites, and this causes a sense of euphoria and pleasure, followed by depression when the effect wears off. Cocaine and amphetamine affect other neurotransmitters to lesser degrees.

21. C: According to Piaget, **concrete operational** (6–11 years) is the stage at which a child would be expected to understand conservation of physical properties and to think logically about objects and events. During the **sensorimotor stage** (birth–2 years), the child learns about the world through movement and senses. During the **preoperational stage** (2–6 years), the child begins thinking egocentrically but develops some understanding of others' minds and acquires motor skills. During the **formal operational stage**, the child can think logically and abstractly.

22. C: If a time study showed that nursing staff members spent only 25% of their time in direct patient care, 30% of their time documenting, and 45% of their time on other activities, the next step is to closely review the "other activities" that require 45% of their time because correcting this could have the greatest impact on patient care. The time spent documenting is also excessive, so documentation procedures should also be reviewed.

23. B: If a 24-year-old patient with autism spectrum disorder level 1 cannot judge the intention behind commands, often becomes distraught over simple directions ("eat your lunch now"), and ignores important directions ("leave by the fire exit"), the term for this type of deficit is **mind blindness.** This same deficit interferes with patients' abilities to recognize faces. Mind blindness may contribute to impaired social interaction. A **meltdown** may begin with a tantrum, but it is more intense because the patient totally loses control and may endanger himself or others. **Stereotypy** is rigid obsessive behavior. These deficits all result in **impaired social interaction.**

24. D: Staff compliance with best practice guidelines is usually best initially with simple changes in procedures, such as instituting checklists, because the learning curve is rapid and results are generally easily quantified. Because there is no financial outlay for new equipment or a need for extensive training, setting up a pilot program is fairly simple. The PMHNP should provide strong evidence based on research that the new practice is effective, and he or she should disseminate the results of the pilot program.

25. C: If a 12-year-old child dying of leukemia tells the PMHNP that she is worried about how her parents will cope after she dies, the most appropriate response is "Perhaps you can tell your parents what your hopes are for them." Children are often afraid that talking about death with their parents will be too upsetting for the parents, but the child should be encouraged to share feelings and concerns, which can help both the child and the parents cope better.

26. A: If the psychiatric unit is changing from a primary care nursing model with all registered nurses or advance practice nurses to a team nursing model that includes LPNs and psychiatric technicians, to help combat resistance, the PMHNP should focus on the benefits of working in a team. Benefits may include more time for professional duties and assistance in providing basic care needs, such as bathing and feeding.

27. D: For a 35-year-old recently widowed woman with severe anxiety and panic attacks left with few employable skills, little money, and three children, the primary need related to Maslow's hierarchy of needs is likely to be safety/security. Although the patient apparently had a stable and happy marriage, meeting the love/belonging need, and although lower needs must be fulfilled before higher needs, it is not uncommon for people to regress under stress. Now, the patient has real concerns about supporting and providing safety for her family, so she must meet the need for safety/security before she can again progress to the next level.

28. C: When conducting psychoeducation for a patient and family members, the initial action of the PMHNP is to identify and mitigate barriers to learning. For example, if a family member is vision impaired, this will impact the development of materials; or if a member does not want to participate, the individual may not be receptive to learning. Once the PMHNP identifies barriers as well as readiness to learn, he or she can develop lesson plans and materials.

29. B: If a patient is admitted for an extended stay in a rehabilitation facility for drug and alcohol addiction, and the patient's 8-year-old child asks the PMHNP if his mother will be able to come home soon, the most appropriate response is "Not soon because your mom needs to get well first." It's important to be truthful with children and to respect their feelings and concerns rather than trying to pass their concerns off on others or to minimize them.

30. A: The evidence-based therapy recommended for adolescents with anorexia nervosa is family-based therapy. (CBT is used with adults.) Because adolescents with anorexia are not able to make good decisions about food or eating, the family is mobilized to assist the patient and carry out therapeutic interventions, such as refeeding and other efforts to restore the patient's weight to a healthy level. Because caloric intake must be high to increase weight, the family must be physically present and monitor each meal, regardless of the time needed for the adolescent to finish eating.

31. D: Acting. The three steps in the process of valuing are as follows:

1. Choosing: This involves applying the intellect to considering alternative values and then selecting those that seem appropriate for the individual.
2. Prizing: This involves the emotions and positive feelings that the person derives from the values that he or she has chosen to live by.
3. Acting: This involves behavior that supports and is consistent with the values the person espouses.

32. C: Secondary prevention for an at-risk adolescent requires some type of intervention to deal with inappropriate behavior, such as working with the patient to modify negative behaviors. The adolescent patient may receive secondary prevention measures (treatment) in the community or as an inpatient. If the patient is hospitalized, the PMHNP focuses on helping the patient to learn more appropriate problem-solving skills and helping the patient (and family) to stabilize in crisis situations.

33. B: If a patient states, "I don't understand! My daughter said that she had to leave town," an appropriate clarifying question would be "Are you confused because you don't know why she had to leave town?" Clarifying questions are used to ensure that the listener has understood the meaning (as opposed to just the words) of the patient's statement. Clarifying questions often contain some paraphrasing of what the patient has stated and may include such phrases as "Did I understand you to say…?" or "Did you say…?"

34. D: If a 9-year-old girl has vaginal tearing, bruising, and scarring, which the mother claims occurred as a result of horseback riding, and the child seems emotionally stable and repeats that she hurt herself riding, but the PMHNP suspects sexual abuse, the most appropriate response is to report suspected abuse to the appropriate authorities. State reporting laws vary somewhat from state to state, but child protective services should be notified. Children sometimes exhibit little outward emotional indications of abuse and may be coached to explain their injuries.

35. A: If a PMHNP working with a 28-year-old female patient with bulimia nervosa finds a container of laxatives hidden in the patient's bed linens, the best response is to tell the patient directly about finding the laxatives without making a judgmental statement. If consequences for violating rules have been established, then those consequences should be applied. Establishing an honest relationship is essential to the development of trust between the patient and the nurse.

36. C: Memory can be assessed in a young child beginning at about 4 years of age. Immediate memory is evaluated by asking the child to repeat words or numbers. A 4-year-old can usually remember three items. Recent memory is tested by asking the child to remember one word and having the child recall the word in 5 or 10 minutes. Remote memory is tested by asking the child to repeat something the child has learned, such as a rhyme or the child's telephone number or address.

37. D: If a patient has received long-term treatment with haloperidol as an antipsychotic agent and has developed repetitive behaviors, including tongue thrusting, lip smacking, and hair pulling, the most likely cause is tardive dyskinesia (TD), which is related to the use of conventional antipsychotics. TD may result in permanent nonvoluntary movements. Symptoms are often irreversible, but stopping or changing the medication may reduce symptoms. Patients must be monitored carefully for initial indications of TD so that medications can be changed before symptoms become severe.

38. B: If the PMHNP overhears a nurse telling a disruptive patient, "Shut up, stop acting stupid, and go to your room," the best response is to begin by describing what he or she observed without attaching a judgment (rude, inappropriate) to it, "I heard you tell the patient to shut up, stop acting stupid, and go to her room." This approach confronts the problem directly and leaves less leeway for excuses or denial.

39. A: If the PMHNP is gathering information about a patient, a tertiary source of information is medical records as well as information from other healthcare providers, such as rehabilitation therapists. Primary information is only information that is derived directly from statements by the patient. Secondary information is derived from personal observation by the PMHNP or from reports of observations by family members or friends. The PMHNP should never rely on only one source of data, keeping in mind that observations may be biased or dishonest.

40. B: If the PMHNP carries out an assessment of patient satisfaction and then devises a strategy to reduce patient complaints regarding the time required for staff members to respond to patient needs, the competency skill that he or she is exhibiting is conceptual. Conceptual skills involve the ability to analyze and reach conclusions about solving problems. Other competency skills include technical skills and interpersonal skills.

41. D: If a patient with psychosis has been prescribed chlorpromazine hydrochloride (Thorazine), an antipsychotic, the PMHNP should advise the patient to avoid sun exposure because photosensitivity reactions of the skin may occur. When outside or exposed to the sun, patients should wear sunblock and protective clothing. Chlorpromazine is more likely to cause photosensitivity than are other medications in the same class. Patients should also avoid alcohol while taking the drug and should avoid activities that require good coordination, especially in the initial weeks of therapy.

42. C: According to Erikson's stages of human development, the key event during the school-aged stage of childhood (6-12 years) is peer relationships and developing competence as they struggle with industry vs. inferiority. During this stage, the child relies heavily on peer groups to find confidence and self-esteem in their ability to produce and achieve goals.

43. A: With rational emotive behavior therapy (REBT), the model suggests that adversity (A—activating event) and consequences (C) are strongly influenced by beliefs (B) about the event. According to this model of therapy, people innately have both rational and irrational tendencies, so if the person has irrational beliefs about an activating event, then the consequences result in feelings of defeat, whereas if the person has rational beliefs, the consequences are more likely to be seen as constructive.

44. A: If, as part of evidence-based research, the PMHNP finds that one instrument produces the same results whenever it is used to measure a similar behavior, this suggests that the instrument has **reliability**. The three properties that are essential to a good measure are reliability, validity, and power. An instrument has **validity** if it can be shown to measure what was intended. **Power** is the ability to detect a significant effect in a sample of a population if it occurs in the whole population.

45. B: The best response to a patient experiencing auditory hallucinations, saying "Don't you hear them?" is to state "I know the voices seem real to you, but I don't hear them." This response validates the patient's perception and his or her real fear of the voices ("I know the voices seem real to you") while orienting the patient to reality ("I don't hear them"). The PMHNP should speak in a calm voice and avoid standing too close to or touching the patient without permission because these actions may increase the patient's fear and anxiety.

46. D: If the PMHNP is concerned that the state's nurse practice act needs revision to more accurately reflect the competencies of PMHNPs, the best means of promoting revision is to become active in a state nursing organization. In almost all cases, revisions are based on lobbying efforts by state and national nursing associations, such as the American Nurses Association, which can plan campaigns to gather support.

47. A: The statement by a patient that is most likely to indicate suicidal ideation and risk for suicide is "My children would be better off without me." When patients make statements indicating possible suicidal ideation, the PMHNP should address this immediately by asking if the patient has thoughts about dying and if the patient has a plan. Patients who have formulated a plan (such as taking an overdose of medications) are at higher risk than those who simply think about wanting to die.

48. C: Delusion of reference: The patient believes that everything in the environment references her, such as the patient believing that messages are being sent to her in newspapers, magazines, radio, and television and that she must decipher them. **Delusion of persecution:** The patient believes that others intend to harm her. **Delusion of control:** The patient believes that other people or objects control her actions. **Delusion of grandeur:** The patient believes that she is an important person or being, such as God.

49. B: If, when conducting evidence-based research, the PMHNP observes that a natural correlation appears to exist between two variables, he or she should consider that there may be a third-variable correlation. That is, a third variable may be affecting the other two variables and there may, in fact, be no cause-and-effect relationship between the two. Therefore, when assessing natural correlations, a researcher should always look for third-cause variables.

50. D: When using clinical pathways, patient progress is measured in relation to expected outcomes. Clinical pathways outline the expected clinical progress for specific conditions and the expected outcomes. While clinical pathways vary, they typically contain a day-by-day outline of activities (participation in exercise, eating, sleep), treatments (group therapy, medications), and expectations (including the length of stay). While clinical pathways are often used in order to minimize costs of care, their primary purpose is to promote consistent and better-quality care.

51. C: In establishing a therapeutic relationship with a patient, the PMHNP's goal for the patient at the end of the orientation phase is for the patient to develop trust in the PMHNP. The orientation phase is critical if the nurse and patient are to have a productive working phase. During orientation, the patient and the PMHNP should also develop respect for each other, identify the patient's primary problems, and estimate the expected duration of the relationship.

52. B: Intellectualism: Using rational intellectual processes to deal with stress and loss, such as by discussing the positive aspects of being single. **Displacement**: Transferring feelings from one person or thing to another, such as being angry with a boss and taking the anger out on a spouse. **Denial**: Completely refusing to acknowledge a situation that is stressful, such as ignoring a child's drug use. **Rationalization**: Attempting to find excuses for unacceptable behavior or feelings, such as drinking to relieve the stress of work.

53. D: The four essential elements of informed consent before a patient can make a decision about care are as follows:

1. Voluntarism: The patient must be free to make the decision without coercion, manipulation, or threats, although persuasion may be used.
2. Competence: The patient must be mentally competent to make decisions.
3. Disclosure: The healthcare provider must provide full disclosure about a treatment, including what comprises the treatment, any alternate options, and the purpose of the treatment.
4. Comprehension: The patient must be able to understand the implications of the treatment.

54. B: If the PMHNP is interviewing a 20-year-old patient who has a four-year history of cyclothymia but is currently asymptomatic, the maximum period of time during which the PMHNP expects the patient to remain asymptomatic is two months (one month for children and adolescents). Symptoms include alternating periods of hypomania and mild depression. For diagnosis, the symptoms must be present for at least two years for adults and one year for children and adolescents.

55. C: According to Maslow's hierarchy of needs, the nursing diagnoses would be prioritized in the following manner (first to last):

*   Physiological needs: Sleep deprivation.
*   Safety and security needs: Risk for injury.
*   Love and belonging: Social isolation.
*   Esteem (self and from others): Ineffective coping.

The last need is for self-actualization, but Maslow's hierarchy of needs is predicated on the idea that one must meet the needs at one level before progressing to the next level, so many people are never able to meet the needs associated with self-actualization.

56. D: The FDA-approved drug for the treatment of obsessive-compulsive disorder (OCD) that the PMHNP can prescribe is fluoxetine (Prozac). Most selective serotonin reuptake inhibitors (SSRIs), such as fluoxetine, seem to show positive results with OCD, although not all are FDA approved specifically for OCD. If the medication is successful, symptoms are often reduced by 40%–60%. Some antidepressants, such as nefazodone, imipramine, and amitriptyline, show little effect.

57. B: During the stage of toddlerhood, the child should learn to delay gratification and feel satisfied when delaying self-gratification is pleasing to others. According to Peplau's interpersonal relations theory, if patients have not completed tasks of toddlerhood, as adults they may use exploitive and manipulative behavior with others, exhibit envy and suspiciousness toward others, hoard, exhibit miserliness, exhibit inordinate neatness/punctuality, have difficulty relating to others, and alter personality characteristics to fit the situation. A patient who has not completed toddlerhood tasks requires complete acceptance in order to feel safe and secure.

58. A: If, as leader of an interdisciplinary team, the PMHNP notes that one team member who has worked on the unit for more than 20 years frequently criticizes younger and less experienced nurses, the best initial approach to resolving this is to ask the experienced nurse to serve as a mentor. This shows recognition of the nurse's skills and may help to alleviate some anxiety the nurse may have about being displaced by younger nurses.

59. C: The structure in the brain that plays a role in emotional memories and other emotional processes is the amygdala, which is part of the limbic system, which also includes the hippocampus and the hypothalamus. The amygdala triggers reactions, such as laughing, crying, and screaming with fright, and it has a primary role in encoding events as fearful. The amygdala is the brain structure that evaluates stimuli to determine if they are good or bad.

60. D: Most people with reasonable cognitive ability understand that smoking is bad for their health, so threatening them or scaring them is not likely to motivate them to quit. Realistically, success rates for smoking cessation are often low, so the PMHNP should consider that not everyone will be successful at quitting and should provide information as a preventive measure about symptoms of concern, such as increasing cough, purulent or bloody sputum, and increased shortness of breath.

61. D: The behavior that would differentiate aggression from anger is making verbal threats because this often means that the patient's anger is escalating and the person's response may be disproportionate to the situation. Other indications of aggression include restless behavior and pacing back and forth, shouting in a loud voice, and using obscenities. The person may be very suspicious and exhibit disturbed thought processes and increased agitation and overreaction to stimuli. Aggressive patients almost always have an intent to hurt someone or something.

62. A: Under provisions of the Americans with Disabilities Act (ADA) related to people with psychiatric disabilities, employers are required to provide reasonable accommodations. This does not mean that the ADA requires the hiring of people with psychiatric disabilities, holding a position open during an employee's absence, or providing for any and all requests that people make. The employee must still be able to carry out the job for which he or she was hired, although accommodations such as flexible work hours or break time and a quieter space to work are reasonable.

63. B: If, during a severe storm, four psychiatric unit staff members are unable to report for duty, leaving the unit understaffed, the PMHNP should proceed by prioritizing patient care needs to ensure that the most important needs (such as medications) are attended to first. Some needs, such as assistance with bathing, may be bypassed for the day. Asking patients to assist is not appropriate, and the administration may not be able to provide additional staff.

64. C: If a 28-year-old female patient who experienced sexual abuse as a child expresses distorted feelings of guilt and shame, blaming herself for the abuse and exhibiting low self-esteem, the most effective therapeutic approach is likely to be CBT. CBT helps patients to change their patterns of thinking and to feel better about themselves. CBT is a relatively short form of therapy, often taking only a few weeks or months of weekly meetings with a therapist.

65. D: If a patient with a right-sided above-elbow (AE) amputation has become increasingly depressed because of persistent severe phantom limb pain, and the PMHNP suggests the use of a mirror box to create the illusion that the limb has been restored, then this therapeutic treatment is based on neuroplasticity. Viewing the limb as intact helps to create new mapping in the brain, eventually allowing the person to "move" the phantom limb to reduce discomfort.

66. A: If a patient who has been using heroin is admitted to the psychiatric unit, the patient is likely to exhibit withdrawal symptoms within 6 to 12 hours after the last dose of heroin because heroin is relatively short acting. Withdrawal symptoms usually peak within 1 to 3 days and subside by the end of a week. Typical withdrawal symptoms include nausea and vomiting, abdominal cramping, myopathy, dysphoric mood, fever, diarrhea, rhinorrhea, and insomnia.

67. D: If a patient with antisocial personality disorder tells the PMHNP (who is sensitive about her weight) that other staff members are making fun of her appearance and state that she is "fat and lazy," the PMHNP should remain calm, avoid showing a reaction, and advise the patient that his comments are inappropriate. Pathological personality traits common to antisocial personality disorder include antagonism characterized by manipulation, deceit, callousness, and hostility. The patient often uses dishonesty, lack of empathy, and hostility to manipulate others.

68. A: The most appropriate documentation regarding an incident with a disturbed patient is "Patient threw a plate at his father, grabbed him by the shirt, and threw him onto the floor." This statement is objective because it is describing the actions of the patient without attaching labels or interpretations (violent, aggressive, upset). Because this incident involved another person, an incident report must be filed, and any actions that were carried out in response to the incident should be detailed.

69. B: The statement by a patient in CBT for major depressive disorder suggesting that she is applying principles learned in therapy is "I can't fix this situation, so I'm going to think about taking a vacation." One of the goals of CBT is to help patients think differently about situations and to use thought-stopping exercises when they begin to obsess over problems, such as a situation they can't fix. Patients use imagery, such as imagining being on a vacation, to help to have more positive thoughts.

70. A: If the PMHNP notes during a patient interview that the patient consistently expresses surprise at information of which the PMHNP knows that he is already aware, the display rule that this behavior exemplifies is **intensification**. **Deintensification** is muting expression. **Masking** is feeling one emotion and expressing another, and **neutralizing** is feeling an emotion but not expressing it.

71. A: The lithium level for maintenance should be 0.5 to 1.5 mEq/L. If the level increases to 1.5 to 2 mEq/L, then the next dose of medication should be withheld and the serum level of the drug should be tested. A further increase to 2 to 3 mEq/L is of considerable concern because the patient may exhibit moderate signs of toxicity. The patient requires immediate IV fluids as well as withholding of lithium. A level of 3 mEq/L or greater is life threatening and requires emergent intervention, sometimes including dialysis to lower lithium levels.

72. C: If a patient has intellectual disability and an IQ of 45 (moderate disability), a realistic maximal expectation is that the patient may be capable of working in a sheltered workshop because he or she should be capable of performing some activities independently while requiring some supervision. The patient should be able to achieve an academic level comparable to second grade. He or she may exhibit some speech impediments and have difficulty with peer relationships because of an inability to understand or adhere to social conventions.

73. A: A symmetrical pattern of bruising and petechiae up and down the back, chest, and shoulders, and across the forehead probably indicates coining (*cao gio*). This is a practice that is common in Southeast Asia and can appear as severe bruising, but the bruises are not random in the same way that is expected with abuse. An ointment is first applied to the skin, which is then rubbed firmly with a coin (or sometimes a spoon) until discoloration occurs as a method to rid the body of "bad blood" that may be causing illness.

74. B: If the PMHNP is prescribing lithium for a patient with bipolar disorder, a drug that should not be taken concurrently is hydrochlorothiazide because thiazides may increase the risk of lithium toxicity. Lithium interacts with numerous other medications (anticonvulsants, antipsychotics, loop diuretics, angiotensin-converting enzyme [ACE] inhibitors), so the PMHNP should always carefully review medication lists and check with a pharmacist if he or she is unsure about the possibility of a drug interaction.

75. C: An example of feedback that is directed at an action/state that the patient cannot modify is "You have memory problems because of your alcohol abuse" because the patient cannot undue the physical damage that has been caused by any specific action. The patient can modify behavior based on the other feedback. The patient can modify behavior if he has made an inappropriate comment, can try to control or explore the reasons for his anger, and can also attempt to make eye contact with his son during a subsequent visit.

76. D: According to CBT, the type of automatic thought exemplified when a patient states "My mother thinks I'm a failure" is **mind reading** because the patient is assuming to know what is in another person's mind (although this would not hold true if the mother actually stated that the patient was a failure). An example of **discounting positives** is "Of course I passed the test. The teacher made it too easy." **All-or-nothing thinking** leaves no room for another interpretation: "Everyone knows I'm stupid." **Personalizing** brings everything back to the individual, "He's successful because of my advice and help."

77. A: In a group process, the three major types of roles that group members assume within the group are:

1. **Completing group tasks:** Roles may include coordinating, evaluating, energizing, orienting, and elaborating.
2. **Supporting the group process:** Roles may include compromising, encouraging, following, harmonizing, and gatekeeping.
3. **Fulfilling personal needs**: Roles may include being aggressive, dominating, blocking, help-seeking, monopolizing, seeking recognition, and seducing.

Although completing group tasks and supporting group processes function to make the group effective, roles involved in fulfilling personal needs may interfere with the overall functioning of the group.

78. D: If a 68-year-old patient with Alzheimer's disease has been showing only mild symptoms on rivastigmine (Exelon) and suddenly had a marked increase in confusion, the medication that may be causing this confusion is oxybutynin. Rivastigmine is a cholinergic drug, and oxybutynin is an anticholinergic drug. Cholinergic drugs mimic the effect of acetylcholine and stimulate cholinergic receptors, but anticholinergic drugs block these receptors, decreasing the effect of the rivastigmine and similar drugs used to treat Alzheimer's.

79. D: The most appropriate intervention for severe confusion and agitation in a patient with dementia related to Alzheimer's disease is nonpharmacological measures, such as altering the environment, using distraction, allowing the patient to pace, and identifying triggers. Numerous studies have shown that antipsychotics are no better than placebos and that their use results in increased risk and adverse effects. Anticonvulsants also show no benefit. SSRIs have not been shown to reduce agitation, confusion, or depression in patients with Alzheimer's disease.

80. C: If a new member of a team on the psychiatric unit failed to follow unit safety protocols when a patient became aggressive and, as a result, sustained injuries when attacked by the patient, in a just culture model, the appropriate response would be coaching and further training because the PMHNP engaged in at-risk behavior by ignoring safety protocol. Human error and unintentional mistakes are dealt with by consolation and support, whereas reckless behavior requires punitive action.

81. B: According to the four phases of alcoholic drinking behavior (Jellinek), blackouts are a characteristic of phase II, early alcoholic. Phases of alcoholic drinking behavior include the following:

- Phase I, prealcoholic: Using alcohol to relieve stress (often learned behavior from childhood).
- Phase II, early alcoholic: Sneaking drinks, experiencing blackouts, and reacting defensively about drinking.
- Phase III, crucial alcoholic: Binge drinking, losing control to physiological dependence, displaying anger and aggression, and showing a willingness to sacrifice almost everything for alcohol.
- Phase IV, chronic alcoholic: Disintegrating physically and emotionally, being intoxicated most of the time, and experiencing life-threatening adverse effects.

82. A: Because of constant need, homeless people are most likely to be motivated by self-interest, so offering free food, water, and hygiene products is probably the best method to use to encourage participation. Although funding may be limited, sometimes community members or organizations, such as the Salvation Army, will contribute, so the PMHNP may need to consider partnering with or working with other community resources, including homeless shelters and food kitchens, because these organizations can refer the homeless.

83. B: If a patient is undergoing opioid withdrawal, the medication that is often prescribed to relieve symptoms is clonidine (Catapres). Although the medication does not reduce the cravings associated with withdrawal, it helps to relieve the patient's anxiety, agitation, and discomfort (muscle aches, cramping, diaphoresis, rhinorrhea). Patients who experience fewer withdrawal symptoms are less likely to relapse. Patients also often receive other drugs during withdrawal, including methadone or buprenorphine, which are also used for maintenance.

84. D: If a patient who was voluntarily committed to a psychiatric facility wants to leave and is restrained from doing so by the PMHNP, this may constitute **false imprisonment** because the patient has the legal right to leave, even against medical advice. **Assault and battery** may occur if a patient was treated without consent or threatened. **Intentional torts** are voluntary purposeful actions intended to bring about a physical or mental consequence. **Negligence** is providing substandard care.

85. A: The electrolyte imbalance of most concern with polydipsia, which is characterized by excessively drinking water (more than 3 liters per day), is hyponatremia because of the diluting effect that the water has on the blood and the inability of the kidneys to excrete urine fast enough. Polydipsia may occur with schizophrenia as well as in those with developmental disabilities. If untreated, the patient may develop seizures and experience cardiac arrest. Treatment of polydipsia generally requires hospitalization. Clozapine is often used to control symptoms.

86. C: If a 55-year-old patient complains of increasing memory loss, a drug that may induce memory impairment is atorvastatin (Lipitor). The FDA added cognitive impairment, including memory loss and confusion, to the list of safety information regarding statins. Research has found that patients taking cholesterol-lowering drugs have about four times the risk of developing cognitive impairment compared to those not taking the drugs, although symptoms tend to recede if the medication is discontinued.

87. B: If, during a patient interview, the PMHNP notes the patient rubbing her hands together, sitting tensely, answering abruptly, and avoiding eye contact and tells the patient, "I can see that you are upset," this therapeutic technique is called observing. The PMHNP is stating a factual observation about what is seen or heard from the patient in order to encourage the patient to verbalize her feelings and concerns.

88. D: If a Mexican immigrant suffering from depression and multiple health complaints agrees to take an antidepressant but insists that he also needs to receive treatment by a *curandero* for *susto* (loss of soul), the best response is to be supportive and facilitate *curandero* treatments. The *curandero* is a healer who is believed to heal the body and the soul using various rituals, herbs, and massage. The PMHNP should review any herbs used in the rituals to make sure they don't interact with the patient's prescription medications.

89. C: If a patient with bulimia nervosa is very angry at the PMHNP because of the restrictions that the PMHNP has prescribed after meals to prevent the patient from purging, but the patient denies she is angry and accuses the PMHNP of being angry with her, this is an example of projection. Projection is a defense mechanism in which the patient projects her own feelings, which she may find unacceptable, onto someone else.

90. C: Inconsistencies in social, medical, and functional data are not uncommon, so the PMHNP should first consult with the source of inconsistent data to try to determine the reason for the inconsistency. In some cases, the inconsistency may result from errors or misstatements. In other cases, the patient's condition may have changed from one assessment to another. The patient usually serves as the primary source of information, but other sources can include family, friends, employers, physicians, other healthcare providers (such as home health nurses and physical therapists), and medical records

91. B: The **Mini-Cog test** requires the person to remember and later repeat the names of three common objects and to draw the face of a clock with all 12 numbers and with the two hands indicating a specified time. The **MMSE** requires a number of tasks, including counting backward from 100 by 7s, providing the patient's current location, repeating phrases, following directions, and copying a picture of interlocking shapes. The **IADL** test measures eight activities necessary for adults to function independently (including shopping, food preparation, telephone use, and managing finances). The **Confusion Assessment Method** is used to assess development of delirium, not dementia.

92. D: If the PMHNP is the manager of the unit and has hired two new graduate nurses to work on the unit, the PMHNP should expect that the nurses will likely need the most guidance related to delegating tasks. New graduate nurses often feel insecure about delegating and tend to try to do everything by themselves, especially if they are unsure of the skills and roles of other staff members.

93. C: If the PMHNP has discovered that Medicare and Medicaid are routinely being charged for services that patients have not received and records are being falsified, the most appropriate action is for the PMHNP to file a *qui tam* lawsuit. This is a whistleblowing action under the False Claims Act against those defrauding the federal government. Many states have similar laws. With a *qui tam* lawsuit, the person who files the complaint is entitled to a percentage of the recouped funds.

94. A: Psychogenic nonepileptic seizures are best treated with antianxiety medications and psychological counseling because they are related to emotional trauma and stress rather than abnormalities in electrical discharges. Indications of pseudoseizures include inconsistent motor movements (such as bilateral asynchronous motions and shaking the head from one side to the other), normal electroencephalogram (EEG) findings, specific triggering events (pain, lights), and a lack of seizure activity during sleep. A primary indication of psychogenic nonepileptic seizure is resistance to antiepileptic drugs. Pseudoseizures may also have organic causes, such as migraines.

95. B: Anorexia and weight loss associated with topiramate (Topamax) may exacerbate the patient's tendency toward anorexia. Sedation may occur initially but usually subsides. Dulling of cognition may occur, but starting with a low dose and increasing it gradually may negate this effect. Many other anticonvulsants are associated with weight gain and increased appetite, and this is sometimes a concern for adolescents. Generalized clonic-tonic seizures can occur at any age and usually have abrupt onset with loss of consciousness for 1 to 2 minutes.

96. A: The theory of cognitive dissonance (Festinger) states that individuals attempt to escape dissonance and avoid inconsistencies between their beliefs and actions. If dissonance occurs, then beliefs and ideas are more likely to change than actions or behavior. To avoid dissonance, people may avoid individuals or situations in which dissonance occurs. When faced with dissonance, the person can:

- Change one cognition (piece of knowledge) to match others or change all to bring them in line.
- Eliminate one cognition or add more to bring about consonance.
- Alter the importance of the cognitions.

97. C: The PMHNP should monitor adolescents taking atypical antipsychotics, such as olanzapine and risperidone, for weight gain. Patients' baseline weights should be noted and monitored frequently because patients may gain up to 20 pounds in the first months of treatment. Adolescents may need nutritional counseling and should be encouraged to participate in physical exercise. Adolescents are often concerned about body image issues, so weight gain is one of the reasons that adolescents may be noncompliant with treatment.

98. B: The PMHNP prescribes antipsychotic medications for patients, even though the PMHNP is aware that the medications have numerous adverse effects that may impair overall health, basing treatment on the ethical principle of beneficence because the intent is to do good and the good overcompensates for the bad. This corresponds to the principle of double effect, wherein the principles of beneficence and nonmaleficence appear to be in conflict.

99. D: These symptoms—depression, lethargy, weight gain, hair loss, dry skin, sensitivity to cold, and slow pulse—are consistent with hypothyroidism, so the initial diagnostic tests that are indicated to determine potential causes for depression include thyroid-stimulating hormone (TSH), T3, and free T4. Normal free T4 values range from 0.8 to 1.5 ng/dL. Normal TSH values range from 0.4 to 4.0 mIU/L. The TSH value is especially important because it often increases first to compensate for a decrease in the free T4 value, so the free T4 value may stay within normal range for a while. Normal free T3 values range from 2.6 to 4.8 pg/mL.

100. A: If the PMHNP is basing her leadership style on expectancy theory (Vroom), which deals with motivation, she is expected to focus on positive reinforcement. Expectancy relates to how the person perceives that his or her needs will be met based on previous experience. According to this theory, motivation in the workplace is associated with positive feedback and the positive relationship between performance and outcomes. Feedback should be positive and specific.

101. C: Activism should begin with knowledge, so the first step that a PMHNP should take if he wants to become a leader in healthcare reform and the role of the PMHNP is to become knowledgeable about the current healthcare system. From this knowledge base, the PMHNP can determine what area or areas of health care he wants to focus on and which organization(s) might be the best fit.

102. A: The ethnic group with the highest rates of suicide in the United States is Caucasians, whose rates are double that of other ethnic groups. The ages at which patients are most at risk of suicide are 15 to 24 and 65 and older. Males have a higher rate of completed suicide, probably because they often choose more lethal methods (such as gunshots), whereas females have a higher rate of attempted suicide. Females, who often choose overdoses of pills, are more likely to be rescued.

103. D: Examples of **decisional responsibilities** include allocation of resources, employee evaluations, hiring and firing staff members, planning, job analysis, and job design. **Informational responsibilities** include serving as a spokesperson, monitoring staff and activities, and disseminating information. **Interpersonal responsibilities** include conflict negotiation/resolution, networking, staff development, and provision of rewards (salaries) and punishments (disciplinary action).

104. B: If the PMHNP is the project manager for a quality improvement project that requires multiple activities and stages of development over a 12-month period, the best method of illustrating the sequence of tasks is by developing a program evaluation and review technique (PERT) flowchart. Events are ordered, activities supporting those events are coded (A–Z), durations are assigned to each event, and a flowchart is developed that visually represents the project flow from beginning to end.

105. C: If a patient being treated for antisocial personality disorder became very agitated and refused to participate in activities, the PMHNP best engages in reflective thinking by reviewing interactions to determine how to better deal with the patient. Reflective thinking may be carried out during or after an event or activity, and it involves thinking about the steps the PMHNP takes and evaluating them to determine if they are effective or if other steps would be more effective.

106. A: The type of organizational structure in which the PMHNP would likely need to report to more than one manager is the matrix structure. For example, the PMHNP may need to report to a functional manager (nursing) as well as a project manager (substance abuse or Alzheimer's). Problems can arise with managers competing for the individual's time.

107. D: Virtual reality allows patients to experience an environment in the digital world and in the relative safety of the treatment facility, so it is best used for exposure therapy. For example, a flight simulation program can allow patients who have a fear of flying to experience entering an airplane and taking off, but the patient can remain in control of the degree of exposure she can tolerate and can terminate the experience if desired.

108. C: If the PMHNP discovers that a coworker has posted information on a social media site about a patient who is well known in the community, giving the person's name and diagnosis and describing the patient's condition, the PMHNP should immediately notify the administration of a breach in confidentiality and should not attempt to deal with this personally. This is a serious Health Insurance Portability and Accountability Act of 1996 (HIPAA) violation that requires notification of the patient and the Department of Health and Human Services that will best be handled by the organization's risk management personnel.

109. C: If the PMHNP has been offered a leadership position but feels unprepared, the best solution is to find a mentor, especially someone that the individual has worked with and respects. Most new leaders are apprehensive and recognize that they will have learning curves, but having someone to discuss situations with on a regular basis and to ask for guidance can be invaluable. Asking subordinates for guidance signals a lack of confidence.

110. A: If a 16-year-old patient with diabetes mellitus, type 1, since age 4 has been hospitalized three times for failing to follow dietary and medication protocols because of peer pressure to conform, the patient may benefit from assertiveness training to learn how to address her diabetes with her friends so that they can better understand her medical needs. The patient should also be assessed for depression and anxiety, which are common findings in adolescents trying to deal with developmental issues and a serious illness because these factors may lead to dietary and medication noncompliance.

111. D: Because the Patient Self-Determination Act ensures that patients have access to health information, the PMHNP can withhold information about a patient's diagnosis from the patient only if the patient has requested the PMHNP do so or the patient has been found to be mentally incompetent and unable to comprehend the information. The PMHNP must evaluate each individual to determine the best method of sharing bad news with him or her.

112. C: Under the doctrine of *respondeat superior*, if the PMHNP is an employer, then the PMHNP is legally responsible for the employee's actions and can be held liable because the employee administered the incorrect dose of the medication during employment and the act was within the realm of employment. For this reason, it's especially important to train and supervise staff well and to ensure that all communications are clear and well understood.

113. B: The best collaborative response is the one that includes "you": "Let's talk about ways to allow you to get more rest." The patient has a legitimate concern and should be encouraged to provide input rather than the PMHNP simply stating a solution or lack of a solution. In some cases, simply rescheduling medications or treatments may help to resolve the issue. If, in fact, there is no real solution, discussing the issue with the patient can help the person feel that his or her concerns are at least being acknowledged.

114. D: **Duty owed to the patient** is the element of malpractice that is violated if the PMHNP gives a patient a sedative and fails to monitor the patient's response. **Breach of duty owed** is failing to adequately communicate changes in the patient's condition to the primary healthcare provider. **Foreseeability** is failing to ensure that minimum standards of care are met. **Causation** is failing to provide necessary education to the patient.

115. A: Although all of these are important, in communicating with an interdisciplinary group, the most critical skill is listening. The other actions, such as making eye contact, using attentive body language to show interest, and verbal tracking, are used to support listening and are part of active listening in which the listener gives feedback to the speaker. Verbal tracking includes keeping track of the conversation and paraphrasing or summarizing to indicate attention to the speaker's words.

116. C: If the organization has flattened the chain of command and widened the span of control (often done as a cost-cutting measure to reduce the layers of authority), as a supervisor, the PMHNP should expect that this will mean increased numbers of staff to manage. The span of control represents the number of staff the individual manages. A wider span of control can make adequate supervision more difficult.

117. D: The **Revised Children's Manifest Anxiety Scale (RCMAS)** assesses anxiety in children and adolescents (6–19) with 37 yes–no questions, and it can be read to young children. The **Hamilton Anxiety Scale (HAS)** provides an evaluation of overall anxiety and its degree of severity for children and adults. This scale is frequently used in psychotropic drug evaluations. The **Beck Anxiety Inventory (BAI)** is a tool for adolescents and adults that ranks 21 common symptoms related to anxiety, according to the degree that they have bothered the client in the previous month. The **Beck Depression Inventory (BDI)** is a widely used, self-reported, multiple-choice questionnaire consisting of 21 items, which measures the degree of depression for persons ages 17 to 80 years.

118. B: SWOT analysis is used to evaluate internal and external factors that can affect work. Opposing factors are considered with strengths (S) and weaknesses (W) focused on internal factors and opportunities (O) and threats (T) focusing on external factors. During SWOT analysis, a diagram is developed that outlines positive and negative opposing factors. Internal factors to consider include human resources, financial resources, processes, physical resources, and historical events. External factors to consider include the general economy, rules and laws, national/international events, demographics, sources of finances, and nursing trends.

119. C: According to Rogers' Innovation–Decision Process, individuals can bring about personal change and accept innovations in the following five stages: (1) knowledge, (2) persuasion, (3) decision, (4) implementation, and (5) confirmation. However, individuals may reject change at any stage in the process, so it is important for an agent of change to remain vigilant and ensure that individuals are apprised of benefits of change at every stage and are encouraged to persist.

120. B: If an observant Muslim patient is hospitalized during the month of Ramadan, staff members should expect the patient to refuse to eat or drink from sunup to sundown as part of observance. Otherwise, the patient will generally carry on as usual. Although people who are ill are excused from the requirement to fast, many patients will insist on remaining observant. The staff should make arrangements for food to be served to the patient before dawn and later in the evening.

121. A: In a recovery-oriented system of care, a patient who is discharged after treatment for drug or alcohol addiction should expect referral to community resources. The recovery-oriented system may involve multiple treatment approaches (because what works for one patient may not work for another), and it makes use of community agencies and resources to help the patient with recovery while recognizing that multiple episodes of treatment may be needed.

122. D: When helping individuals to resolve conflicts, the PMHNP realizes that the most difficult conflicts to resolve are value-based because people are often unwilling to consider a change in values or belief systems. Additionally, values are subjective, so it can be difficult to provide objective evidence to convince people. Because of this, value-based conflicts often remain unresolved. Other types of conflicts include goal based, fact based, and approach based.

123. A: If the administration has asked the PMHNP for guidance on eliminating lateral violence (bullying among coworkers) from the workplace, the initial recommendation should be to conduct an anonymous survey. Lateral violence is almost always underreported because of the fear of reprisal, and many staff members will not talk openly about the problem but may be more forthcoming in an anonymous survey. The results can show the extent of lateral violence and help to determine appropriate interventions.

124. C: Staring. The STAMP acronym is used to identify behaviors that pose the risk of violence, as follows:

- **S**taring: Prolonged glaring at an individual.
- **T**one and voice volume: Increased volume and sarcastic or sharp retorts.
- **A**nxiety: Flushed, hyperventilating, dilated pupils, rapid speech, confusion, disorientation, and physical indications of pain.

- **M**umbling: Slurred, incoherent speech, criticizing just loud enough to be overheard, and repeating the same statements or questions.
- **P**acing: Walking back and forth, flailing, and being resistive of healthcare interventions.

125. A: Illusion: The patient misinterprets real external stimuli, such as perceiving the picture of the red roses as a monster with blood dripping from its mouth. **Delusion:** The patient has false personal beliefs despite evidence to the contrary, such as a somatic delusion in which he or she has false ideas about the functioning of his/her body. **Hallucination:** The patient experiences false sensory perceptions (auditory, visual, tactile, gustatory, and olfactory). **Magical thinking:** The patient believes that thoughts have power to control people, situations, or things.

126. C: Most aggressive acts are committed against people who are known to the aggressor, usually family members. The exceptions to this general rule are male adolescents, who may act violently against acquaintances who they know only slightly or against complete strangers.

127. D: The important first step is a thorough assessment of the situation, i.e., asking lots of questions before making any suggestions. Subsequently, the practitioner can assess the client's level of education and vulnerability concerning high-risk behaviors, determine whether separate therapists are indicated, and determine the degree to which the behavior is normative or pathological.

128. B: Toluene is a constituent of solvents that are abused through inhalation. Like most of the substances abused through inhalation, toluene is not detected by urine drug screenings. Other means of assessing inhalant abuse, such as detecting the odor of the inhalant on the subject's breath (where it may persist for many hours) or finding products of abuse stored in unusual locations, must be sought.

129. A: Given this history, the patient is unlikely to have a strong grasp of the English language, adding an additional degree of difficulty to developing his "health literacy," that is, his "capacity to obtain, process, and understand basic health information and services needed to make appropriate health decisions." Being able to provide information and education in a language that he can understand is the first step, preceding even an assessment of his understanding.

130. B: The majority of studies show a concordance of 40% for monozygotic twins and 0 to 10% for dizygotic twins. When unipolar depression and bipolar I disorder are considered, the risk is 69% for identical twins and is 19% for fraternal twins when the index twin has bipolar I disorder.

131. B: The response of TSH to TRH is blunted in a significant proportion of patients with major depressive disorder. The dexamethasone suppression test is positive (that is, cortisol is not suppressed) in only about 50% of patients with major depressive disorder. CSF levels of the serotonin metabolite 5HIAA are significantly reduced in patients who commit suicide. MHPG is elevated in the urine of patients with delusional depression compared with patients without delusional depression.

132. C: Either depressed mood or loss of interest or pleasure must be present for 2 weeks. Suicidal ideation need not be present for the diagnosis, but at least 5 of the listed symptoms must be present for 2 weeks. There must be clinically significant distress or impairment of function caused by the symptoms.

133. A: Patients may remain conscious during unilateral, partial motor seizures; however, the spread of the seizures to both cerebral hemispheres (indicated by bilateral tonic/clonic movements) is always associated with loss of consciousness. The other symptoms are frequently seen during seizure disorders.

134. D: Munchausen by proxy (factitious disorder by proxy) usually involves a parent who presents a child repeatedly for treatment with physical complaints or conditions that turn out to be fabricated or produced by the parent, who is motivated by a wish to adopt a sick role vicariously through the child. Malingering would usually be manifest by the adoption of feigned or exaggerated symptoms in order to obtain nursing home admission, when the patient has minimal signs and symptoms. If the patient has an occult substance abuse problem that causes serious impairment at home but not when sober, as here when seen by the physician, it could explain the disconnect. However, the family is usually aware of and reports the substance abuse. "Granny dumping," the attempt to offload a burdensome elder onto the healthcare system, must be considered prominently in the differential diagnosis, given the limited information.

135. D: Antisocial Personality Disorder requires evidence of a disregard for the rights and feelings of others with onset before age 15 years.

136. B: Patients with this degree of behavioral dyscontrol should not be managed by a solo practitioner in a private office setting. The NP needs to terminate services and help her find an alternative venue that will more comprehensively manage her neediness and dilute her transference over a wider group of clinicians.

137. A: Many incarcerated individuals have antisocial personality disorders and will attempt to manipulate or con susceptible prison staff, often seeking drugs or diagnoses that will gain them special treatment. Malingering (making up symptoms to gain an advantage) is common in this population. Individuals feigning symptoms for this purpose will generally be uninterested in non-medical approaches, allowing some differentiation between a malingering population and those with a genuine problem.

138. D: The PMHNP is not required to expose herself to undue risk of injury or even abuse from a potentially violent patient. The compassionate and correct way to terminate services is to speak with the patient directly, by telephone if an office visit will present too great a risk, and inform them of the decision and why she is making it, offering to help arrange additional treatment for substance abuse issues. Full documentation in the medical record and in a registered letter and the offer to be available on an emergency basis for 1 month will protect the NP against any accusation of abandonment. Offering to help arrange in-patient detoxification will protect her against any liability should the patient refuse and then have withdrawal complications.

139. A: If state confidentiality statutes are more restrictive than the federal guidelines of HIPAA, the former take precedence. Here, there has been no compelling reason presented to the NP that would supersede his explicit contract of confidentiality with the patient about his privileged information. Although the consequences of sharing information without his permission may be greater, given his paranoid personality disorder, that alone should not be the rationale for deciding to share confidential information or not. Also, attempting to speak with the patient if he has not requested it would generally be too involved or intrusive to be positive for the treatment alliance with this type of patient.

140. C: Both flurazepam and diazepam have long elimination half-lives and are not recommended for use in patients over the age of 65 years. Eszopiclone is likely to be more expensive than the other agents listed, which are available in generic form. Temazepam has an intermediate half-life, is FDA-approved for insomnia, and is well-tolerated and inexpensive.

141. B: Deterioration of kidney function with long-term lithium use is a significant risk, requiring BUN and creatinine to be monitored at least annually. Whereas lithium can cause T wave changes in the ECG and can exacerbate or precipitate psoriasis in some patients, there is no need to monitor these areas in any regular way. Lithium has been associated with elevations in serum parathyroid hormone and serum calcium, but not frequently enough to be routinely monitored.

142. A: The newer second-generation antipsychotic medications have demonstrated a tendency to significantly increase appetite, weight, and glucose intolerance. Clozapine and olanzapine are the most likely, risperidone and quetiapine are less likely, and ziprasidone (Geodon) and aripiprazole are least likely to be associated with these adverse effects.

143. C: Although Obsessive Compulsive Disorder is clearly an Axis I condition mediated by abnormalities in brain function and neurotransmitter balance, good empirical evidence indicates that the application of behavioral techniques such as exposure and response inhibition are effective in motivated patients for improving symptom control.

144. D: The hazard of psychotherapeutic informed consent is that it interferes with the establishment of initial rapport and therapeutic alliance by fostering discouragement and a negative suggestion about the possible outcome of the treatment. The other choices are the benefits of informed consent for psychotherapy.

145. B: Patients in restraints or seclusion must be observed and assessed every 10 to 15 minutes for circulation, respiration, nutrition, hydration, and elimination. Orders for restraints or seclusion must be reissued by a physician every 4 hours for adults (every 2 hours for those aged 9 to 17 years and every 1 hour for children younger than 9 years), and a physician must evaluate the patient while in restraints or seclusion every 8 hours (18 years and older) or every 4 hours (younger than 18 years). (The Joint Commission Guidelines)

146. A: In the absence of any stated or implied suicidal ideation or intent and without evidence of very significant self-neglect, involuntary hospitalization in this case would have been beyond the scope of the usual statutes governing such interventions, which usually require "likelihood of serious harm" or "substantial risk" of injury to self or others. If the patient is assessed as competent, the clinician cannot be held liable for the patient's deliberate withholding of suicidal ideation or intent and of information about possession of lethal means or for the patient's failure to seek help when such suicidal ideation or intention arose.

147. C: The CDC provides information for health protection and disease prevention, including environmental health and occupational health and safety and infectious disease monitoring. The NCHS compiles health statistics to guide policy formation in the health care field. The AHRQ develops clinical guidelines and promotes evidence-based medical practices. The Joint Commission performs periodic reviews of hospital care, including areas of operations, staff performance, physical facilities, and standard operating procedures. If the institution meets standards of practice in these areas, it is given initial or ongoing accreditation. The Joint Commission is a non-profit organization that has been accrediting institutions since 1951. Accreditation by the Joint Commission is often required by health insurance plans for coverage of services.

148. C: The elements of answer A are those of the Implementation component of nursing process. The elements of answer B are those of the Assessment component of the nursing process. The elements of answer D are those of the Documentation aspect of the nursing process.

149. D: Although family members might be willing to "take responsibility," they are not trained mental health professionals and the NP will be liable for any adverse outcome resulting from delaying the admission overnight. Even expecting the mother to follow through on taking her son to the community hospital is risky, because she could decide to drive him home instead. An involuntary commitment without discussion with the family would be needlessly challenging to the therapeutic alliance, unless the assessment is that the patient would run away if he knew that he would be taken to the community hospital immediately, instead of waiting for a bed to become available at the university hospital. Sending the patient voluntarily by ambulance is the best route, if the family agrees, with involuntary commitment as the fallback option.

150. A: When both the subject and the investigator are "blind" to the treatment option being given, it is a "double-blind" trial. When only the subject is unaware of which treatment is being given, it is a "single blind" trial, which is considered to be subject to investigator bias because the latter knows the treatment being given and may be influenced to assess it as more effective in the subjects receiving it. Cross-sectional studies make observations in subjects at a single point in time, whereas a case-control study identifies subjects with the condition and compares them with a sample of subjects without the condition to determine which other factors are associated with the difference in outcomes.

151. D: Suicide risk increases with age and is highest in persons older than 65 years. Whites have the highest rate of suicide, followed by Native Americans, African Americans, Hispanic Americans, and Asian Americans. Women attempt suicide at a higher rate than do men, but men succeed more often.

152. D: Motivational interviewing is a client-centered approach that involves "rolling with the resistance" rather than confronting it, expressing empathy and viewing the situation from the client's perspective, supporting self-efficacy by explicitly embracing client autonomy, and developing discrepancy.

153. C: Some of the many factors that increase stress levels are social isolation, financial instability, job loss, divorce or separation, and physical illness. Signs of stress include irritability, loss of interest, sleep disturbance, weight loss, increased use of alcohol or drugs, increased use of sick time from work, and increased levels of physical complaints and symptoms.

154. B: The correct form of question "b" is "Have people annoyed you by criticizing your drinking?" The others are correct formats from the CAGE (Cut down, Annoyed, Guilty, Eye opener) assessment for alcohol problems.

155. B: The prevalence of schizophrenia among non-twin siblings of a schizophrenic patient is 8%. Being a dizygotic twin of a schizophrenic patient raises the prevalence rate to 12%, and being a monozygotic twin of a schizophrenic patient raises the prevalence rate to 47%.

156. B: Opioid Withdrawal Syndrome is associated with severe muscle cramps and bone aches, profuse diarrhea, abdominal cramps, rhinorrhea, lacrimation, piloerection or gooseflesh, yawning, fever, pupillary dilation (mydriasis), hypertension, tachycardia, and temperature dysregulation.

157. A: If a patient binges and purges only during periods of time when other signs and symptoms qualify the patient for a diagnosis of Anorexia Nervosa, Bulimia Nervosa will not be diagnosed additionally. The correct diagnosis in this situation is Anorexia Nervosa, Binge Eating-Purging Type.

158. B: In both Factitious Disorder and malingering, false or grossly exaggerated physical or psychological symptoms are intentionally reported. Careful assessment both excludes other causes and often allows documentation of direct evidence of fabrication based on the non-physiological or non-anatomical nature of the symptoms, changes in symptoms, or observations (e.g., witnessing a patient deliberately contaminate a wound that mysteriously refuses to heal). There may be a pattern of such "illnesses" in both cases. Malingering (which has the V code of V65.25) is associated with a clear external incentive or secondary gain from assuming a sick role, such as avoiding military service or incarceration, avoiding work, obtaining financial rewards such as disability payments or other financial compensation, obtaining drugs, or evading criminal prosecution. Factitious Disorder is associated with a more internal motive, that is, to assume the sick role.

159. A: Deficits in cognition can be similar in delirium and dementia, but the distinguishing characteristics are twofold: delirium manifests with an alteration in alertness or level of consciousness and with a reduced capacity for cognitive processing, both of which appear within a short time frame; most dementias are slower in onset, and cognitive decline usually takes place in the setting of clear sensorium (although dementia with Lewy Bodies can be characterized by altered sensorium and prominent perceptual distortions, such as hallucinations).

160. C: Despite evidence of resolve and appropriate self-care in dealing with difficult ex-boyfriends, a pattern of involvement in abusive relationships may exist that bears examination and intervention.

161. B: There are no absolute rules about self-disclosure, accepting small gifts, or touch, because the diverse cultural backgrounds and sociocultural situations of clients may make an action appropriate in one situation but inappropriate in another. However, it is never appropriate to allow romantic feelings or thoughts to interfere with clinical care. In such cases, supervision should be sought, and the situation should be monitored closely; it may become necessary for the client to be referred to another practitioner.

162. C: Any member of the family who prepares meals should be educated about the potential tyramine reaction that can occur with the ingestion of aged cheeses, certain sausages and other fermented protein products, and some alcoholic beverages (beer and wine). The presence of these products in food may be masked during preparation; therefore, both the food preparer and the patient should be aware of the risk.

163. A: A number of adequately designed and controlled studies have demonstrated the efficacy of stimulant medications, BPT, BCM, and peer-focused behavioral interventions in recreational settings in both children and adults with ADHD.

164. B: MAO inhibitor antidepressants—such as phenelzine, tranylcypromine, and isocarboxazid—are reserved for use until at least 3 or 4 other antidepressant options have failed to be helpful, because of the risk of toxic interactions with dietary items and other medications. The MAO inhibitor selegiline, applied as a patch, may circumvent some of these issues and may be categorized as a third- or fourth-line treatment.

165. B: No evidence indicates that lithium levels worsen psoriasis at the high end of the therapeutic range or are associated with improvement in psoriatic lesions at the lower end of the therapeutic range; therefore, blood monitoring is not helpful for managing lithium-associated psoriasis.

166. A: The aim of supportive psychotherapy is to help the patient through a difficult period by strengthening, supporting, and highlighting the patient's already existing strengths and assets. The duration of both the sessions themselves and of the course of therapy may be brief. Techniques of psychoanalysis meant to foster free association or even to provoke anxiety and uncertainty, such as the therapist presenting a "blank screen," tend to undermine or diminish usual defense mechanisms rather than strengthen them, as is the goal of supportive psychotherapies.

167. D: Phototherapy works better by increasing the intensity of light exposure rather than by increasing its duration, appears to be most effective when administered in the morning, and can have positive effects with as little as 30-45 minutes of exposure per day. Blue-green light may be the most effective part of the visual spectrum for treating depression.

168. C: The courts now require that practitioners relate sufficient information about alternative treatments that may be advantageous to the patient, discuss the possible risks and benefits associated with them, and discuss the option of no treatment.

169. B: The principle of autonomy holds that adults have the ability and the right to make reasonable and responsible choices for themselves. An adult woman in an abusive relationship may request counseling and even shelter, but the health practitioner is not mandated to report the situation to any civil or criminal authority, independent of the patient's willingness or consent. Doing so without the patient's consent would be a violation of confidentiality.

170. D: Financial indiscretion is not considered a reason for involuntary commitment for mental illness in most jurisdictions.

171. A: Piaget's 4 stages of cognitive development are Sensorimotor (birth to 2 years), Preoperational (ages 2-6 years), Concrete Operations (ages 6-12 years), and Formal Operations (ages 12-15+ years); Kohlberg's levels of moral development are Preconventional (ages 4-10 years), Conventional (ages 10-13 years and into adulthood), and Postconventional (from adolescence onward); Peplau's stages of personality development are Infancy (learning to count on others), Toddlerhood (learning to delay satisfaction), Early Childhood (identifying oneself), and Late Childhood (developing skills in participation); and Mahler's theory of separation-individuation includes the Autistic Phase (birth to 1 month), the Symbiotic Phase (ages 1-5 months), and the Separation-Individuation Phase (ages 5-36 months).

172. B: PHI does not include the name of the patient's physician, because this is not information that "identifies the individual or with respect to which there is a reasonable basis to believe the information can be used to identify the individual" (U.S. Department of Health and Human Services, 2003).

173. C: Veracity is the duty to tell the truth and not intentionally deceive or mislead clients. Occasions when the truth would produce harm or interfere with the recovery process are rare. The principle of autonomy holds that the patient is presumed rational and responsible, retaining the right to determine their own destiny and to be fully informed about their condition. Withholding the truth would violate this principle as well. In this case, the nurse is attempting to act under the principles of nonmaleficence (to do no intentional harm to the client), beneficence (to benefit or promote the good of others), and justice (to treat all individuals, including the family, equally and fairly); however, the primary duty is to the patient.

174. D: The chief reason to obtain consultation is to determine a professional assessment of whether a patient's situation is beyond the NP's experience or knowledge to handle properly. Another reason to obtain consultation would be to honor the patient's requests for a second opinion, which should generally be facilitated. Although a second opinion provides a sharing of medical-legal responsibility, this is not the primary reason to obtain such.

175. C: Analytical Precision is not concerned with statistics and instruments. It refers to the decision-making process by which researchers synthesize concrete data (words of the subjects) into an abstract that clarifies the meaning and the importance of the study. The last of the 5 criteria is Heuristic Relevance: The researcher clarifies the significance of the study, its applicability to public health or community nursing, and its likely influence on future research.

NP Practice Test #2

To take this additional NP practice test, visit our online resources page:
mometrix.com/resources719/nppmh-27810

How to Overcome Test Anxiety

Just the thought of taking a test is enough to make most people a little nervous. A test is an important event that can have a long-term impact on your future, so it's important to take it seriously and it's natural to feel anxious about performing well. But just because anxiety is normal, that doesn't mean that it's helpful in test taking, or that you should simply accept it as part of your life. Anxiety can have a variety of effects. These effects can be mild, like making you feel slightly nervous, or severe, like blocking your ability to focus or remember even a simple detail.

If you experience test anxiety—whether severe or mild—it's important to know how to beat it. To discover this, first you need to understand what causes test anxiety.

Causes of Test Anxiety

While we often think of anxiety as an uncontrollable emotional state, it can actually be caused by simple, practical things. One of the most common causes of test anxiety is that a person does not feel adequately prepared for their test. This feeling can be the result of many different issues such as poor study habits or lack of organization, but the most common culprit is time management. Starting to study too late, failing to organize your study time to cover all of the material, or being distracted while you study will mean that you're not well prepared for the test. This may lead to cramming the night before, which will cause you to be physically and mentally exhausted for the test. Poor time management also contributes to feelings of stress, fear, and hopelessness as you realize you are not well prepared but don't know what to do about it.

Other times, test anxiety is not related to your preparation for the test but comes from unresolved fear. This may be a past failure on a test, or poor performance on tests in general. It may come from comparing yourself to others who seem to be performing better or from the stress of living up to expectations. Anxiety may be driven by fears of the future—how failure on this test would affect your educational and career goals. These fears are often completely irrational, but they can still negatively impact your test performance.

Elements of Test Anxiety

As mentioned earlier, test anxiety is considered to be an emotional state, but it has physical and mental components as well. Sometimes you may not even realize that you are suffering from test anxiety until you notice the physical symptoms. These can include trembling hands, rapid heartbeat, sweating, nausea, and tense muscles. Extreme anxiety may lead to fainting or vomiting. Obviously, any of these symptoms can have a negative impact on testing. It is important to recognize them as soon as they begin to occur so that you can address the problem before it damages your performance.

The mental components of test anxiety include trouble focusing and inability to remember learned information. During a test, your mind is on high alert, which can help you recall information and stay focused for an extended period of time. However, anxiety interferes with your mind's natural processes, causing you to blank out, even on the questions you know well. The strain of testing during anxiety makes it difficult to stay focused, especially on a test that may take several hours. Extreme anxiety can take a huge mental toll, making it difficult not only to recall test information but even to understand the test questions or pull your thoughts together.

Effects of Test Anxiety

Test anxiety is like a disease—if left untreated, it will get progressively worse. Anxiety leads to poor performance, and this reinforces the feelings of fear and failure, which in turn lead to poor performances on subsequent tests. It can grow from a mild nervousness to a crippling condition. If allowed to progress, test anxiety can have a big impact on your schooling, and consequently on your future.

Test anxiety can spread to other parts of your life. Anxiety on tests can become anxiety in any stressful situation, and blanking on a test can turn into panicking in a job situation. But fortunately, you don't have to let anxiety rule your testing and determine your grades. There are a number of relatively simple steps you can take to move past anxiety and function normally on a test and in the rest of life.

Physical Steps for Beating Test Anxiety

While test anxiety is a serious problem, the good news is that it can be overcome. It doesn't have to control your ability to think and remember information. While it may take time, you can begin taking steps today to beat anxiety.

Just as your first hint that you may be struggling with anxiety comes from the physical symptoms, the first step to treating it is also physical. Rest is crucial for having a clear, strong mind. If you are tired, it is much easier to give in to anxiety. But if you establish good sleep habits, your body and mind will be ready to perform optimally, without the strain of exhaustion. Additionally, sleeping well helps you to retain information better, so you're more likely to recall the answers when you see the test questions.

Getting good sleep means more than going to bed on time. It's important to allow your brain time to relax. Take study breaks from time to time so it doesn't get overworked, and don't study right before bed. Take time to rest your mind before trying to rest your body, or you may find it difficult to fall asleep.

Along with sleep, other aspects of physical health are important in preparing for a test. Good nutrition is vital for good brain function. Sugary foods and drinks may give a burst of energy but this burst is followed by a crash, both physically and emotionally. Instead, fuel your body with protein and vitamin-rich foods.

Also, drink plenty of water. Dehydration can lead to headaches and exhaustion, especially if your brain is already under stress from the rigors of the test. Particularly if your test is a long one, drink water during the breaks. And if possible, take an energy-boosting snack to eat between sections.

Along with sleep and diet, a third important part of physical health is exercise. Maintaining a steady workout schedule is helpful, but even taking 5-minute study breaks to walk can help get your blood pumping faster and clear your head. Exercise also releases endorphins, which contribute to a positive feeling and can help combat test anxiety.

When you nurture your physical health, you are also contributing to your mental health. If your body is healthy, your mind is much more likely to be healthy as well. So take time to rest, nourish your body with healthy food and water, and get moving as much as possible. Taking these physical steps will make you stronger and more able to take the mental steps necessary to overcome test anxiety.

Mental Steps for Beating Test Anxiety

Working on the mental side of test anxiety can be more challenging, but as with the physical side, there are clear steps you can take to overcome it. As mentioned earlier, test anxiety often stems from lack of preparation, so the obvious solution is to prepare for the test. Effective studying may be the most important weapon you have for beating test anxiety, but you can and should employ several other mental tools to combat fear.

First, boost your confidence by reminding yourself of past success—tests or projects that you aced. If you're putting as much effort into preparing for this test as you did for those, there's no reason you should expect to fail here. Work hard to prepare; then trust your preparation.

Second, surround yourself with encouraging people. It can be helpful to find a study group, but be sure that the people you're around will encourage a positive attitude. If you spend time with others who are anxious or cynical, this will only contribute to your own anxiety. Look for others who are motivated to study hard from a desire to succeed, not from a fear of failure.

Third, reward yourself. A test is physically and mentally tiring, even without anxiety, and it can be helpful to have something to look forward to. Plan an activity following the test, regardless of the outcome, such as going to a movie or getting ice cream.

When you are taking the test, if you find yourself beginning to feel anxious, remind yourself that you know the material. Visualize successfully completing the test. Then take a few deep, relaxing breaths and return to it. Work through the questions carefully but with confidence, knowing that you are capable of succeeding.

Developing a healthy mental approach to test taking will also aid in other areas of life. Test anxiety affects more than just the actual test—it can be damaging to your mental health and even contribute to depression. It's important to beat test anxiety before it becomes a problem for more than testing.

Study Strategy

Being prepared for the test is necessary to combat anxiety, but what does being prepared look like? You may study for hours on end and still not feel prepared. What you need is a strategy for test prep. The next few pages outline our recommended steps to help you plan out and conquer the challenge of preparation.

STEP 1: SCOPE OUT THE TEST

Learn everything you can about the format (multiple choice, essay, etc.) and what will be on the test. Gather any study materials, course outlines, or sample exams that may be available. Not only will this help you to prepare, but knowing what to expect can help to alleviate test anxiety.

STEP 2: MAP OUT THE MATERIAL

Look through the textbook or study guide and make note of how many chapters or sections it has. Then divide these over the time you have. For example, if a book has 15 chapters and you have five days to study, you need to cover three chapters each day. Even better, if you have the time, leave an extra day at the end for overall review after you have gone through the material in depth.

If time is limited, you may need to prioritize the material. Look through it and make note of which sections you think you already have a good grasp on, and which need review. While you are studying, skim quickly through the familiar sections and take more time on the challenging parts. Write out your plan so you don't get lost as you go. Having a written plan also helps you feel more in control of the study, so anxiety is less likely to arise from feeling overwhelmed at the amount to cover.

STEP 3: GATHER YOUR TOOLS

Decide what study method works best for you. Do you prefer to highlight in the book as you study and then go back over the highlighted portions? Or do you type out notes of the important information? Or is it helpful to make flashcards that you can carry with you? Assemble the pens, index cards, highlighters, post-it notes, and any other materials you may need so you won't be distracted by getting up to find things while you study.

If you're having a hard time retaining the information or organizing your notes, experiment with different methods. For example, try color-coding by subject with colored pens, highlighters, or post-it notes. If you learn better by hearing, try recording yourself reading your notes so you can listen while in the car, working out, or simply sitting at your desk. Ask a friend to quiz you from your flashcards, or try teaching someone the material to solidify it in your mind.

STEP 4: CREATE YOUR ENVIRONMENT

It's important to avoid distractions while you study. This includes both the obvious distractions like visitors and the subtle distractions like an uncomfortable chair (or a too-comfortable couch that makes you want to fall asleep). Set up the best study environment possible: good lighting and a comfortable work area. If background music helps you focus, you may want to turn it on, but otherwise keep the room quiet. If you are using a computer to take notes, be sure you don't have any other windows open, especially applications like social media, games, or anything else that could distract you. Silence your phone and turn off notifications. Be sure to keep water close by so you stay hydrated while you study (but avoid unhealthy drinks and snacks).

Also, take into account the best time of day to study. Are you freshest first thing in the morning? Try to set aside some time then to work through the material. Is your mind clearer in the afternoon or evening? Schedule your study session then. Another method is to study at the same time of day that you will take the test, so that your brain gets used to working on the material at that time and will be ready to focus at test time.

STEP 5: STUDY!

Once you have done all the study preparation, it's time to settle into the actual studying. Sit down, take a few moments to settle your mind so you can focus, and begin to follow your study plan. Don't give in to distractions or let yourself procrastinate. This is your time to prepare so you'll be ready to fearlessly approach the test. Make the most of the time and stay focused.

Of course, you don't want to burn out. If you study too long you may find that you're not retaining the information very well. Take regular study breaks. For example, taking five minutes out of every hour to walk briskly, breathing deeply and swinging your arms, can help your mind stay fresh.

As you get to the end of each chapter or section, it's a good idea to do a quick review. Remind yourself of what you learned and work on any difficult parts. When you feel that you've mastered the material, move on to the next part. At the end of your study session, briefly skim through your notes again.

But while review is helpful, cramming last minute is NOT. If at all possible, work ahead so that you won't need to fit all your study into the last day. Cramming overloads your brain with more information than it can process and retain, and your tired mind may struggle to recall even previously learned information when it is overwhelmed with last-minute study. Also, the urgent nature of cramming and the stress placed on your brain contribute to anxiety. You'll be more likely to go to the test feeling unprepared and having trouble thinking clearly.

So don't cram, and don't stay up late before the test, even just to review your notes at a leisurely pace. Your brain needs rest more than it needs to go over the information again. In fact, plan to finish your studies by noon or early afternoon the day before the test. Give your brain the rest of the day to relax or focus on other things, and get a good night's sleep. Then you will be fresh for the test and better able to recall what you've studied.

STEP 6: TAKE A PRACTICE TEST

Many courses offer sample tests, either online or in the study materials. This is an excellent resource to check whether you have mastered the material, as well as to prepare for the test format and environment.

Check the test format ahead of time: the number of questions, the type (multiple choice, free response, etc.), and the time limit. Then create a plan for working through them. For example, if you have 30 minutes to take a 60-question test, your limit is 30 seconds per question. Spend less time on the questions you know well so that you can take more time on the difficult ones.

If you have time to take several practice tests, take the first one open book, with no time limit. Work through the questions at your own pace and make sure you fully understand them. Gradually work up to taking a test under test conditions: sit at a desk with all study materials put away and set a timer. Pace yourself to make sure you finish the test with time to spare and go back to check your answers if you have time.

After each test, check your answers. On the questions you missed, be sure you understand why you missed them. Did you misread the question (tests can use tricky wording)? Did you forget the information? Or was it something you hadn't learned? Go back and study any shaky areas that the practice tests reveal.

Taking these tests not only helps with your grade, but also aids in combating test anxiety. If you're already used to the test conditions, you're less likely to worry about it, and working through tests until you're scoring well gives you a confidence boost. Go through the practice tests until you feel comfortable, and then you can go into the test knowing that you're ready for it.

Test Tips

On test day, you should be confident, knowing that you've prepared well and are ready to answer the questions. But aside from preparation, there are several test day strategies you can employ to maximize your performance.

First, as stated before, get a good night's sleep the night before the test (and for several nights before that, if possible). Go into the test with a fresh, alert mind rather than staying up late to study.

Try not to change too much about your normal routine on the day of the test. It's important to eat a nutritious breakfast, but if you normally don't eat breakfast at all, consider eating just a protein bar. If you're a coffee drinker, go ahead and have your normal coffee. Just make sure you time it so that the caffeine doesn't wear off right in the middle of your test. Avoid sugary beverages, and drink enough water to stay hydrated but not so much that you need a restroom break 10 minutes into the test. If your test isn't first thing in the morning, consider going for a walk or doing a light workout before the test to get your blood flowing.

Allow yourself enough time to get ready, and leave for the test with plenty of time to spare so you won't have the anxiety of scrambling to arrive in time. Another reason to be early is to select a good seat. It's helpful to sit away from doors and windows, which can be distracting. Find a good seat, get out your supplies, and settle your mind before the test begins.

When the test begins, start by going over the instructions carefully, even if you already know what to expect. Make sure you avoid any careless mistakes by following the directions.

Then begin working through the questions, pacing yourself as you've practiced. If you're not sure on an answer, don't spend too much time on it, and don't let it shake your confidence. Either skip it and come back later, or eliminate as many wrong answers as possible and guess among the remaining ones. Don't dwell on these questions as you continue—put them out of your mind and focus on what lies ahead.

Be sure to read all of the answer choices, even if you're sure the first one is the right answer. Sometimes you'll find a better one if you keep reading. But don't second-guess yourself if you do immediately know the answer. Your gut instinct is usually right. Don't let test anxiety rob you of the information you know.

If you have time at the end of the test (and if the test format allows), go back and review your answers. Be cautious about changing any, since your first instinct tends to be correct, but make sure you didn't misread any of the questions or accidentally mark the wrong answer choice. Look over any you skipped and make an educated guess.

At the end, leave the test feeling confident. You've done your best, so don't waste time worrying about your performance or wishing you could change anything. Instead, celebrate the successful completion of this test. And finally, use this test to learn how to deal with anxiety even better next time.

> **Review Video: Test Anxiety**
> Visit mometrix.com/academy and enter code: 100340

Important Qualification

Not all anxiety is created equal. If your test anxiety is causing major issues in your life beyond the classroom or testing center, or if you are experiencing troubling physical symptoms related to your anxiety, it may be a sign of a serious physiological or psychological condition. If this sounds like your situation, we strongly encourage you to seek professional help.

Online Resources

Due to our efforts to try to keep this book to a manageable length, we've created a link that will give you access to all of your online resources:

mometrix.com/resources719/nppmh-27810

It's Your Moment, Let's Celebrate It!

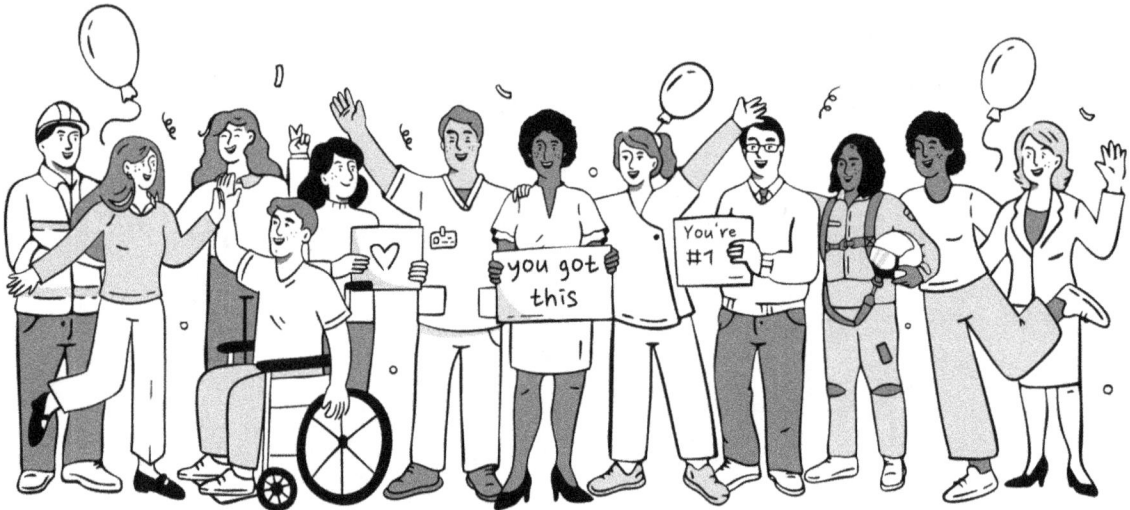

Share your story @mometrixtestpreparation

www.ingramcontent.com/pod-product-compliance
Lightning Source LLC
Chambersburg PA
CBHW081146040426

42445CB00015B/1781